# Applied Respiratory Pathophysiology

# Applied Respiratory Pathophysiology

Edited by
## Louis-Philippe Boulet
Respirologist at Québec Heart and Lung Institute
Professor of Medicine, Laval University (Université Laval)
Québec, Canada

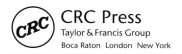

CRC Press is an imprint of the
Taylor & Francis Group, an **informa** business

CRC Press
Taylor & Francis Group
6000 Broken Sound Parkway NW, Suite 300
Boca Raton, FL 33487-2742

© 2018 by Taylor & Francis Group, LLC
CRC Press is an imprint of Taylor & Francis Group, an Informa business

No claim to original U.S. Government works

Printed and bound in India by Replika Press Pvt. Ltd.

Printed on acid-free paper
Version Date: 20170223

International Standard Book Number-13: 978-1-138-19644-5 (Paperback) 978-1-138-19651-3 (Hardback)

This book contains information obtained from authentic and highly regarded sources. While all reasonable efforts have been made to publish reliable data and information, neither the author[s] nor the publisher can accept any legal responsibility or liability for any errors or omissions that may be made. The publishers wish to make clear that any views or opinions expressed in this book by individual editors, authors or contributors are personal to them and do not necessarily reflect the views/opinions of the publishers. The information or guidance contained in this book is intended for use by medical, scientific or health-care professionals and is provided strictly as a supplement to the medical or other professional's own judgement, their knowledge of the patient's medical history, relevant manufacturer's instructions and the appropriate best practice guidelines. Because of the rapid advances in medical science, any information or advice on dosages, procedures or diagnoses should be independently verified. The reader is strongly urged to consult the relevant national drug formulary and the drug companies' and device or material manufacturers' printed instructions, and their websites, before administering or utilizing any of the drugs, devices or materials mentioned in this book. This book does not indicate whether a particular treatment is appropriate or suitable for a particular individual. Ultimately it is the sole responsibility of the medical professional to make his or her own professional judgements, so as to advise and treat patients appropriately. The authors and publishers have also attempted to trace the copyright holders of all material reproduced in this publication and apologize to copyright holders if permission to publish in this form has not been obtained. If any copyright material has not been acknowledged please write and let us know so we may rectify in any future reprint.

Except as permitted under U.S. Copyright Law, no part of this book may be reprinted, reproduced, transmitted, or utilized in any form by any electronic, mechanical, or other means, now known or hereafter invented, including photocopying, microfilming, and recording, or in any information storage or retrieval system, without written permission from the publishers.

For permission to photocopy or use material electronically from this work, please access www.copyright.com (http://www.copyright.com/) or contact the Copyright Clearance Center, Inc. (CCC), 222 Rosewood Drive, Danvers, MA 01923, 978-750-8400. CCC is a not-for-profit organization that provides licenses and registration for a variety of users. For organizations that have been granted a photocopy license by the CCC, a separate system of payment has been arranged.

**Trademark Notice:** Product or corporate names may be trademarks or registered trademarks, and are used only for identification and explanation without intent to infringe.

---

**Library of Congress Cataloging-in-Publication Data**

Names: Boulet, Louis-Philippe, 1954- editor.
Title: Applied respiratory pathophysiology / [edited by] Louis-Philippe Boulet.
Description: Boca Raton : CRC Press, [2017] | Includes bibliographical references.
Identifiers: LCCN 2017001550| ISBN 9781138196445 (pbk. : alk. paper) | ISBN 9781138196513 (hardback : alk. paper) | ISBN 9781315177052 (Master eBook)
Subjects: | MESH: Respiratory Tract Diseases--physiopathology | Respiratory Physiological Phenomena
Classification: LCC RC702 | NLM WF 140 | DDC 616.2--dc23
LC record available at https://lccn.loc.gov/2017001550

---

**Visit the Taylor & Francis Web site at**
http://www.taylorandfrancis.com

**and the CRC Press Web site at**
http://www.crcpress.com

# Contents

| | | |
|---|---|---|
| Preface | | vii |
| Acknowledgments | | ix |
| Contributors | | xi |
| 1 | Embryology, anatomy, and histology of the lung<br>*Christian Couture* | 1 |
| 2 | Physiology of the respiratory system<br>*Pierre LeBlanc* | 15 |
| 3 | Laboratory techniques to study the cellular and molecular processes of disorders<br>*Catherine Laprise* | 33 |
| 4 | Acute respiratory insufficiency<br>*Mathieu Simon* | 55 |
| 5 | Pathophysiology of asthma<br>*Louis-Philippe Boulet* | 67 |
| 6 | Chronic obstructive pulmonary disease<br>*Julie Milot and Mathieu Morissette* | 97 |
| 7 | Pulmonary vascular diseases<br>*Annie C. Lajoie, Vincent Mainguy, Sébastien Bonnet and Steeve Provencher* | 119 |
| 8 | Respiratory infections<br>*Noël Lampron* | 149 |
| 9 | Sleep-related breathing disorders<br>*Frédéric Sériès and Wenyang Li* | 163 |
| 10 | Interstitial lung diseases<br>*Geneviève Dion, Yvon Cormier and Louis-Philippe Boulet* | 177 |
| 11 | Lung cancer<br>*Christian Couture* | 207 |
| 12 | Occupational respiratory diseases<br>*Louis-Philippe Boulet and Marc Desmeules* | 223 |
| 13 | Diseases of the pleura<br>*Jean Deslauriers* | 243 |
| 14 | Cystic fibrosis (mucoviscidosis)<br>*Lara Bilodeau* | 259 |
| 15 | Bronchiectasis<br>*Louis-Philippe Boulet* | 271 |
| Index | | 283 |

# Preface

Respiratory diseases affect about 20% of the population and are responsible for a marked human and socio-economic burden. Since the latter part of the twentieth century, there has been impressive progress in understanding the mechanisms of these conditions and developments in their assessment and treatment, with many new agents now offered to treat those ailments. It is of utmost importance for the clinician and those interested in respiratory diseases to know the etiologic factors and pathophysiology of the latter, to better understand the rationale for assessments and therapeutic interventions, and to know the various factors influencing their outcomes. The aim of this book is therefore to gather the most updated notions about mechanisms and determinants of the most common respiratory diseases. It does not aim to provide an in-depth discussion of basic molecular mechanisms but to synthetize them in a practical way, to provide clinicians with what is needed to better define the various forms of disease and the targets of therapy. Treatments are not discussed in detail but their mechanisms of action and indications are described.

We hope that this publication will be helpful to all those interested in respiratory conditions, including students, researchers, physicians, and other health professionals.

–Louis-Philippe Boulet, MD, FRCP(C)
Québec Heart and Lung Institute, Québec, Canada

# Acknowledgments

We sincerely thank the following people for their comments and suggestions for specific sections of this edition: Doctors Élyse Bissonnette, James G. Martin, Parameswaran Nair, David Bernstein, Yves Berthiaume, Charlene Fell, Antoine Delage, Denis O'Donnell, Michel Laviolette, and John Kimoff. We also thank Karine Tremblay for the elaboration of several figures, as well as Sylvie Carette for her help with the preparation of this book. We also thank the pulmonologists of the Quebec Heart and Lung Institute, Laval University for their comments and suggestions.

# Contributors

**Lara Bilodeau** has been a respirologist at the Institut universitaire de cardiologie et de pneumologie de Québec (Quebec Heart and Lung Institute) since 2009. She completed a fellowship in adult cystic fibrosis at the Université de Montréal. Currently a director of the cystic fibrosis clinic of her institution, Dr. Bilodeau frequently lectures on the management of CF.

**Sébastien Bonnet** is a professor of medicine at the department of medicine at Laval University. He holds a Canadian Research Chair in translational research in pulmonary vascular diseases and is cofounder of the Pulmonary Hypertension Research Group at Laval University. He has made breakthrough findings in several types of diseases, including pulmonary arterial hypertension and cancer, and has received numerous research scholarships, prestigious awards, and grants. He is also an associate editor for leading journals, including *Circulation* and *AJP Lung*, as well as an active member of numerous national peer review committees. His main research interests are mechanisms leading the pulmonary vascular remodeling that characterizes pulmonary arterial hypertension. Dr. Bonnet has published more than 100 scientific papers and has presented at more than 200 provincial, national, and international congresses or symposia.

**Louis-Philippe Boulet** is a respirologist at the Institut de cardiologie et de pneumologie de Québec (Quebec Heart and Lung Institute). He is a professor of medicine at the department of medicine at Laval University and holds a chair in knowledge translation, education and prevention in respiratory and cardiorespiratory health at Laval University. He is a past chair of the Canadian Thoracic Society, Canadian Thoracic Society Respiratory Guidelines Committee and he is a member of many Canadian and international medical societies. He has been a founding member of the Quebec Respiratory Health Education Network. In addition to his clinical practice and teaching, Dr. Boulet conducts a research program mainly on the themes of asthma phenotypes, airway responses, inflammation and remodeling, respiratory allergy, respiratory health of athletes, knowledge translation, and health education. He is an assistant editor of many respiratory journals and has written more than 500 medical publications, in addition to 600 abstracts, 35 book chapters, and edited/authored six books.

**Yvon Cormier** is a retired respirologist from Institut de cardiologie et de pneumologie de Québec (Quebec Heart and Lung Institute). He is a professor emeritus at the department of medicine at the Faculty of Medicine at Laval University. He is a past president of Quebec and Canadian Thoracic Societies, past director of Laval Hospital Research Center, and past director of the Quebec Respiratory Health Network of the FRQS. He has also been vice dean for research at the superior studies school of the Faculty of Medicine in Laval University. His main research interests are on allergic alveolitis and all other respiratory diseases caused by organic dust.

**Christian Couture** is a pulmonary and cardiovascular pathologist at the Institut de cardiologie et de pneumologie de Quebec (Quebec Heart and Lung Institute) and a clinical professor at Laval University in Quebec City. His main research interests are lung cancer biomarkers, emerging pulmonary infections and heart valvulopathies. He has co-authored 75 publications and 2 book chapters.

**Jean Deslauriers** is a currently retired thoracic surgeon who spent his entire professional career at the Institut universitaire de cardiologie et de pneumologie de Québec (Quebec Heart and Lung Institute). He is a graduate of Laval University medical school in Quebec City and did his post-graduate thoracic surgical training at the University of Toronto under the tutorship of Dr. F.G. Pearson. In 1992, he became professor of surgery at Laval University and in 2016, was named Professor Emeritus. In 2008-2009, he spent a full year as an international consultant in thoracic surgery at Jilin University in the People's Republic of China. He is an honorary member of several international thoracic surgery associations and was the first Canadian ever to be on the board of directors of the Society of Thoracic Surgeons ( STS, USA). He has edited or co-edited 16 textbooks on thoracic surgery in addition to authoring more than 250 articles in peer-reviewed medical journals and specialty textbooks. In 2010, he was the recipient of the Career Teaching Award from Laval University and in 2011 was named member of the Order of Canada. In 2015, he was honored as a Legend in Thoracic Surgery by the American Association of Thoracic Surgery (AATS), and in 2016, he received the Canadian Association of Thoracic Surgeons (CATS) Lifetime Achievement Award.

**Marc Desmeules** is a retired respirologist at the Institut universitaire de cardiologie et de pneumologie de Québec (Quebec Heart and Lung Institute) and professor of medicine at the department of medicine at Laval University. He studied at the Faculty of Medicine at Laval University and completed a fellowship in France under the direction of Professor Paul Sadoul. He was certified in internal medicine and respirology by the Quebec College of Physicians and Royal College of Physicians and Surgeons of Canada. He is specialized in occupational respiratory diseases, and he has worked for more than 30 years as a clinician, teacher, and researcher. He served as president of the Workmen's Compensation Board for the Province of Quebec from 1982 to 2011. He has also held many administrative positions at Laval University and was previously the director of the department of medicine and the dean of the Faculty of Medicine at this university.

**Geneviève Dion** is a respirologist at the Institut universitaire de cardiologie et de pneumologie de Québec (Quebec Heart and Lung Institute). She has completed a fellowship in the field of interstitial lung disease at the hospital Avicenne de Bobigny (France) and in cystic fibrosis at the Hôpital Cochin de Paris (France). She is the medical director of the interstitial lung disease clinic of the Institut universitaire de cardiologie et de pneumologie de Québec and actively provides care at the cystic fibrosis clinic. Her research focusses on the investigation of interstitial lung diseases.

**Annie C. Lajoie** is a third year medical resident in the General Internal Medicine Residency Program at Laval University, Québec. She is also completing a masters degree in clinical epidemiology at Laval University under the supervision of Drs. Steeve Provencher and Yves Lacasse, both respirologists at the Institut universitaire de cardiologie et de pneumologie du Québec.

**Noël Lampron** is a respirologist and internist at the Institut universitaire de cardiologie et de pneumologie de Québec (Quebec Heart and Lung Institute). He served as director of the intensive care unit from 1997 to 2001. He is a clinical professor at the department of medicine at Laval University. His main interests are in respiratory infections, sleep apnea, and interventional bronchoscopy. He has contributed to the development of Canadian guidelines for the prevention of community-acquired pneumonia and acute exacerbation of COPD.

**Catherine Laprise** is a professor of genetics at the University of Quebec at Chicoutimi. She is a member of AllerGen Network of Centers of Excellence and director of the Asthma Strategic Group Committee of the Respiratory Network of the FRQS. She is a researcher for the project GABRIEL and takes part in the research consortium on lactic acidosis. She has held a Canada chair in environment and genetics of respiratory disorders and allergy since January 2015. Her research work centers on the identification of genetic determinants of asthma, gene–gene and gene–environment interactions, as well as on the study of these gene functions and their roles in asthma. She also contributes to various projects in the field of genetics in collaboration with international groups. Dr. Laprise has published more than 100 scientific papers and more than 50 educational tools in genetics for the general public including a book on genetics and exhibition.

**Pierre LeBlanc** is a respirologist at the Institut de cardiologie et de pneumologie de Québec (Quebec Heart and Lung Institute). He is a professor at the department of medicine at Laval University. His main interest is exercise physiology, and he has collaborated on more than 50 medical publications. He is in charge of teaching respiratory physiology to the medical students at Laval University. He served as vice dean at Laval University from 2002 to 2010 and has been the director of the department of medicine at Laval University from 2011 to 2017.

**Wenyang Li** completed her postgraduate studies in 2012 at China Medical University under the direction of Professor Jian Kang and is now completing a fellowship on sleep disordered breathing diseases at Institut universitaire de cardiologie et de pneumologie de Québec Research center under the direction of Dr. Frédéric Sériès. Her main fields of interest include the pathophysiology of obstructive sleep apnea with a particular focus of upper airway physiology.

**Vincent Mainguy** completed his postgraduate studies in 2012 at the Institut universitaire de cardiologie et de pneumologie de Québec (Quebec Heart and Lung Institute) under the direction of Dr. Steeve Provencher, respirologist. His research concerned the mechanisms of exercise intolerance in patients with lung arterial high blood pressure. On completing his studies as a medical resident, he will practice family medicine.

**Simon Martel** has been a respirologist at the Institut de cardiologie et de pneumologie de Québec (Quebec Heart and Lung Institute) since 1995 and is an associate clinical professor at the department of medicine at Laval University. He is a medical director in respiratory endoscopy sector at the Institut universitaire de cardiologie et de pneumologie de Québec. His research interests include pulmonary hypertension, lung cancer, and interventional bronchoscopy.

**Julie Milot** is a respirologist at the Institut de cardiologie et de pneumologie de Québec (Quebec Heart and Lung Institute). She is the director of the chronic obstructive pulmonary disease clinic at the Institut universitaire de cardiologie et de pneumologie de Québec. Her research focuses on the pathophysiology of emphysema, especially the role of apoptosis in the destruction of the lung parenchyma. She is also involved in a project to improve chronic obstructive pulmonary disease management and quality of life.

**Mathieu Morissette** completed his postgraduate studies in 2010 at the Institut universitaire de cardiologie et de pneumologie de Québec (Quebec Heart and Lung Institute) Research center under the direction of Dr. Julie Milot. He then completed a fellowship on obstructive airway diseases at McMaster University under the direction of Dr. Martin Stämpfli. His main fields of interest include the environmental factors and immune mechanisms involved in lung and airways damage in chronic obstructive pulmonary disease.

**Steeve Provencher** is a respirologist at the Institut de cardiologie et de pneumologie de Québec (Quebec Heart and Lung Institute). He is a professor of medicine at the department of medicine at Laval University, medical director of the pulmonary vascular diseases clinic of the Institut universitaire de cardiologie et de pneumologie de Québec, and cofounder of the Pulmonary Hypertension Research Group at Laval University. He chairs the pulmonary vascular clinical assembly of the Canadian Thoracic Society and is a TASK force member of the World Symposium on Pulmonary Hypertension. In 2011, Dr. Provencher received the *Prix reconnaissance Marc Julien*, awarded by the internal medicine residents in recognition of outstanding work done in teaching hospitals, dedication to his patients, clinical skills, and quality of care. He is also on the editorial board of leading journals in respirology as well as an active member of numerous peer review committees. His main research interests are exercise pathophysiology and epidemiology of pulmonary arterial hypertension, as well as mechanisms leading the pulmonary vascular remodeling that characterizes this disease. Over his short career, Dr. Provencher has published more than 100 scientific papers and has been invited to speak at over 150 provincial, national, and international congresses or symposia.

**Frédéric Sériès** completed his specialist training in France, after which he began his practice of respirology and research in Quebec in 1985 by setting up the sleep laboratory at the Laval Hospital dedicated to the clinical investigation and research on sleep disorders. He developed, at the same time, a research program on the investigation and the treatment of the respiratory anomalies connected to sleep and physiology of the upper airways. He was named national researcher of the FRSQ in 2004 and is a full professor at Laval University Faculty of Medicine. He is director of the Institut universitaire de cardiologie et de pneumologie de Québec sleep laboratory. His research focuses on upper airway physiology, sleep apnea-related metabolic disturbances, and sleep apnea treatment.

**Mathieu Simon** has practiced pneumology for more than 10 years. He holds a fellowship in intensive care and is a director of the intensive care unit at the Institut universitaire de cardiologie et de pneumologie de Québec. He is also responsible for the medical students' curriculum on respiratory system at the Faculty of Medicine of Laval University where he is a clinical professor.

# 1

# Embryology, anatomy, and histology of the lung

CHRISTIAN COUTURE

| | |
|---|---|
| Introduction | 1 |
| Embryology | 2 |
|     Embryonal stage | 2 |
|     Pseudoglandular stage | 3 |
|     Canalicular stage | 3 |
|     Saccular stage | 4 |
|     Alveolar stage | 4 |
| Anatomy and histology | 4 |
|     Conducting airways | 4 |
|     Exchange surfaces | 9 |
|     Vasculature | 11 |
|     Lymphatic drainage | 12 |
|     Innervation | 12 |
|     Ultrastructure | 13 |
| References | 14 |

## Introduction

The respiratory system allows gas exchanges between ambient air and blood circulation by extracting oxygen from inhaled air into blood and rejecting carbon dioxide from the blood into exhaled air. This function is accomplished by the interplay of the three functional components of the respiratory system: conducting airways, exchange surfaces, and a ventilatory apparatus (Figure 1.1).

Conducting airways do not simply conduct air between the external environment and the exchange surfaces. They also humidify and warm inhaled air, and eliminate inhaled dusts and microorganisms. Upper airways include the nasal cavity, nasal sinuses, nasopharynx, oropharynx, and larynx. Lower airways extend from the trachea to the bronchi and their successive ramifications down to terminal bronchioles. Exchange surfaces are specialized in the rapid gas exchange between inhaled air and blood circulation. They are made of respiratory bronchioles, alveolar ducts, alveolar sacs, and alveoli. The ventilatory apparatus includes bones and muscles of the thoracic cage, diaphragm, and abdomen as well as elastic tissues from the pleura and the lungs, and finally respiratory centers in the brainstem and afferent/efferent nerves. Approximately

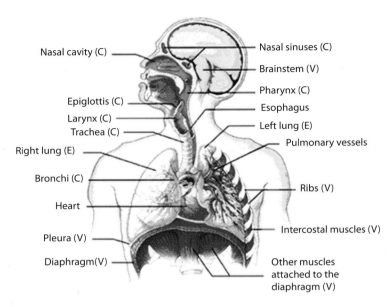

Figure 1.1 Anatomic structures of the respiratory system. Function indicated in parentheses: conducting airways (C), exchange surfaces (E), and ventilatory apparatus (V).

10–12 times per minute, the brainstem sends an automatic inspiratory signal to the diaphragm via the phrenic nerves and to other muscles of the thoracic cage. Their contraction causes an expansion of the thoracic cage and lungs, which drives external air containing 21% oxygen and less than 1% carbon dioxide into airways, down to the exchange surfaces. Then, the inspiratory signal ceases and the thoracic cage passively returns to its resting position. In doing so, the inhaled air, now containing only 16% of oxygen and 6% of carbon dioxide, is then exhaled. This chapter describes the embryology, anatomy, and histology of the respiratory system. It is based on major reference textbooks on the subject [1–6].

## Embryology

The lungs do not perform a respiratory function during intrauterine life. Instead, they are responsible for the production of amniotic fluid. Lung development is classically divided into five stages, which partially overlap one another and correspond to the successive establishment of conducting airways, transition airways (respiratory bronchioles), and exchange surfaces. This process results in an average of 16 successive dichotomic ramifications of the conducting airways, and in seven additional levels in the transition airways and exchange surfaces, resulting in a total of about 23 levels of ramification from the trachea to the alveoli. Extrauterine life is only possible from the 24th week of gestation, when a functional pulmonary vasculature appears and the production of surfactant begins. Figure 1.2 summarizes the development of the respiratory system.

## Embryonal stage

At days 26–28 after conception, two pulmonary buds form at the distal extremity of the laryngotracheal groove on the ventral pharynx. They will become the right and left mainstem bronchi. The right bronchial bud is oriented vertically whereas the left bronchial bud is almost horizontal. Bronchial buds also subdivide inequally into three lobar bronchi on the right side and only two on the left side. The pulmonary asymmetry of adult age is thus established early in the development. At the end of the embryonal stage, all the segmental bronchi of the pulmonary lobes are formed.

# Embryology

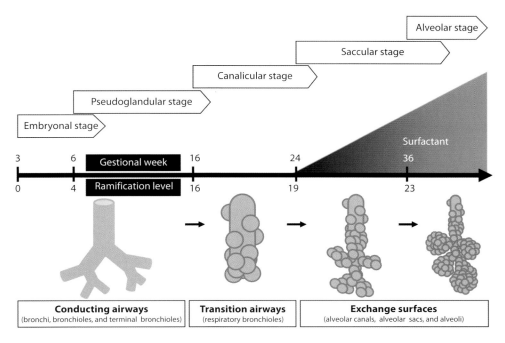

Figure 1.2 Development of the respiratory system. Embryonal and pseudoglandular stages are marked by the establishment of conducting airways. Canalicular stage is characterized by the formation of respiratory bronchioles, a transition between conducting airways and exchange surfaces. During saccular and alveolar stages, the first exchange surfaces develop and surfactant production starts, marking the beginning of a potential for extrauterine fetal viability. At the 36th week of gestation, a definitive ramification level of 23 is reached from the trachea to respiratory bronchioles but alveolar acquisition continues after birth and until the age of 8 years.

## Pseudoglandular stage

From the 6th to the 16th gestational weeks, the entire conducting airways are formed by a succession of ramifications culminating in the terminal bronchioles. These ramifications are under the control of the primitive mesenchymal tissue surrounding the airways in which proliferation genes are activated at the ramification points. This primitive mesenchymal tissue will later differentiate into bronchial cartilage, blood vessels, smooth muscle, and connective tissue.

## Canalicular stage

From weeks 16 to 26, canalicules originating from the terminal bronchioles begin to constitute the pulmonary parenchyma. All respiratory units derived from a specific terminal bronchiole form an acinus, which includes 3–4 generations of respiratory bronchioles, extended by alveolar ducts that then bud into alveolar sacs. The milestone of canalicular stage is the modification of both the primitive mesenchymal tissue and the epithelial lining into a conformation allowing a potential for respiratory function. Specifically, along all terminal bronchioles and other structures derived from them, the primitive mesenchyma develops as a delicate network of capillaries that brings the blood circulation into intimate contact with exchange surfaces. Also, the lumen of the canalicules, and later of their derivatives, enlarges while part of their epithelial lining flattens, thin (squamous) type I pneumocytes differentiating from cubic type II pneumocytes. At the end of canalicular stage and the beginning of saccular stage, type II pneumocytes also begin to secrete pulmonary surfactant (**surf**ace **act**ing **a**gent). The chemical composition of this substance (mainly glycerophospholipids, proteins, neutral fats, and cholesterol) prevents alveolar collapse during expiration from birth and thereafter by reducing the surface tension of the alveolar surfaces it covers. These changes are pivotal as they mark the beginning of a potential for extrauterine viability for the fetus around the 24th week of gestation. Pulmonary maturation can be measured by the ratio between surfactant lecithin and amniotic fluid sphingomyelin, with the lecithin/sphingomyelin ratio increasing as the lungs mature. The administration of steroids can accelerate pulmonary maturation and surfactant production in premature neonates.

## Saccular stage

Between 24 and 38 weeks of gestation, additional exchange surfaces are generated by alveolar sacs forming at the end of alveolar ducts, hence the name saccular.

## Alveolar stage

During the last weeks of pregnancy, new alveolar sacs continue to form, eventually leading to their final and smallest subdivisions, the alveoli. This "alveolarization," or alveolar development, continues massively during the first 6 months after birth, and to a lesser extent until the age of 8 years, after which the alveolar count culminates at 300 millions. In adulthood, the total alveolar surface is estimated to reach 80 m$^2$, the equivalent of a badminton court.

## Anatomy and histology

### Conducting airways

Airways not only do "conduct" but also "clean," warm, and humidify inhaled air. Hairs at the very entrance of upper airways in the nasal vestibule filter dust particles. The nasal cavity, nasal sinuses, and nasopharynx are richly vascularized to humidify and warm inhaled air. These structures have glands that secrete mucus containing mucinous glycoproteins, lipids, proteoglycans, immunoglobulins, lysozyme, lactoferrin, peroxidase, and other substances forming an effective arsenal against microorganisms. The columnar ciliated (respiratory) epithelial lining of the conducting airways propels and evacuates the mucus on which dust particles and bacteria are deposited. Both the respiratory and digestive systems share the oral cavity, oropharynx, and larynx. The epithelial lining of these anatomic structures is of the pseudostratified squamous type, which is adapted to resist the mechanical trauma of solid food swallowing. Under the vocal cords of the larynx, the epithelium becomes of the respiratory type again. The epiglottis of the larynx acts as a valve preventing food aspiration in the airways. The cricothyroid ligament located between the thyroid cartilage and cricoid cartilage is the site for emergency cricothyroidotomy to ventilate a suffocating individual in situations such as accidental food bronchoaspiration or epiglottitis (Figures 1.3 and 1.4).

As mentioned in the "Embryology" section, the conduction airways successively and dichotomously branch 23 times from the trachea to the respiratory bronchioles. This represents an average as the number of branchings actually varies from 10 to 30 depending on the exact location. The first dichotomy, located in the distal part of the trachea, is called the carina and gives rise to the right and left mainstem bronchi. On the right side, a second dichotomous branching generates the right upper lobe (RUL) bronchus and the *bronchus intermedius* (intermediary bronchus) which after a third branching generates the right middle lobe (RML) bronchus and the right lower lobe (RLL) bronchus. On the left side, the second dichotomous separation directly gives rise to the left upper and left lower lobar (LUL and LLL) bronchi. There is no middle lobe bronchus of the left. Rather, there is a rudimentary bronchus of the LUL

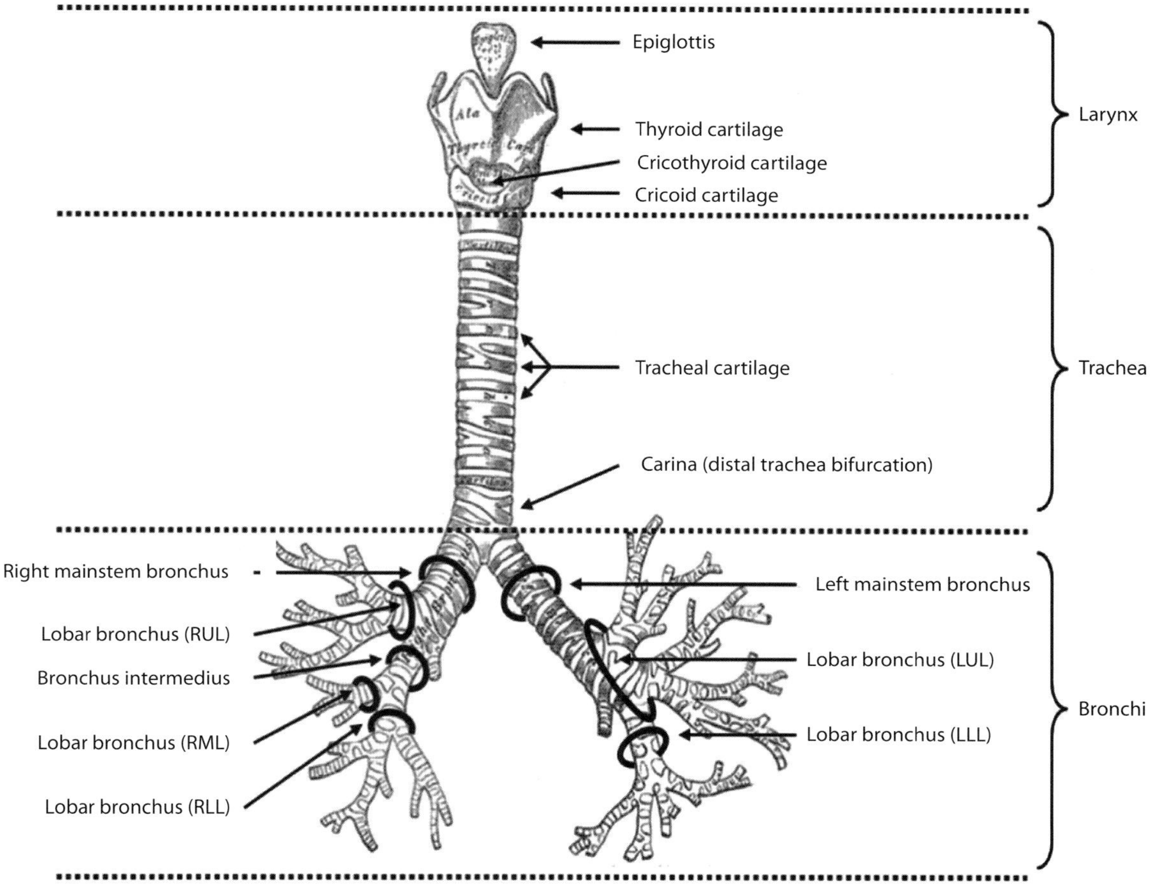

Figure 1.3 Anatomy of the larynx, trachea, and bronchi. LLL, left lower lobe; LUL, left upper lobe; RLL, right lower lobe; RML, right middle lobe; RUL, right upper lobe.

bronchus called the lingula. The five lobar bronchi divide into 18 segmental bronchi that define the 18 bronchopulmonary segments. Their knowledge and nomenclature is essential in locating pathological lesions (Table 1.1).

The wall of the trachea and bronchi contains cartilage that acts as an exoskeleton keeping their lumen open. In the trachea and mainstem bronchi, the cartilage is horseshoe-shaped with two posterior ends interconnected by a muscle strip. In the lobar bronchi and their subsequent ramifications, the cartilage rather organizes in the form of irregularly interconnected circular rings. Thus, in cross sections, the lumen of the trachea and mainstem bronchi is semicircular and that of the more distal bronchi circular (see Figure 1.4a). Gradually, as the bronchi branch, their diameter decreases and eventually the cartilage disappears, which influences the terminology as follows:

- *Bronchi:* presence of cartilage; diameter >1 mm
- *Bronchioles:* absence of cartilage; diameter <1 mm
- *Nonrespiratory bronchioles:* bronchioles proximal to respiratory bronchioles
- *Terminal bronchioles:* bronchioles immediately proximal to the first respiratory bronchioles
- *Respiratory bronchioles:* bronchioles with alveoli originating from their wall

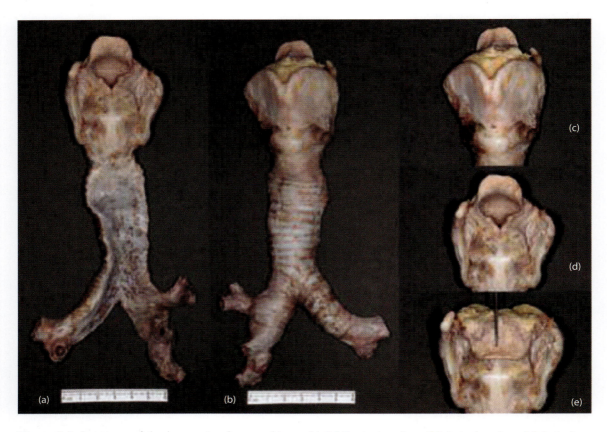

Figure 1.4 Anatomy of the larynx, trachea, and bronchi. (a) Posterior view. (b) Anterior view. (c) Anterior view of the larynx. (d and e) Posterior views of the larynx illustrating the valve movement of the epiglottis in the open position for ventilation (d) and closed position for swallowing (e).

Table 1.1 Bronchopulmonary segments

| RUL | LUL |
|---|---|
| 1. Apical | 1. Apical posterior |
| 2. Posterior | 2. Anterior |
| 3. Anterior | |
| RML | Lingula (of the LUL) |
| 4. Lateral | 3. Superior |
| 5. Medial | 4. Inferior |
| RLL | LLL |
| 6. Superior dorsal | 5. Apical posterior |
| 7. Medial basal | 6. Basal anteromedial |
| 8. Anterior basal | 7. Basal lateral |
| 9. Lateral basal | 8. Basal posterior |
| 10. Posterior basal | |

LLL, left lower lobe; LUL, left upper lobe; RLL, right lower lobe, RML, right middle lobe; RUL, right upper lobe.

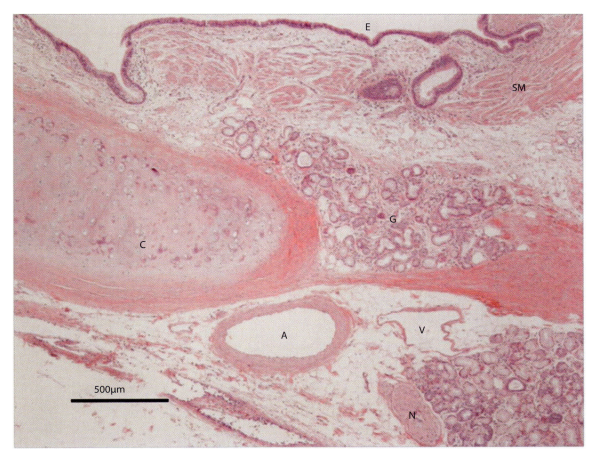

Figure 1.5 Histology of bronchi at low magnification on hematoxylin-eosin stain. A, artery; C, bronchial cartilage; E, bronchial epithelium; G, bronchial glands; N, nerve; SM, smooth muscle; V, vein.

The histology of bronchi is presented in Figures 1.5 through 1.7. The bronchial epithelium lies on a basement membrane resting on loose connective tissue that contains blood capillaries and small lymphatic vessels. Together, the bronchial epithelium, the basal membrane, and the loose connective tissue constitute the bronchial mucosa. The submucosa is, as its name indicates, located underneath the bronchial mucosa but there is no straightforward demarcation between the two. The submucosa comprises bronchial glands, smooth muscle, cartilage, nerves, arteries, veins, and lymphatic vessels. The bronchial glands are partly of the serous type and partly of the mucinous type. Their secretions are collected in excretory ducts opening into the bronchial lumen. Smooth muscle regulates airflow in the conducting airways by contracting (bronchoconstriction) or by relaxing (bronchodilation). Bronchial cartilage is largely made of a cartilaginous extracellular matrix produced by chondrocytes. The bronchial epithelium is of the columnar pseudostratified ciliated type. It contains ciliated cells, basal cells, goblet cells, and rare neuroendocrine cells. Columnar ciliated cells are found on the surface and cuboid basal cells are located adjacent to the basement membrane. The nuclei of these two cell types appear often arranged in two superimposed layers on histological sections but they are all in contact with the basement membrane. Mucous cells are rare. They have a goblet

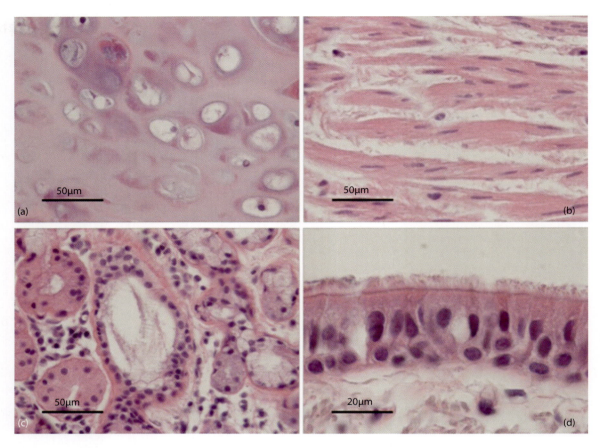

Figure 1.6 Histology of bronchi at high magnification on hematoxylin-eosin stain. (a) Bronchial cartilage with chondrocytes and cartilaginous matrix. (b) Smooth muscle. (c) Bronchial glands of the serous type with pink cytoplasm (left) and mucinous type with pale cytoplasm (right) and an excretory duct (center). (d) Bronchial mucosa with the pseudostratified ciliated columnar epithelium resting on a basement membrane (imperceptible) and underlying loose connective tissue.

appearance and their cytoplasm is completely occupied by a large vacuole of mucin. Although rare, neuroendocrine cells are also present. They occasionally form small clusters called neuroepithelial bodies.

Nonrespiratory bronchioles have a histology similar to bronchi except that their wall is thinner and contains neither cartilage nor glands. The height of the respiratory epithelium gradually decreases as the bronchioles diminish in size, their shape changing from cylindrical to cubo-cylindrical then to cuboid. Concomitantly, the ciliated cells and goblet cells are gradually replaced by Clara cells, which are nonciliated and whose apical cytoplasmic portion is enlarged. Clara cells have a secretory role as they produce a surfactant-like substance. They are also the progenitors of the bronchiolar epithelium. The transition from conduction airways to exchange surfaces occurs in the respiratory bronchioles. Respiratory bronchioles lined by respiratory epithelium begin to have alveoli budding from their wall. In addition to the normal ventilation from the trachea to the bronchi to the bronchioles to the alveoli, three structures allow a collateral ventilation. First, pores of Köhn connect adjacent alveoli. Second, Lambert canals directly connect nonrespiratory bronchioles to alveoli. Third, interbronchiolar communications of Martin occasionally connect a bronchiole to another (Figure 1.8).

Anatomy and histology 9

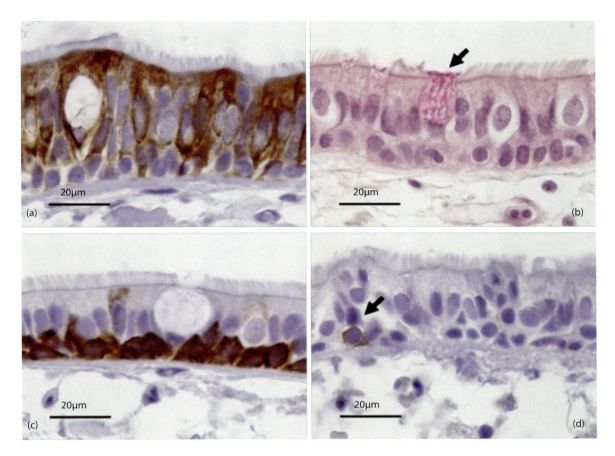

Figure 1.7 Cells of the bronchial epithelium at high magnification as depicted using immunohistochemical and histochemical stains. **(a)** Columnar ciliated cells immunostained with cytokeratin 7. **(b)** Goblet cell containing mucus stained by mucicarmin stain (arrow). **(c)** Basal cells immunostained with cytokeratin 5/6. **(d)** Neuroendocrine cell immunostained with neural cell adhesion molecule CD56 (arrow).

## Exchange surfaces

The average weight of the two lungs is 850 g in men and 750 g in women. The right lung has three lobes (upper, middle, and lower) and the left lung has two lobes (upper and lower). The pleura lines the surface of both lungs. This thin translucent, smooth, and shiny envelope histologically corresponds to a fibroelastic membrane covered by flattened or cuboidal mesothelial cells, often imperceptible on histology. Mesothelial cells secrete the pleural fluid that lubricates the external surface of the lungs and the internal surface of the chest wall to allow gentle sliding without friction between the two surfaces during inspiration–expiration cycles. The lung lobes are defined by folds of the visceral pleura called fissures. Each lobe has its own pleural lining while a bronchopulmonary segment has neither its own pleura nor fissure and is only recognizable by virtue of the segmental bronchus ventilating it. The pulmonary lobule is the smallest anatomical lung compartment that is visible to the naked eye, each lobule measuring 1–2 cm in diameter. Histology of the lung is depicted in Figures 1.9 and 1.10.

Each pulmonary lobule is delimited by the pleura and/or interlobular septa. It has a central bronchovascular bundle consisting of a bronchiole and an arteriole of similar caliber. The septa and visceral pleura

10  Embryology, anatomy, and histology of the lung

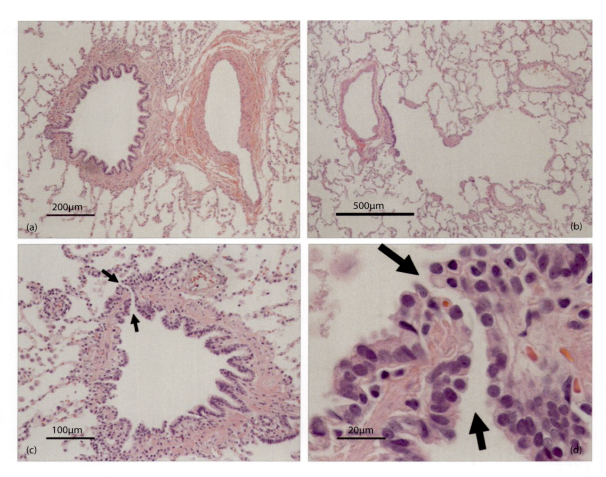

Figure 1.8 Histology of the bronchioles on hematoxylin-eosin stain. **(a)** Bronchovascular bundle comprising a bronchiole without cartilage (left) and an artery of similar caliber (right). **(b)** From left to right: arteriole, respiratory bronchiole with ciliated columnar epithelial lining disappearing with the onset of alveoli projecting from the bronchiolar wall and transition to air ducts and sacs. **(c** and **d)** Lambert canal (arrows) directly connecting a nonrespiratory bronchiole to an alveolus. Ciliated columnar cells and Clara cells (nonciliated cylindrical) are also identified.

contain veinules and lymphatic vessels. Small lymphatic vessels also drain bronchovascular bundles. Between the center and the periphery of the lobule, the lung parenchyma includes alveolar ducts, alveolar sacs, alveoli, and alveolar capillaries. If the lobule is the smallest visible pulmonary anatomical unit, *the acinus* is the functional unit of the lung, defined as the airways distal to the terminal bronchioles. Acini include multiple respiratory bronchioles and their alveolar ducts and sacs and alveoli. There are about 25,000 acini of 187 mm$^3$ on average for a total lung volume of 5.25 L. In the acinus, gas exchanges occur through a very thin membrane at the interface between air and blood. The alveolar septa consist of the cytoplasm of pneumocytes covering the alveolar surface, endothelial cells, and their fused basement membranes. Type I pneumocytes are flat and cover over 90% of the alveolar surface. Their cytoplasm is so thin and it is almost imperceptible in conventional optical microscopy. This reflects the specialization of type I pneumocytes for gas exchange. Rarer type II pneumocytes are more readily identifiable because of their cuboid shape. They produce pulmonary surfactant, which, by reducing the alveolar surface tension, prevents alveolar collapse

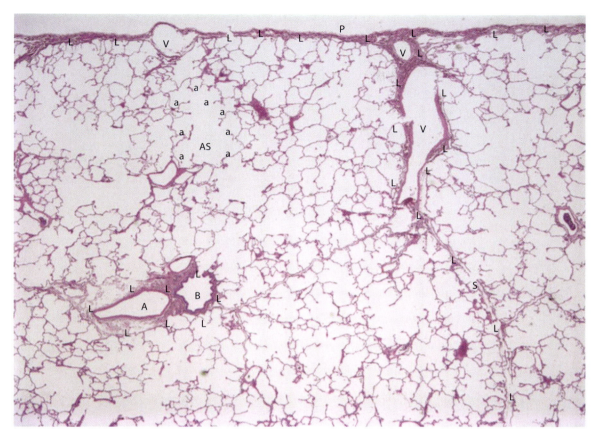

Figure 1.9 Histology of the lung at low magnification on hematoxylin-eosin stain. a, alveoli; A, artery; AS, alveolar sac; B, bronchiole; L, lymphatics; P, pleura; S, interlobular septa; V, veins.

during exhalation. Type II pneumocytes are also the progenitors of type I pneumocytes. In other words, cuboid type II pneumocytes become flat type I pneumocytes after cell division.

## Vasculature

The lungs have a dual blood supply: pulmonary and systemic. The pulmonary circulation is a low-pressure system (on average about 15 mmHg), which is dependent on the right side of the heart and whose role is to oxygenate blood. In contrast, the systemic circulation is a high-pressure system (100 mmHg) that depends on the left side of the heart and whose role is to distribute oxygenated blood to the whole body. The pulmonary arteries are part of the pulmonary circulation and accompany bronchi in their subdivisions to achieve a rich capillary network that surrounds the alveolar walls to maximize the gas exchange area between blood and air. Bronchial arteries are part of the systemic circulation and come either from the aorta or intercostal arteries. They form a plexus in the bronchial wall, which extends to the terminal bronchioles. Proximally, they anastomose to the inferior thyroid artery-dependent tracheal arterial network. Branches of the bronchial arteries also provide vascularization of the visceral pleura. Pulmonary veins start when efferent pulmonary capillaries form small veins (venules) in the interlobular septa. On histological sections, pulmonary arteries are centrobular accompanying a bronchiole having approximately the same size and veins are at the lobule periphery either in interlobular septa or the pleura.

## 12 Embryology, anatomy, and histology of the lung

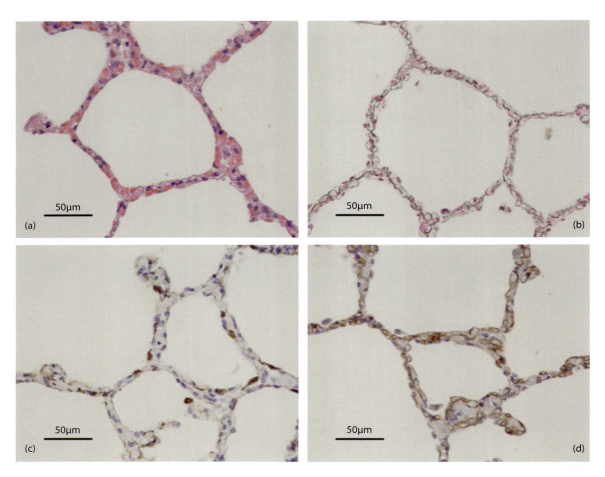

Figure 1.10 Histology of the lung at high magnification. (a) Lung alveoli with red blood cells in the capillaries of the alveolar septa (hematoxylin-eosin stain). (b) Shared basement membranes of pneumocytes and endothelial cells (Laidlaw stain). (c) Alveolar pneumocyte type I (cuboidal) and type II (flat) lining (cytokeratin 7 immunostain). (d) Endothelial cells of alveolar capillaries (CD34 immunostain).

## Lymphatic drainage

The lungs have a network of lymphatic vessels running along bronchovascular bundles, the pleura, and interlobular septa. Macrophages patrol the alveolar surfaces and engulf debris, dust, and microorganisms. They are the first line of immune defense and enter lymphatic vessels to stimulate an inflammatory response when necessary. Lymphoid tissue and histiocyte collections form along the lymphatic vessels to eventually organize into lymph nodes along the bronchi and sometimes in the lung parenchyma. Lymphoid tissue can also be directly associated with bronchi forming the bronchus-associated lymphoid tissue (BALT).

## Innervation

The phrenic nerves transmit the signal from the respiratory centers of the brainstem to the diaphragm to initiate the inspiratory movement. The trachea and bronchi include an external nerve plexus and an internal peribronchial plexus between the bronchial mucosa and the bronchial cartilage. In the bronchioles, where cartilage is absent, the internal and external nerve plexus are indistinguishable and can simply be called "peribronchiolar plexus." The vagus nerve provides parasympathetic innervation of the muscles, bronchial tree (bronchoconstriction), pulmonary vessels (vasodilation), and bronchial glands (secretomotor effect). Impulses from the paravertebral sympathetic chain antagonize these effects. If these effects on the bronchial muscles are easily observable, their mechanism is not fully understood because the airway smooth muscle is not innervated directly. The vagus nerve is also involved in the transmission of nerve impulses related to the cough reflex, bronchial muscle mechanoreceptors sensitive to stretch, pulmonary artery baroreceptors, and pulmonary veins chemoreceptors sensitive to the concentration of gas in the blood. Nociceptive signals (pain and noxious stimuli) are transmitted with sympathetic fibers to the pleura and bronchi but with the vagus nerve in the trachea and the respiratory system globally.

## Ultrastructure

Some subcellular components of the cells of the respiratory system are worth mentioning (Figure 1.11). These elements cannot be identified by conventional optical microscopy and require the use of an electron

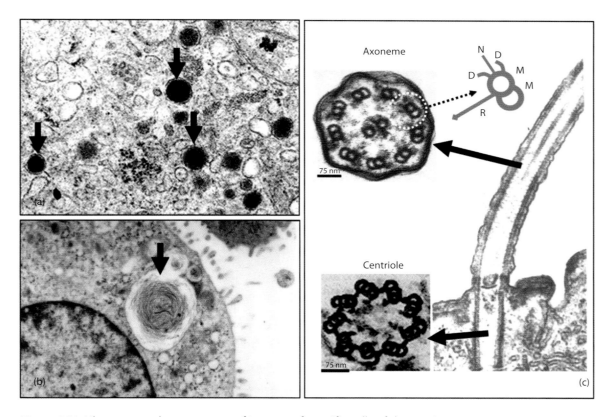

Figure 1.11 Ultrastructural components of interest of specific cells of the respiratory system. **(a)** Neurosecretory granules of neuroendocrine cells of the bronchial epithelium. **(b)** Lamellar body of a type II pneumocyte (surfactant). **(c)** Bronchial cilium. Cross sections of axoneme (top) and centriole (bottom). In the axoneme, there are nine peripheral microtubule doublets (M) and one central pair whereas in the centriole, the arrangement is rather nine peripheral triplets without central doublet. The main proteins that provide stability and coordination for the movement of microtubules during ciliary beat are illustrated. Radial spokes (R) stabilize and connect each peripheral doublet to the central doublet. Dynein arms (D) actively help adjacent peripheral doublets slide over one another and nexin (N) slows this movement.

microscope, for which the term *ultrastructure* is used. First, the secretory products of neuroendocrine cells of the bronchial epithelium appear in electron microscopy as round, dense cytoplasmic granules called dense core granules. Second, type II pneumocytes of the alveolar epithelium show microvilli, and lamellar bodies corresponding to surfactant. Finally, electron microscopy allows visualization of the complexity and elegance of the respiratory epithelium cilia. In cross section of their upper extracellular portion called the axoneme, the cilia include nine microtubule doublets and a central microtubule doublet whereas in their basal intracytoplasmic portion, called the centriole, the arrangement is rather nine microtubule triplets without central doublet. The ciliary beat results from the sliding of the peripheral microtubule doublets over one another in the axoneme. Several proteins provide stability and coordination of this movement. Radial spokes stabilize the axoneme by connecting each peripheral doublet to the central doublet. Dynein arms actively help adjacent peripheral doublets slide over one another and nexin slows this movement.

## References

1. Kuhn C III. Normal anatomy and histology. In: Churg AM, Myers JL, Tazelaar HD, Wright JL, editors. *Thurlbeck's Pathology of the Lung*. 3rd edition. New York, NY: Thieme; 2005:1–38.
2. De Paepe ME. Lung growth and development. In: Churg AM, Myers JL, Tazelaar HD, Wright JL, editors. *Thurlbeck's Pathology of the Lung*. 3rd edition. New York, NY: Thieme; 2005:39–84.
3. Wright JL, Thurlbeck WM. Quantitative anatomy of the lung. In: Churg AM, Myers JL, Tazelaar HD, Wright JL, editors. *Thurlbeck's Pathology of the Lung*. 3rd edition. New York, NY: Thieme; 2005:85–94.
4. Colby TV, Yousem SA. Lungs. In: Mills SS, editor. *Histology for Pathologists*, 3rd edition. New York, NY: Lippincott-Raven; 2007:473–504.
5. Travis WD, Colby TV, Koss MN, Rosado-de-Christenson ML, Müller NL, King TE Jr. Non-neoplastic disorders of the lower respiratory tract. In: King DW, editor. *Atlas of Nontumor Pathology*. First Series. Fascicle 2. Washington, DC: Armed Forces Institute of Pathology; 2002:1–15.
6. Moore KL, Dalley AF. *Anatomie Médicale. Aspects Fondamentaux Et Applications Cliniques*. Éditions De Boeck Université. 2ème édition de la traduction française. Bruxelles: De Boeck Université; 2007:74–135.

# 2

# Physiology of the respiratory system

PIERRE LEBLANC

| | |
|---|---|
| Functional anatomy of the cardio-respiratory system | 16 |
|     Functional structure of the respiratory system | 16 |
|     Functional structure of the circulatory system | 16 |
| Respiratory mechanics | 17 |
|     Elastic properties of the respiratory system: The pressure–volume curve | 17 |
|     The sequential unfolding of inspiration and expiration | 18 |
|     Resistive characteristics of the respiratory system | 19 |
|     Dynamic compression of airways | 21 |
|     Tissue oxygenation | 22 |
|     Respiratory manoeuvres | 22 |
|     Ventilation | 22 |
|     Ventilation/perfusion ratio | 22 |
|     Diffusion | 23 |
|     Oxygen transport | 24 |
|     Cellular respiration | 24 |
| Carbon dioxide physiology | 26 |
|     $CO_2$ production | 26 |
|     Alveolar ventilation | 26 |
|     $CO_2$ transport | 26 |
|     Acid–base status | 27 |
|     pH concept | 28 |
|     Acid and base concept | 29 |
|     The "buffer" concept | 29 |
|     pK | 29 |
|     Henderson–Hasselbalch equation | 30 |
|     Acid homeostasis | 31 |
|     Acid–base equilibrium disturbance | 31 |
|     Acid–base equilibrium disturbance compensation | 31 |
| Suggested readings | 32 |

This chapter describes the lung mechanical properties and their function as a transfer organ for gases such as oxygen and carbon dioxide. The reader is invited to consult the suggested readings list and general references related to the topic.

# Functional anatomy of the cardio-respiratory system

## Functional structure of the respiratory system

From a functional point of view, the respiratory system can be divided into three components: the ventilatory pump, an air distribution network, and a blood and gases exchange zone.

The ventilatory pump includes thoracic structures such as ribs, vertebrae, sternum, and the respiratory muscles. The diaphragm is the main respiratory muscle that performs most of the inspiratory work. Its innervation comes from the third, fourth, and fifth cervical nerves *via* the phrenic nerve. During inhalation, the diaphragm moves downward in the abdominal cavity in much the same manner as a piston. The abdominal organs stabilize this contraction and enable the ribs upward movement, similar to a bucket handle. It also contributes in increasing the thoracic volumes in its three axes. The intercostal muscles are at rest during normal breathing; they contract when the ventilation increases under certain conditions such as exercise or in respiratory diseases. The inner part of the thoracic cavity and the lung are both covered by thin membranes called the parietal and the visceral pleura, respectively. Between these two membranes, there is a virtual space containing a small amount of fluid which behaves as a lubricant and allows both membranes to slide smoothly on each other. Any outward movement of the thoracic cage initiated by inspiratory muscles is thus transmitted to the lung, which in turn increases its volume.

The distribution network of air encompasses the upper and lower airways dedicated to the filtration, heating, and humidification of ambient air to play a major role in smelling, swallowing, and speech. The upper airways include the nose, the para-nasal sinuses, the pharynx, and the larynx. The lower airways start at the junction between the larynx and the trachea at the level of the vocal cords and include the trachea, bronchi, bronchioles, and alveoli. The lower airways may be divided into two components: (1) the conduction zone, which is proximal to the terminal bronchioles and forms the anatomical dead space and not involved in gaseous exchanges. From the trachea to the terminal bronchioles, the bronchi dichotomically divide about 16 times. This contributes to increase the transversal area from 2 to 5 cm$^2$ in the trachea to 300 cm$^2$ at the terminal bronchioles level and (2) the respiratory zone, distal to the respiratory bronchioles down to the alveoli. This respiratory zone is responsible for the alveolar ventilation that contributes to the gas exchange of oxygen and carbon dioxide.

The gas exchange area includes the alveoli, whose number is about 300 million. At this level, the exchange area of the membrane reaches close to 80 m$^2$; the equivalent of a tennis court. The walls of the alveoli accommodate a capillary network where the exchange of oxygen and carbon dioxide occurs through a diffusion process, as the result of a pressure gradient across the alveolo-capillary membrane.

## Functional structure of the circulatory system

From a functional point of view, the circulatory system can also be divided into three components: the circulatory pump, a blood distribution network, and an exchange zone for gas transfer.

The circulatory pump is the consequence of the rhythmic contraction of the ventricules and results in the convective transport of inspired gases between the pulmonary capillary and the tissues. The pulmonary valve prevents the blood regurgitation toward the right ventricule during its relaxation period (diastole). The pulmonary vascular system operates at a mean pressure of 15 mmHg, namely at a pressure five times lower than the mean systemic pressure.

The blood distribution network is different from the previously described airway conduction network due to the double blood input to the lung from both the bronchial and the pulmonary arteries. The bronchial arteries originate from the aorta and carry oxygenated blood. They irrigate the trachea and bronchi down to the respiratory bronchioles. The division of these arteries follows the bronchial divisions. The bronchial veins drain mostly into the azygos veins in the venous circulation, but a part of the drainage includes anastomoses between the bronchial veins and the pulmonary veins and thus, contributing to the right-to-left physiological shunt with the Thebesian coronary veins. The pulmonary artery originates from the right ventricle and divides in parallel to the bronchi, to the terminal bronchioles, after which they develop a capillary network down to the alveoli. Once the blood has been oxygenated, it comes back to the left atrium through the pulmonary veins at the level of the terminal bronchioles. These veins drain a portion of the bronchial circulation and they anastomose with the pulmonary veins close to the left atrium. For more details, refer to Chapter 1.

The exchange zone includes a blood volume approximating, at rest about 100 mL, which is transported to the alveolar capillaries. The red blood cells have to remain in contact with air during a 0.25-second period to enable complete oxygen saturation of hemoglobin and an equilibration of the $CO_2$ and partial pressure of oxygen ($PaO_2$) between both compartments. At rest, the 0.75-second transit time of red blood cells is sufficient for these exchanges to take place.

## Respiratory mechanics

### Elastic properties of the respiratory system: The pressure–volume curve

The elastic properties of the lung depend of the fibroelastic tissue network constituting the lung parenchyma and, in turn, provides structural support to the alveolar walls. When lung volume increases during inspiration, the elastic recoil pressure of the lung increases. This pressure is not only generated by elastic fiber stretching, but also depends on the surface tension of the air–liquid interface of the alveoli and of the integrity of the surfactant coat that covers their inner wall. Therefore, the lung tends to empty completely when it is not submitted to external pressure. At the completion of a normal expiration, at the functional residual capacity (FRC), the lung tends to collapse. This movement is opposed by the tendency of the rib cage to increase its volume at FRC. Therefore, it can be said that the resting position of the lung outside of the thorax is volume 0 whereas the resting or relaxation volume of the rib cage without the lung is around 1 L above the FRC. When these structures interact within the thorax, the lung and the rib cage volume at FRC is around 3 L in a normal adult, equivalent to 50% of the total lung capacity (TLC).

There is a pressure–volume relationship for the lung, another one for the rib cage and another for the total (combined) respiratory system globally, which is in fact the sum of the first two curves (see Figure 2.1). It is thus possible to measure, for the lung and the rib cage, a change in pressure for a given change in volume ($\Delta P/\Delta V$). The opposite of this relation ($\Delta V/\Delta P$) is designated as the *compliance curve* and allows us to assess the capacity of a structure to be distended.

In performing such measurements, we will observe that the pressure inside an isolated lung is 0 (equal to the atmospheric pressure) and that the lung is completely deflated. When it is inflated, the inner pressure increases curvilinearly. At TLC, which is the maximal volume that can be inhaled by an individual, the pressure in the lung is +30 cm $H_2O$ (Figure 2.1).

Otherwise, if we could close the rib cage after having removed the lungs, the volume of the rib cage would be 1 L above the volume that would be present had the two lungs been intact. If we could decrease the rib cage volume (without lung) at a volume corresponding to the residual volume (RV), namely the minimal volume that the lung contains when an individual makes a maximal effort to empty his lung, the pressure inside the rib cage would be −20 cm $H_2O$. If we could increase the rib cage at a volume corresponding to the TLC, the pressure inside the rib cage would be around +10 cm $H_2O$.

Therefore, when the lung and the rib cage are coupled and no respiratory muscle is active, the lung is at FRC. At this volume, the elastic pressure of the lung and the rib cage is equal and opposite in direction: the algebraic sum is zero. The inspiratory muscles will have to generate a 40 cm $H_2O$ pressure to inflate

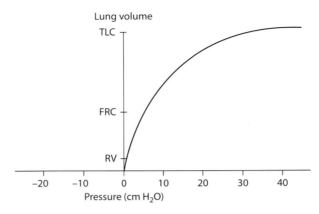

Figure 2.1 Pressure–volume curve of the lung. The elastic recoil pressure of the lung is null under the residual volume and increases at 30 cm H₂O at total lung capacity.

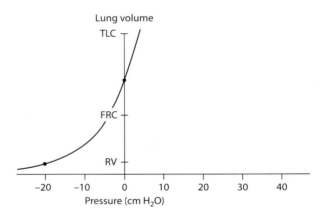

Figure 2.2 Pressure–volume curve of the rib cage. The elastic recoil pressure of the rib cage is negative up to 1 L under the total lung capaciy which means that it has a natural trend to expand, in opposition to the lung.

the respiratory system to TLC (30 cm H₂O to expand the lung and 10 cm H₂O to expand the rib cage) and the expiratory muscles will have to generate a 20 cm H₂O pressure to deflate the respiratory system to RV (20 cm H₂O to compress the rib cage; Figure 2.2).

## The sequential unfolding of inspiration and expiration

Inspiration is an active process that requires the contraction of inspiratory muscles. This contraction leads to a negative intrapleural pressure and creates a pressure gradient between the inside and the outside of the alveoli. The pressure inside the alveoli becomes more negative than the atmospheric pressure and air penetrates into the alveoli. By increasing its volume, it accumulates an elastic recoil pressure that is equal and opposite of the pleural pressure. When equilibrium is reached, the air flow in the alveoli stops. The intra-alveolar pressure is then equal to the atmospheric pressure. Therefore, the stronger the inspiratory muscle contraction, the more negative the intrapleural pressure will be and more air will flow into the alveoli (Figure 2.3).

# Respiratory mechanics 19

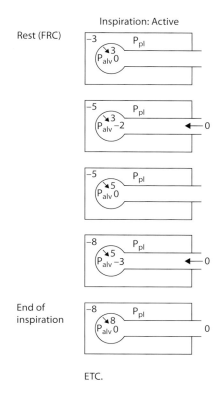

Figure 2.3 Sequential unfolding of inspiration. During inspiration, pleural pressure becomes more negative from −3 to −8 cm H₂O. This ends up in a negative pressure inside the alveoli and the aspiration of air from outside which inflates the alveoli.

At the end of an inspiratory manoeuver, the alveoli have stored elastic energy. The inspiratory muscles stop their activity. The intrapleural pressure becomes less negative, the elastic recoil of the alveoli becomes more positive than the atmospheric pressure, and the air flows outside. This lasts as long as the equilibrium between the elastic recoil of the alveoli and the intrapleural pressure is not reached (Figure 2.4). This is a passive process that does not require any expiratory muscle contraction. At the end of an inspiratory manoeuvre, it is possible to contract expiratory muscles and increase the air flow out of the lung. During this contraction, the transpulmonary pressure remains the same as during normal expiration, but the pressure gradient between the inside and outside of the alveoli increases. The expiratory flow is then higher than during a normal expiration.

## Resistive characteristics of the respiratory system

During inspiration, the respiratory muscles work against the elastic resistance to stretching and also against the frictional resistance when air flows from the mouth to the alveoli. This resistance is mostly located in larger airways where the flow is turbulent.

Many factors limit the expiratory flow. The pressure that generates a given flow $P$ (A-ao) is the difference between alveolar pressure ($P_A$) and the pressure at the aperture of the airways ($P_{ao}$). The resistance ($R_{aw}$) is then calculated by this equation:

$$R_{aw} = \frac{P_A - P_{ao}}{\dot{V}}$$

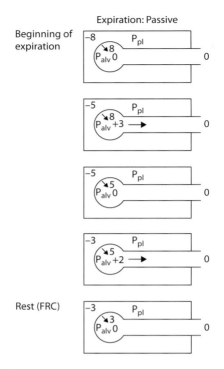

Figure 2.4 Sequential unfolding of expiration. During expiration, pleural pressure becomes less negative. The pressure becomes positive inside the alveoli, driving air outside.

where $\dot{V}$ is the expiratory flow.

The driving pressure necessary to overcome the resistance depends on the type of flow. When it is laminar, the flow ($\dot{V}$) is proportional to the driving pressure and complies with Poiseuille law according to this relation:

$$\dot{V} = \frac{P\pi r^4}{8 nL}$$

where "n" is gas viscosity, "l" length of the tube, "$\dot{V}$" flow, "R" tube radius, and "P" pressure. The resistance is inversely proportional to the radius at the power of four. There is a strong relationship between flow and radius.

When turbulent, the driving pressure is proportional to the flow squared and the pressure required to generate a given flow is higher than when the flow is laminar. The Reynolds number is used to classify the nature of the flow, a value under 2000 producing a laminar flow and a value over 2000, a turbulent flow. Furthermore, the airway caliber is in inverse proportion to the lung volume. Therefore, at high lung volume such as TLC, the airway radius is longer than at RV. Airway resistance is thus higher at RV. At this volume, the flow may become turbulent, requiring a higher pressure to generate a given flow.

Moreover, expiratory muscles are stronger close to TLC and weaker as we approach RV. It is at TLC that the optimal conditions are met to generate high airflow: airways are larger, flow is laminar and expiratory muscles are stronger. When the lungs empty, the conditions become disadvantageous, with smaller airways and higher resistance to airflow in addition to weaker expiratory muscles. These mechanisms explain why you fully expand your lungs before blowing out candles on a cake.

## Dynamic compression of airways

To understand the factors limiting expiratory airflow, the *equal pressure point (EPP)* and the *critical transmural pressure* (Ptm1) concepts must be understood. At the completion of a normal inspiratory manoeuver, the intrapleural pressure ($-10$ cm $H_2O$) counterbalances the elastic recoil pressure of the lung ($+10$ cm $H_2O$). During the passive expiration that follows, the pleural pressure becomes less negative. Air flows from the alveoli to the mouth whereas part of the pressure inside the bronchi is dissipated by the resistance generated by the flow which is about 1 L/sec. During forced expiration, the pleural pressure becomes positive and this pressure is transmitted to the whole respiratory system. The driving pressure increases and the pleural pressure around the bronchi increase by the same amount. The expiratory flow increases and once again, a portion of the pressure inside the bronchi is lost through resistance. At a moment during expiration, there will be a zone along the bronchi where the pressure inside the bronchi will be equal to the pressure outside. This is the equal pressure point (EPP). Downstream to the mouth, the pressure inside the bronchi keeps on decreasing whereas the pressure outside remains high. A compression of the bronchi happens and may progress to complete obstruction of the airway. This is the critical transmural pressure (Ptm1), the pressure that causes a collapse of the bronchi. There is transitory absence of flow, a decrease in resistance, an increase of the airway pressure and a flow recovery. An additional expiratory effort will produce more compression whereas the flow remains constant (Figure 2.5).

We may conclude that expiratory flow depends on three factors: elastic recoil of the lung, the critical closing pressure of airways, and the airway resistance upstream of the compressible segment. The upper airflow resistance is located between the alveoli and the ptm1 zone. When the pressure is higher than the Ptm1, airflow is effort independent and depends of the elastico-resistive properties of the lung. Therefore, airflow decreases with lung volume because the elastic recoil of the lung decreases and the airway resistance increases. For example, airflow decreases in asthma as the airway resistance is increased. In emphysema, it decreases because elastic recoil is diminished and the airway resistance is increased.

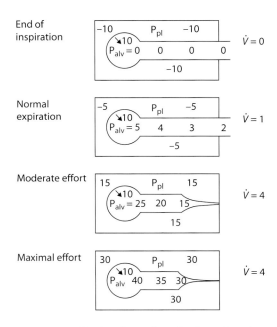

Figure 2.5 Forced respiratory sequence. During forced expiration, the pleural pressure becomes more positive than the pressure inside the bronchi causing a collapsus and a flow limitation. At a given flow, an increase in pleural pressure has no effect on flow.

## Tissue oxygenation

Oxygenation includes three steps: (1) respiration that brings oxygen molecules from ambient air to the alveoli before diffusing into the blood through the alveolo-capillary membrane; (2) oxygen transport to the tissues, which needs hemoglobin and an appropriate cardiac output; and (3) cellular respiration, where there is diffusion of oxygen molecules from the capillaries to the tissues and use of oxygen to produce energy.

## Respiration

There are three components contributing to breathing (respiration): (1) the *ventilation*, which allows the turnover of oxygen in alveoli and the washout of $CO_2$; (2) the *ventilation/perfusion ratio* of alveoli, which quantifies the degree of contact between alveoli and capillaries; and (3) the *diffusion*, which depends on contact duration of the red blood cells transported in the capillaries and the integrity of the alveoli-capillary membrane.

## Ventilation

The oxygen volume that reaches alveoli is dependent on ventilation. Ventilation is driven mostly by the arterial $CO_2$ ($PaCO_2$) and arterial $O_2$ ($PaO_2$). $CO_2$ is a powerful ventilatory stimulus; also, any increase in $PaCO_2$ causes a stimulation of ventilation (through the central chemoreceptors that also allows an increase in $O_2$ delivery to the alveoli (Figure 2.6).

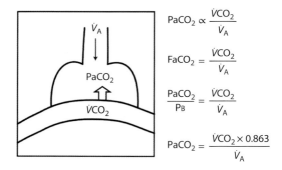

Figure 2.6 Alveolar ventilation equation. $PaCO_2$ is directly proportional to $CO_2$ production and indirectly proportional to alveolar ventilation.

## Ventilation/perfusion ratio

In a normal adult, alveolar ventilation is about 4 L/min and the total lung perfusion is 5 L/min. The ventilated zones must be perfused; a right lung ventilated and a left lung perfused would be useless without $O_2$ and $CO_2$ exchange. Perfusion in the lung is dependent on gravity, which creates perfusion inhomogeneity. The vertical gradient of pressure in the vessel varies by 1 cm $H_2O$ for each centimeter of height. The hydrostatic hemodynamic reference point is located at the level of the right atrium. In standing position, the lower part of the lung is more perfused than the apex. The ratio of perfusion between the base and the apex of the lung may reach 20/1. There is also an inhomogeneity in ventilation that varies according to the difference in compliance and resistance of the different pulmonary zones. To understand this concept, one must understand the transpulmonary pressure ($P_L$) concept. It is the difference between the alveolar pressure ($P_A$) and the pleural pressure ($P_{pl}$).

$$P_L = P_A - P_{Pl}$$

The pleural pressure is not the same everywhere within the thorax. At the end of a normal inspiration, the basal pleural pressure is 8 cm $H_2O$ higher than the apical pleural pressure. Pleural pressure increases linearly at a rate of 0.25 cm $H_2O$ for each centimeter from the top to the bottom of the lung. Therefore, the pleural pressure varies from −2 cm $H_2O$ at the bottom to −10 cm $H_2O$ at the top of the lung. As the alveolar pressure is 0 within the entire lung, the transpulmonary pressure varies from +2 at the bottom to +10 cm $H_2O$ at the top. At the end of a normal inspiration, the alveoli at the top of the lung are more inflated than those at the bottom. During inhalation, the pleural pressure uniformly diminishes into the entire thoracic cavity and decreases from −2 to −7 cm $H_2O$ at the bottom and from −10 to −15 cm $H_2O$ at the top. Due to the pressure–volume relationship of the alveoli, those at the top will have a lesser change in volume than those at the bottom, because they are less compliant, being initially more inflated. During a normal inhalation, ventilation will preferentially be distributed to the alveoli of the bottom. The ventilation in the lower part is twice that of the upper part of the lung.

A simple method to evaluate the relationship between the ventilation and the perfusion in the lungs is to establish a ratio of both components. It is called the *ventilation/perfusion ratio* ($\dot{V}_A/\dot{V}_Q$). In a normal individual, this ratio is at 3.3 at the top of the lung and at 0.63 at the bottom. The average $\dot{V}/\dot{Q}$ ratio of the lung is at 0.8 which corresponds to the ratio of the alveolar ventilation (4 L) to the perfusion (5 L).

According to the circumstances, a pulmonary zone may be well ventilated but not perfused. This may occur with pulmonary emboli, when a pulmonary vessel is occluded by a clot while the ventilation is preserved. The $\dot{V}/\dot{Q}$ ratio is then infinite. Such a zone behaves like a dead space in which the ventilation is lost, not participating in gas exchange. Conversely a pulmonary zone may be well perfused but not ventilated. This may occur in pneumonia when the alveoli are filled with the inflammatory fluid that precludes ventilation although perfusion is preserved. The $\dot{V}/\dot{Q}$ ratio is then at 0. Such a zone behaves like a right to left shunt, where the blood goes through the capillary without being oxygenated and refers to shunt.

In a normal individual, 30% of total ventilation does not reach alveoli: a portion of the inspired gas resides in large airways without participating in gas exchange. This lost ventilation is called "anatomic" dead space. Of the 6 L/min of ventilation at rest, 4 L reach the alveoli and 2 L are lost (dead space). Between 3% and 5% of the blood flowing into the thorax goes back to the left atria without being oxygenated. This is the blood coming from some pulmonary veins and Thebesius veins. This tiny right-to-left shunt contributes to the small difference between the alveolar $PO_2$ and the arterial $PO_2$. In some diseases of the lung, the dead space and the shunt may increase significantly and cause major abnormalities in gas exchange, mostly hypoxemia.

## Diffusion

The alveolo-capillary surface behaves like a semi-permeable membrane where gas exchange occurs as determined by pressure gradients. Diffusion is defined by the Fick law.

$$\dot{V}\text{gas} = \frac{A \times D \times (P1 - P2)}{T}$$

The transfer of a gas through a tissue is proportional to the surface of the tissue (*A*), to the solubility coefficient of the gas through the membrane (*D*), and the partial pressure difference from one side to the other (*P1−P2*) and is inversely proportional to the thickness of the membrane. $CO_2$ has a diffusion capacity 20 times greater than the oxygen. To diffuse through a membrane, a gas needs an equilibrium time long enough to allow equilibrium between the alveoli and the capillary and enough alveoli to allow an adequate volume of gas exchange. The transit time into the pulmonary capillary is 0.75 sec at rest and 0.25 sec during exercise. The necessary time to equilibrate transfer gradients between the alveoli and the capillary is 0.25 sec. The equilibrium is reached during the first third of the transit into the capillary. Oxygen diffusion is then limited partly by the perfusion and the speed of the binding of hemoglobin and oxygen. During the oxygen passage into the pulmonary capillary blood, the pressure difference ($P1-P2$) decreases and the transfer is less efficient. This may be counteracted by increasing the pulmonary perfusion; an example of this is the increase in cardiac output during exercise.

The factors that can contribute to the decreased diffusion or preclude the equilibration are the thickening of the alveolo-capillary membrane (pulmonary fibrosis), the decrease in the pressure gradient (altitude), intense exercise, and the decrease in the surface area for gas exchange (emphysema, pneumonectomy).

## Oxygen transport

Oxygen is carried in the blood in two forms: dissolved and bound to hemoglobin. The amount dissolved is dependent on the solubility constant of oxygen in the plasma at 37°C namely 0.003 mL/mmHg/100 mL of blood. There is a linear relationship between the $PaO_2$ and the dissolved volume. When $PaO_2$ is 100 mmHg, 0.3 mL of oxygen is dissolved per 100 mL of blood (3 mL/L); this volume of oxygen is inadequate to satisfy the energy requirements of humans. We would need a 100 L/min cardiac output to do so. Hemoglobin increases the efficiency of oxygen transport. This is a high molecular weight molecule (64,500 daltons) made up of heme and globin. Globin is made of four amino acid chains: two alpha chains of 141 amino acids each and two beta chains of 146 amino acids each. Each chain is bound to a heme group that is made of a porphyrin group and an iron molecule. This last fixes oxygen. Each hemoglobin molecule can combine with four molecules of oxygen and its affinity increases as more oxygen molecules fix to hemoglobin. The percentage of the oxygen transport sites occupied by oxygen molecules defines the percentage of hemoglobin saturation in oxygen ($SaO_2$). One gram of hemoglobin has the capacity to carry 1.39 mL of oxygen, when 100% saturated. The blood contains 15 g of hemoglobin per 100 mL and thus has the capacity to carry 200 mL of oxygen per liter when the hemoglobin is 100% saturated.

There is a relationship, although not linear, between $PaO_2$ and $SaO_2$. This relationship has a sigmoid shape and is defined as the *hemoglobin desaturation curve* (Figure 2.7). On this curve, there is a critical zone between 20 and 60 mmHg where a small change in $PaO_2$ leads to a considerable change in $O_2$ saturation. Therefore, at a normal $PaO_2$ of 100 mmHg, $SaO_2$ is at 97% whereas at a $PvO_2$ (the partial pressures in the venous blood) of 40 mmHg, $SaO_2$ is at 75% (Figure 2.7).

The hemoglobin dissociation curve may shift to the right or to the left in some conditions (Figure 2.8). The curve shifts to the right when the pH is acid, when $PaCO_2$ increases (respiratory acidosis) or when the temperature increases. Under these conditions, the hemoglobin saturation is lower for a given $PaO_2$ and promotes the oxygen release. This occurs in tissues like muscle during exercise. Otherwise, the curve may shift to the left when pH is alkaline, when the $PaCO_2$ decreases (respiratory alkalosis) or when the temperature decreases. Under these conditions, the hemoglobin saturation is higher for a given $PaO_2$ and promotes the oxygen capture. This occurs in alveoli. These peculiarities of the hemoglobin dissociation curve are well adapted for oxygen transport.

## Cellular respiration

The arterial blood is distributed into the body at a given oxygen concentration. Oxygen uptake ($\dot{V}O_2$) varies between organs and the degree of extraction is variable. For example, heart muscle extracts more oxygen

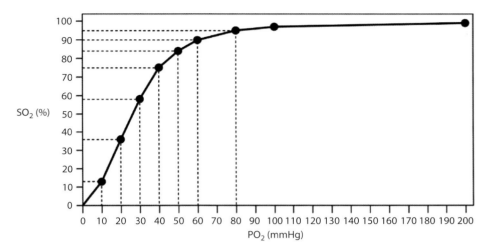

Figure 2.7 Oxyhemoglobin dissociation curve. The relationship between partial pressure of oxygen and hemoglobin saturation is not linear.

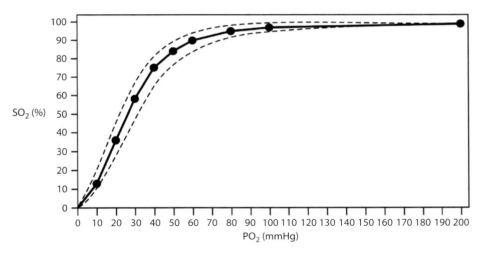

Figure 2.8 Displacement of the oxyhemoglobin dissociation curve. The relationship between partial pressure of oxygen and hemoglobin saturation may move to the right or to the left according to metabolic conditions.

than skin by a coefficient of 10. Organs that consume less oxygen usually use the blood flow for duties other than oxygenation such as thermic regulation for the skin or the filtration for the kidney glomeruli. In the mitochondria, oxygen is mostly used to oxidize the pyruvic acid into the Krebs cycle and to produce adenosine triphosphate (ATP) molecules that hold high energy links, necessary to the global operation of the body. In the absence of oxygen, the body must rely more on anaerobic metabolism. This mechanism is ineffective and generates few ATP molecules that result in acidemia. Hypoxia occurs when oxygen is not sufficient to satisfy the metabolic needs of the tissues. We consider that this occurs when $PaO_2$ inside the mitochondria is lower than 7 mmHg.

## Carbon dioxide physiology

### CO$_2$ production

CO$_2$ production ($\dot{V}CO_2$) depends on the intensity of energy expenditure and the substrate of metabolism. At rest, an individual consumes about 250 mL/min of oxygen and produces 200 mL/min of CO$_2$. The $\dot{V}CO_2/\dot{V}O_2$ ratio at 0.8 is defined as the respiratory quotient. The $\dot{V}O_2$ and the $\dot{V}CO_2$ may increase by a coefficient of 15–20 in a normal individual during exercise. $\dot{V}O_2$ and $\dot{V}CO_2$ increase to 3000–4000 mL/min. The lung is not only the source of entry of oxygen, but also the exit for CO$_2$. Contrary to oxygen, the CO$_2$ produced by tissue metabolism must be carried to the lung to be exhaled during expiration. There is an equilibrium between the CO$_2$ produced by the tissue, the amount of CO$_2$ carried in the blood (PaCO$_2$) and the amount of CO$_2$ excreted, or exhaled by the lung. The regulation system between the tissue production and the elimination depends on rate of alveolar ventilation. When there is hypercapnia (increase in PaCO$_2$ in venous blood), a larger amount of CO$_2$ reaches the lung and the arterial blood carries more CO$_2$. This stimulates the central bulbo-pontine respiratory centers to increase ventilation. The faster renewal of air in alveoli allows a decrease in PaCO$_2$ and promotes CO$_2$ diffusion from the blood to the alveoli. Therefore, there is a greater removal of CO$_2$.

There is a proportional relationship between alveolar ventilation ($\dot{V}A$), $\dot{V}CO_2$ and PaCO$_2$ in arterial blood; it is described by the alveolar ventilation equation:

$$PaCO_2 = \frac{\dot{V}CO_2 \times 0.863}{\dot{V}A}$$

According to this equation, the only way to maintain a constant PaCO$_2$ when $\dot{V}CO_2$ increases is to increase ventilation. It is crucial for the body to maintain PaCO$_2$ constant as any variation brings major changes in the H$^+$ ion concentration in the blood and has a direct impact on pH and acid–base balance.

### Alveolar ventilation

Alveolar ventilation must be differentiated from total ventilation. We calculate total ventilation by multiplying tidal volume ($\dot{V}t$), the volume expired at each respiration, by the frequency of breathing in breath/min *(Bf)*:

$$\dot{V}E = \dot{V}t \times Bf.$$

Only a part of the total volume of air breathed reaches the alveoli to participate in gas exchange. The best way to evaluate if ventilation is appropriate for $\dot{V}CO_2$ is to measure PaCO$_2$. As previously shown, in the alveolar ventilation equation, PaCO$_2$ is inversely proportional to the alveolar ventilation. $\dot{V}E$ includes the alveolar ventilation ($\dot{V}A$) and the dead space ventilation ($\dot{V}D$) that includes the volume of air that remains in dead space zones without participating in gas exchange. In a normal individual, $\dot{V}t$ is around 500 mL, $\dot{V}D$ 150 mL, and $\dot{V}A$ 350 mL. With a breathing frequency of 12/min, total ventilation at rest is 6 L, but alveolar ventilation is only 4.2 L.

### CO$_2$ transport

Although related to oxygen, CO$_2$ transport shows peculiar characteristics, mostly due to its close relationship to acid–base balance. CO$_2$ is carried under four forms: (1) dissolved, (2) carbonic acid (H$_2$CO$_3$), (3) carbonic anhydrase ion (HCO$_3^-$), and (4) as carbamino compounds.

The $CO_2$ volume dissolved into the blood obeys Henry's law and is proportional to the partial pressure of the gas ($PaCO_2$) and to its solubility coefficient. Normal $PaCO_2$ is 40 mmHg and the solubility coefficient 0.072 mL/mm Hg/100 mL. The dissolved arterial $CO_2$ content is therefore 2.9 mL/100 mL of blood. This volume may be expressed in mEq/mmHg. A coefficient of 0.03 mEq/L/mmHg means the dissolved $CO_2$ is 1.2 mEq/L (miliequivalent/liter). One mEq of $CO_2$ corresponds to 2.23 mL of $CO_2$. Eight percent of the $CO_2$ is carried in dissolved form.

Dissolved $CO_2$ may combine with water to make carbonic acid from the action of carbonic anhydrase (c.a):

$$CO_2 + H_2O \xrightleftharpoons{\text{(c.a)}} H_2CO_3 \xrightleftharpoons{\text{(c.a)}} HCO_3^- + H^+$$
$$(340) \quad (1)$$

Although $H_2CO_3$ is a major intermediate product of this reaction, it is found in tiny quantities throughout the body. There is 0.006 mL of $H_2CO_3$/100 mL in the plasma. It is 340 times less than the dissolved form. $H_2CO_3$ is an unstable product but it is the center of the reaction.

The previous equation shows that equilibrium exists between dissolved $CO_2$ and $H_2CO_3$. $HCO_3^-$ ion accounts for 80% of $CO_2$ transport in the body. This is possible thanks to two reactions: one with carbonic anhydrase and another with chloride transfer. Carbonic anhydrase is an enzyme found in red cells and that activates the reaction.

$$CO_2 + H_2O \xrightleftharpoons[\text{(c.a)}]{\text{(hydration)}} H_2CO_3 \xrightleftharpoons[\text{(c.a)}]{\text{(dissociation)}} HCO_3^- + H^+$$

Carbonic anhydrase displaces the reaction to the right and promotes $HCO_3^-$ production by increasing the reaction speed by a factor of 13,000. The amount of $HCO_3^-$ in the blood is always expressed in mEq/L. The normal $HCO_3^-$ concentration in the plasma is 24 mEq/L namely 53.3 mL of $CO_2$/100 mL.

When $CO_2$ diffuses from the tissues, it accumulates in the plasma. It diffuses into the red cells where it is quickly transformed in $H_2CO_3$ under the action of carbonate anhydrase and immediately in $HCO_3^-$ and $H^+$ ions. $H^+$ ion will not accumulate in the cell and will quickly bind to hemoglobin, which acts as a buffer. Simultaneously, bicarbonate ion is carried from inside blood cells to the plasma. The transfer of $HCO_3^-$ ion in the plasma creates an electrostatic gradient between the red cell and the plasma. This results in a movement of chloride ion from the plasma into the red cell cytoplasm to maintain red cell electroneutrality (Figure 2.9).

A small volume of $CO_2$ is carried in the plasma, where it binds to proteins. $CO_2$ interacts with an amino group. A protein that carries $CO_2$ is called *carbamino group*. Two percent of $CO_2$ is transported this way. $CO_2$ may also combine with the globin protein on hemoglobin to make a carbamino-hemoglobin group. This binding between $CO_2$ and hemoglobin takes place on different sites than for oxygen, which binds to the heme component of hemoglobin. The hemoglobin affinity for $CO_2$ increases when the quantity of oxygen binding to hemoglobin decreases, which means that desaturated hemoglobin has a higher affinity for a given $PaCO_2$ (Haldane effect). Conversely, hemoglobin that carries $CO_2$ has less affinity for oxygen (Bohr effect). Ten percent of $CO_2$ is carried as carbamino-hemoglobin groups.

## Acid–base status

The human body is an environment that maintains its stability (homeostasis) despite multiple external assaults. After a copious meal, after ingesting a large quantity of liquid including alcohol, after intense

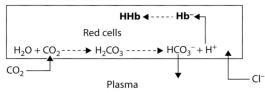
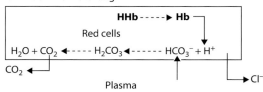

Figure 2.9 Chloride and bicarbonates exchanges to maintain cell electroneutrality. Entrance of chloride in red cell in exchange of bicarbonate ions allows the maintenance of cell electroneutrality and promotes $CO_2$ transport.

exercise, or after exposition to inhospitable conditions under extreme temperatures or altitude, the body remarkably succeeds in maintaining acid–base homeostasis. One of many parameters that can be used to evaluate this stability is the acid–base status. Indeed, there is a tight equilibrium between acids and bases in the body. Humans have many mechanisms to maintain this equilibrium throughout the entire lifespan. Small changes may give rise to important disturbances to the physiology of many organs.

Acid–base status is usually evaluated by measuring the $H^+$ ion concentration in the body. This measurement may be done on a blood sample with an electrode. The normal concentration of $H^+$ ion is 40 $n$Mol/L or $40 \times 10^{-9}$ mol/L.

## pH concept

$H^+$ ion is present in the blood in very small quantity and we express its concentration by reversing the concentration logarithm:

$$[H+] = 40 \ n\text{Mol}/L$$
$$= 40 \times 10^9 \ \text{mol}/L$$
$$pH = -\log 40 - \log 10^{-9}$$
$$= (-1.6) - (-9.0)$$
$$= -1.6 + 9.0$$
$$= 7.4$$

Normal pH is 7.40. Therefore, when $[H^+]$ increases, pH decreases and when $[H^+]$ decreases, pH increases. Due to the logarithmic relationship, a large change in $[H^+]$ gives rise to a small change in pH. When we double $[H^+]$, the pH decreases by 0.3.

| pH | 6.80 | 7.10 | **7.40** | 7.70 | 8.00 |
|---|---|---|---|---|---|
| $[H^+]$nMol/L | 160 | 80 | **40** | 20 | 10 |

The pH range compatible with life is quite narrow, particularly when the pH is higher than 7.40. A pH lower than 6.9 (0.5 under normal) or higher than 7.7 (0.3 greater than normal) is not compatible with life. The [H$^+$] compatible with life varies between 20 and 130 nMol/L. Between a pH of 7.28 and 7.45, a change in pH of 0.01 corresponds to a change in [H$^+$] of 1 *n*Mol/L. At a pH of 7.28, [H$^+$] = 52 *n*Mol/L. At a pH of 7.45, [H$^+$] = 35 *n*Mol/L.

## Acid and base concept

Acid is a substance that releases [H$^+$] ions in solution.

$$HCl \rightarrow [H^+] + [Cl^-]$$
$$H_2CO_3 \leftrightarrow [H^+] + [HCO_3^-]$$

An acid is strong when it completely dissociates in solution whereas it is weak when it incompletely dissociates. HCl is a strong acid and $H_2CO_3$ is a weak acid. A base is a substance that absorbs [H$^+$] ion in solution. In the previous equation, $HCO_3^-$ is a low. When we dissolve a weak acid in a solution, one part remains under the acid form and the other remains under base form. There is equilibrium between both components.

## The "buffer" concept

A buffer solution is one in which the pH strives to remain stable. The pH in a buffer solution is less affected by the addition of [H$^+$] than a solution without a buffer. The buffer minimizes the change in pH by converting strong acids or bases into weak ones. A buffer solution is usually made of a weak acid and a salt of its conjugated base.

$$H_2CO_3 \leftrightarrow NaHCO_3$$

When a strong acid is added to a buffer solution, it reacts with the salt of its conjugated base.

$$\frac{HCl + H_2CO_3}{NaHCO_3} \rightarrow NaCl + H_2CO_3$$

There are many buffer systems in the body. The most familiar that is used in the acid–base status evaluation is the bicarbonate system. There are extracellular (bicarbonate, plasma proteins such as albumin and globulins, inorganic phosphates, etc.) and intracellular (bicarbonates, hemoglobin and oxyhemoglobin, and organic and inorganic phosphates) buffers. The bicarbonate system provides 50% of the buffer activity in the body.

## pK

The efficacy of a buffer system depends on three characteristics: the quantity of available buffer, the pK of the solution, and the operating mode in an open or a closed system. The pK of a weak acid is the pH at which 50% of the acid is dissociated and 50% correct; it is its optimal efficacy pH.

$$H_2CO_3 \leftrightarrow H^+ + HCO_3^-$$

The pK of the bicarbonate system is at a pH of 6.1 that is to say that at this pH, [$H_2CO_3$] = [$HCO_3^-$]. Because a strong acid is buffered by the dissociated part of the buffer solution [$NaHCO_3$] and a strong base is buffered by the nondissociated part of a solution [$H_2CO_3$], at a pH of 6.1, a base or an acid can be buffered equally. At a normal pH of 7.4, 95% of bicarbonates are in dissociated form, which makes them more efficient to buffer acids than bases. The bicarbonate system is open because it communicates externally through the lung. Accordingly, there is no accumulation of weak acids in the system. $H_2CO_3$ transforms to $CO_2$ that can be washed out of the lung through ventilation.

$$\text{Ventilation} \leftarrow CO_2 + H_2O \leftarrow H_2CO_3 \leftarrow H^+ + HCO_3^-$$

## Henderson–Hasselbalch equation

There is a mathematical constant relationship between the components of the acid dissociation reaction (Henderson equation). For a given acid, there is a constant, describing the components of the acid on the left side of the equation and its dissociation production on the right side.

$$Kc = \frac{[H+][HCO_3^-]}{[H_2CO_3]}$$

Kc is the constant of the carbonic acid dissociation.

$$H+ = \frac{Kc[H_2CO_3]}{[H_2CO_3^-]}$$

Hasselbalch modified this first equation using a logarithmic transformation:

$$pH = pKc + \log\frac{[HCO_3^-]}{[H_2CO_3]}$$

where pK is the logarithmic reciprocal of the carbonic acid dissociation constant. For practical purposes, it is difficult to measure very small concentrations of [$H_2CO_3$]. Therefore we substitute the concentration of dissolved $CO_2$ for [$H_2CO_3$] to obtain the modified Henderson–Hasselbalch equation.

$$pH = pKc + \log\frac{[HCO_3^-]}{[CO_2 \text{ diss}]}$$

In this equation, [$HCO_3^-$] = 24 mEq/L and [$CO_2$ diss] = 1.2 mEq/L. According to Henry's law, [$CO_2$ diss] = 40 mmHg × 0.03 mEq/L/mmHg = 1.2 mEq/L.

$$pH = 6.1 + \log\frac{24 \text{ mEq/L}}{1.2 \text{ mEq/L}}$$
$$pH = 6.1 + \log 20$$
$$pH = 6.1 + 1.3$$
$$pH = 7.4$$

## Acid homeostasis

Human metabolism mostly generates acid excess that the body has to eliminate to maintain homeostasis. The principal organs to eliminate acid are the lung and the kidney. In humans, the lung excretes 13,000 mEq/L of $CO_2$ daily whereas the kidney excretes only 80 mEq. Due to disproportion, these two organs are essential and the lung is not able to guarantee acid homeostasis by itself. The lung excretes the volatile acids, namely those that can be transformed from a liquid to a gaseous phase. Carbonic acid is the only acid that can be excreted by the lung under normal conditions. The kidneys eliminate fixed acids such as sulfuric acid or phosphoric acid that cannot be transformed into gas and must be excreted in their liquid form in urine.

## Acid–base equilibrium disturbance

When we refer to the Henderson-Hasselbalch equation, pH will be modified if there is a change in the $[HCO_3^-]/PaCO_2$ ratio. If the ratio increases, pH increases—that is to say the $[H^+]$ decreases. If the ratio decreases, pH decreases then $[H^+]$ increases. The increase in $[HCO_3^-]/PaCO_2$ ratio may be due to an increase in $[HCO_3^-]$ or to a decrease in $PaCO_2$. The reduction in the $[HCO_3^-]/PaCO_2$ ratio may be the result of a decrease in $[HCO_3^-]$ or an increase in $PaCO_2$. When the variation is the result of a change in $PaCO_2$, it suggests the presence of an underlying respiratory disorder. When the variation is the result of a change in $[HCO_3^-]$, we are talking about a metabolic problem (Table 2.1).

Table 2.1 Acid–base equilibrium disturbances

| Acidosis | Respiratory | ↑ $PaCO_2$ |
|---|---|---|
|  | Metabolic | ↓ $[HCO_3^-]$ |
| Alkalosis | Respiratory | ↓ $PaCO_2$ |
|  | Metabolic | ↑ $[HCO_3^-]$ |

## Acid–base equilibrium disturbance compensation

Any acid–base equilibrium disturbance initiates compensatory mechanisms that aim to restore equilibrium to the system. This compensation intends to bring back the $[HCO_3^-]/PaCO_2$ ratio to normal. This compensation is never complete and the pH never comes back to its normal value of 7.0. When the disturbance results from a decrease in $PaCO_2$, the body reacts by regenerating bicarbonate in the kidney. If there is an increase in $PaCO_2$ like in alveolar hypoventilation, there is an increase in $[HCO_3^-]$. Otherwise, when the disturbance is the result of a decrease in $[HCO_3^-]$ such as in renal failure, the body reacts by decreasing $PaCO_2$ whereas when there is an increase in $[HCO_3^-]$, the body reacts by increasing $PaCO_2$.

The lung is responsible for $CO_2$ regulation. When the production increases, central respiratory centers stimulate an increase in minute ventilation. Alveolar ventilation increases and $PaCO_2$ remains constant. If $[HCO_3^-]$ increases or decreases, alveolar ventilation is modified, driving a change in $PaCO_2$ that will aim to normalize the $[HCO_3^-]/PaCO_2$ ratio. The ventilatory response is usually fast and occurs within minutes following the disturbance.

In conclusion, the respiratory system has specific properties that have a direct influence on ventilation and gas exchange. Its direct input to acid–base equilibrium contributes to the complexity of the multiple functions required to properly understand the pathophysiology of respiratory diseases discussed in Chapters 4, 5, 6 and 10 of this book.

## Suggested readings

1. Cotes JE. *Lung Function*. 5th ed. Oxford: Blackwell, 1993.
2. Crystal RG, West JB, Weibel ER, Barns PJ, eds. *The Lung: Scientific Foundations*. 2nd ed. New York, NY: Raven Press, 1997.
3. Leff AR, Schumacher PT. *Respiratory Physiology: Basics and Applications*. 1st ed. Philadelphia, PA: WB Saunders Company, 1993.
4. Levizky MG. *Pulmonary Physiology*. 4th ed. New York, NY: McGraw-Hill, 1996.
5. Murray JF. *The Normal Lung: The Basis for Diagnosis and Treatment of Pulmonary Disease*, Philadelphia, Saunders, 1976.
6. Murray JF, Nadel JA. *Textbook of Pulmonary Medicine*. 4th ed. Philadelphia, PA: Elsevier, 2005.
7. Nunn JF. *The Normal Lung*. 2nd ed. Philadelphia, PA: WB Saunders, 1986.
8. West JB. *Pulmonary Pathophysiology: The Essentials*. 5th ed. Baltimore, MD: Williams and Wilkins, 1997.
9. Flenley DC. Another non-logarithmic acid-base diagram? *Lancet* 1971;1:961–965.
10. Weibel ER. Morphological basis of alveolar-capillary gas exchange. *Physiol Rev* 1973;53:419–495.
11. West JB. Ventilation-perfusion relationships. *Am Rev Respir Dis* 1977;116:919–943.
12. West JB, Wagner PD. Pulmonary gas exchange. In: West JB ed. *Bioenginnering Aspects of the Lung*. New York, NY: Marcel Dekker, 1977.

# 3

# Laboratory techniques to study the cellular and molecular processes of disorders

CATHERINE LAPRISE

| | |
|---|---|
| Introduction | 33 |
| Immunocytochemistry | 34 |
| Enzyme-linked immunosorbent assay | 35 |
| Southern blot | 36 |
| Northern blot | 36 |
| Western blot | 36 |
| Quantitative flow cytometry analysis | 38 |
| Polymerase chain reaction | 38 |
|     Multiplex PCR | 41 |
|     Multiplex real-time PCR | 43 |
|     Molecular cloning | 45 |
|     Clustered regularly interspaced short palindromic repeats-associated proteins (CRISPR-Cas9) system | 46 |
|     Cellular and animal model systems | 48 |
|     Perspectives: Precision Medicine - from phenotypes to endotypes | 48 |
| Conclusion | 49 |
| References | 49 |

## Introduction

The goal of this chapter is to succinctly describe the main methodological approaches that are used to study the molecular and cellular processes of respiratory disorders, mainly illustrated through their uses in asthma research. This chapter emphasizes techniques aimed to examine a disease at the cellular and molecular levels, including the study of DNA, RNA, and proteins using asthma as a model when it is applicable. Each technique is described in detail on the Current Protocols in molecular biology website (www.currentprotocols.com).

Asthma is one of the most common chronic inflammatory diseases that affects the airways. This condition affects approximately 300 million people globally and its prevalence, morbidity, and mortality have been increasing since the 1960s in all industrialized countries [1,2]. The definition of asthma is becoming more and more specific (see Chapter 5) and recognizes that the presence of bronchial hyperresponsiveness is associated with the inflammatory responses and bronchial structural changes (remodeling). Asthma is no doubt a complex trait given the multitude of genetic and environmental determinants involved in its development and clinical expression.

## Immunocytochemistry

Histochemistry refers to the identification of cellular components in tissues (*histo*) based on the chemical reactions (*chemistry*) between a reagent and a target such as DNA, glycogen, or lipids. Reagents used in traditional staining methods in tissues were developed from textile dyes and they are still being used in the general staining process for optical microscopy [3]. With the development of new reagents, the staining techniques have improved tremendously to capture specific organelles and even molecules. A reagent is tagged with an enzyme that gives off a detectable signal (e.g., color or fluorescence) after binding to a target. In the case where the reagent being used is an antibody that recognizes a particular molecule (i.e., antigen),

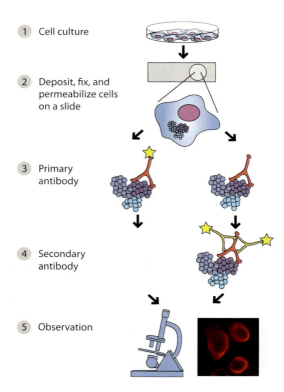

Figure 3.1 Immunocytochemistry. Step 1: Biological samples are prepared (e.g., cells in culture or biopsy tissues). Step 2: Samples are deposited on a microscope slide using centrifugation or cultured on slides previously treated with poly-L-lysine. Permeabilization of samples followed. Step 3: In direct immunofluorescence staining (left path), an antibody conjugated with a fluorochrome and specific to the targeted protein is deposited onto the sample. In indirect immunofluorescence staining (right path), the antibody is not labeled. Step 4: In indirect fluorescence staining, a secondary antibody labeled with a fluorochrome will be added after washing. Several secondary antibodies in turn bind to the primary antibody—targeted protein complex and emit a signal. The signal is amplified given the multiple binding of the secondary antibodies to one primary antibody. Step 5: Targeted protein is detected using fluorescence microscopy. The insert shows the localization of keratine 5 proteins (in red) in keratinocytes. The secondary antibodies used were red fluorochrome Cy3.

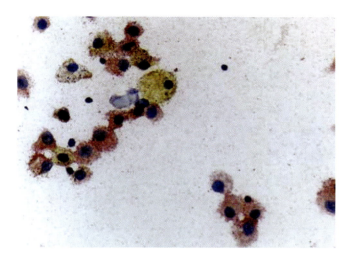

Figure 3.2 Detection of IL-12 and IL-13 in bronchoalveolar lavage cells by double immunohistochemistry (IHC). IL-12 proteins are labeled with brown color stain and IL-13 with red.

specifically, it is called immunohistochemistry (IHC). IHC is very specific and sensitive; it uses either direct or indirect labeling for target recognition (Figure 3.1).

The direct labeling method is carried out by using an antibody specific to an antigen and the antibody is conjugated with an enzyme whose enzymatic reaction can be visually detected under a microscope (e.g., fluorescence, coloring agent, or colloidal matter) [4]. The indirect labeling technique uses an antigen-specific antibody, but the antibody is not directly conjugated to an enzyme. Hence, an additional step is needed with a second antibody that is conjugated to an enzyme. While the antigen-specific antibody is called the primary antibody, the enzyme-conjugated antibody is referred to as the secondary antibody [5]. The recognition and binding of the secondary antibody to the primary antibody allow the visualization of the target under a microscope. One benefit of indirect labeling is signal amplification. By having multiple secondary antibodies bound to a primary antibody–antigen complex, the visual signal emitted is amplified. Both direct and indirect labeling methods are routinely used for the study of allergic asthma, especially to investigate the cellular and tissue distribution of a targeted protein in asthmatic relative to nonasthmatic subjects. For example, various T-helper 2-type (Th2) cytokines (e.g., interleukin (IL)-4, -5, and -13) and receptors have been found to be elevated in the airways of allergic asthmatic relative to nonasthmatic healthy individuals [6–8].

In addition to capturing the distribution of one target, IHC can also be used to detect the multiple targets. In this case, each multiple secondary antibody is conjugated with a different label molecule that would give off different color, and each color corresponds to a target (Figure 3.2). For example, double IHC detected the coexpression of IL-4 and IL-5 in T cells, mast cells, and eosinophils of bronchial tissues from allergic asthmatic subjects [8].

## Enzyme-linked immunosorbent assay

Enzyme-linked immunosorbent assay (ELISA) is commonly used to detect and measure the amount of an antigen of interest in biological fluid [9]. On a microslide, wells are usually coated with an antibody that is specific to an antigen. The coating process is done through electrostatic interactions. After a fluid is added into each well, the antigen, if present, would bind to the coated antibody. A secondary antibody, called the tracer, is also specific to the antigen and is subsequently added into the wells. The tracer recognizes the immobilized antigen and binds to it. Similar to IHC, the detection of the antigen–antibody binding can be done through direct (i.e., the tracer is conjugated with a label molecule) or indirect (i.e., the tracer is not conjugated and a secondary antibody conjugated with an enzyme is added for visualization) method. Any remaining loose tracers are washed away before the addition of the substrate to react with the conjugated enzyme. The enzymatic reaction is then detected and the amount of antigen can be estimated using a calibration curve generated from various known concentrations of the antigen. The intensity of the signal given corresponds to the amount of immobilized antigens originally in the fluid.

ELISA is a useful technique to detect protein expression in blood, serum, and bronchial lavage fluid of asthmatic subjects. Just in the past 5 years alone, hundreds of publications have reported associations between a protein of interest and asthma pathogenesis (www.ncbi.nlm.nih.gov). Most of the studies investigated cytokines production differences using ELISA in different asthma phenotypes or treatment responses [10–12]. By identifying the cytokines which are highly secreted in asthmatic subjects, these cytokines in turn become good candidates for therapeutic development.

## Southern blot

Southern blot technique, developed by Edwin Mellor Southern, is used to detect a specific DNA sequence in a cell [13]. Briefly, double-stranded DNA is first extracted and cleaved into fragments by a restriction enzyme. DNA fragments are denatured by an alkaline treatment into single-stranded DNA and separated on an agarose gel using electrophoresis. The separated fragments are then transferred from an agarose gel onto a nylon membrane by capillarity. The nylon membrane containing DNA fragments is then incubated with radioisotope (e.g., phosphorous 32)-labeled DNA probes with the sequence complementary to the target. The probes bind to the DNA fragments of interest and excess unbound probes are removed by numerous washings. The nylon membrane is then put in contact with an x-ray film for several days before being developed. Black bands on the film represent single-stranded DNA hybridized to the radioactive probes. The location of the bands on the film against a molecular-weight size marker determines the weight of the target [14].

Southern blot technique is used mainly to characterize restriction, insertion, or deletion polymorphisms. For example, by Southern blot a polymorphism on the beta-2 adrenergic receptor gene (*ADRB2*) was discovered and found to be associated with asthma incidence and lower airways response to inhaled salbutamol [15]. This technique also inspired the development of other blotting methods such as Northern blot and Western blot.

## Northern blot

Northern blot is used to detect a specific messenger RNA (mRNA) in a mixture of RNA sample. It is based on the same principles as Southern blot, except that the RNA strands in Northern blot do not need to be fragmented by a restriction enzyme [16].

The ability to detect a specific mRNA sequence by Northern blot allows the characterization of its distribution, relative expression, and length variation (i.e., alternative splicing or intermediate isoforms) in different tissues or cell types. Furthermore, Northern blot is often used to measure changes in gene expression of a targeted gene upon stimulation. For example, more than two decades ago, it was shown by Northern blot that tumor necrosis factor (TNF)-α and IL-1beta could induce an increase in IL-8 mRNA expression in human bronchial epithelial cells, implicating a role of bronchial epithelial cells in asthma pathogenesis [17].

## Western blot

Western blot is used to examine the expression level of a protein of interest in a sample [18]. The technique begins with the isolation of proteins from cells or tissues, followed by denaturation at 100°C in the presence of sodium dodecyl sulfate (SDS) and a reducing agent (e.g., dithiotreitol or b-mercaptoethanol). SDS introduces negative charges to the protein molecule and the reducing agent eliminates any secondary, tertiary, and quaternary structures of proteins. Electrophoresis is used to separate proteins on a polyacrylamide gel based on their molecular weight. After separation, all the proteins on the gel are transferred to a nitrocellulose membrane using electric current passing from gel to membrane in a transfer apparatus. Primary antibody that is specific to the target is added to the membrane and binds to the target forming a complex; a secondary antibody labeled with peroxidase is then added to the membrane. To visualize the protein of interest, luminol, a peroxidase substrate, is added and the luminous energy generated is captured on an autoradiographic film. Targets appear as dark bands on the film. Figure 3.3 schematically illustrates the Western blot technique.

Western blot is useful to examine *in vitro* changes in protein expression of a targeted protein after stimulation. For example, in airway smooth muscle cells, stimulation with TNF-α and interferon (IFN)-γ increased the protein production of IL-33, a pro-inflammatory mediator [7]. These observations revealed that structural cells also exhibit an inflammatory response in asthma pathogenesis.

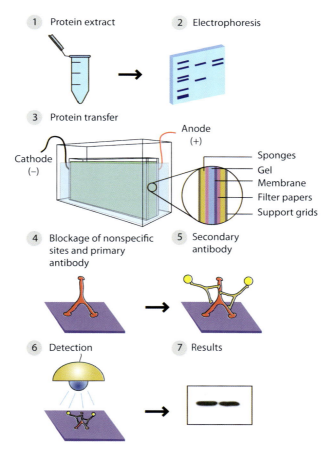

Figure 3.3 Western blot. Step 1: Proteins are isolated from cells or tissues. Step 2: Proteins are separated on a polyacrylamide gel using electrophoresis. Step 3: Inside a transfer apparatus, electric current transfers separated proteins from the polyacrylamide gel onto a nitrocellulose membrane. Step 4: Membrane is incubated with a protein blocker to block all nonspecific sites. Step 5: Membrane is incubated with a primary antibody that specifically recognizes and binds to the target. A secondary antibody labeled with peroxidase is added to the membrane. Step 6: Luminol is added as a peroxidase substrate. The peroxidase enzymatic reaction produced luminous energy and is captured on a radiographic film. Step 7: Targeted proteins are depicted as dark bands on the film.

## Quantitative flow cytometry analysis

Quantitative flow cytometry was first invented in the 1950s and it is commonly used to detect microorganisms, organelles, and cell types in a sample [19,20]. Samples are first suspended in a biological fluid at high speed and subjected to a constant flux. The criteria for target selection may be a general parameter such as size and granularity or molecule-specific. Fluorophore or antibody conjugated with a fluorophore is added into the solution depending on the selection criteria. A single particle or cell is forced through an opening and illuminated by a light source, generally a laser. As each particle passes the light source, the incoming light is scattered and the intensity of the scatter is detected and transformed into a voltage pulse. Scatters can be described as either forward or side. The intensity of the forward scatter is proportional to the size of the particle or cell, and the side scatter is proportional to the granularity or complexity within the cell.

Electrical signals can be represented either as a histogram, which reflects a single parameter (e.g., the distribution of a fluorescence), or a cytogram, a scatter plot that reflects two parameters. Figure 3.4 represents an example of flux cytometry results.

Given that flow cytometry can be linked to a cell sorter that can select a specific cell population in a heterogenous sample, it is extremely useful when there is a need to isolate a specific type of cell for *in vitro* experiments [21]. Figure 3.5 shows the various cell populations in a bronchoalveolar lavage fluid sample obtained from a healthy subject (93% alveolar macrophage cells, 5% lymphocytes, and less than 1% of eosinophils and epithelial cells). In an asthma study that investigated whether B cells produced IL-17 in response to an inflammatory signal, B cells from tonsil samples were isolated and sorted by flow cytometry to remove T cells and macrophages/monocytes from the heterogenous cell population [22]. B cells were subsequently stimulated with IL-23 and production of IL-17A and IL-17F were detected. These observations established a role of B cells in asthma pathogenesis.

## Polymerase chain reaction

Polymerase chain reaction (PCR) was developed by Kary Banks Mullis in 1985 to amplify short DNA sequences [23]. A thermocycler is used to allow temperature to vary for specific steps of the amplification

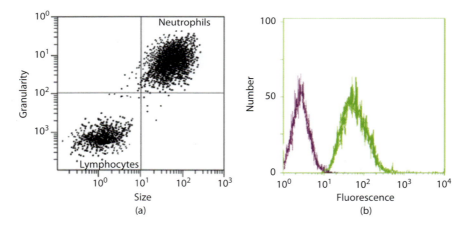

Figure 3.4 Using flow cytometry to distinguish two cell populations in a blood sample. **(a)** Two cell populations in a blood sample can be seen on this cytogram with size on the x-axis and granularity on the y-axis. Lymphocytes are small cells each with a single nucleus (i.e., low granularity) while neutrophils are big cells with numerous granulations. **(b)** The histogram depicted the negative control in purple (represents cell autofluorescence) and the targeted molecules in green. The level of fluorescence is associated with the quantity of the target in a sample.

process. Figure 3.6 illustrates the steps of PCR. Briefly, double-stranded DNA is denatured into single-stranded DNA at 94°C (denaturation step). Primers, oligonucleotides of 20–25 nucleotides long, which are complementary to the sequences flanking the sequence of interest, are added into the master mix. Primers hybridize to the single-stranded DNA at roughly 60°C (hybridization step). After hybridization, complementary nucleotides are incorporated and elongated from the primer in the 5′–3′ end direction by the

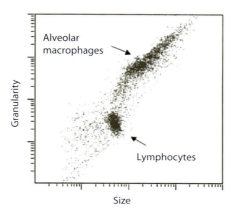

Figure 3.5 Flow cytometric analysis of cell populations in bronchoalveolar lavage cells. This cytogram depicted the results of a flow cytometric analysis in bronchoalveolar lavage cells obtained from a subject with normal lung function. Alveolar macrophages and lymphocytes are distinguishable from each other by their size and granularity.

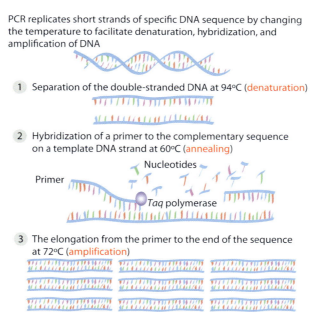

Figure 3.6 Polymerase chain reaction (PCR). Step 1: Denaturation—DNA is denatured at 94°C. Step 2: Hybridization—Forward and reverse primers are short sequences of 20–25 nucleotides long which together frame the region targeted for amplification. Annealing of the primers to template DNA occurs at around 60°C. Step 3: Elongation—*Taq* polymerase (red dot) adds complementary nucleotide in the 5′–3′ end direction at 72°C. A PCR cycle is usually repeated 30 times.

enzyme *Taq* polymerase at 72°C (elongation step). The cycle repeats about 30 times. This method is relatively simple and can be easily automated to sequence and genotype DNA.

The advance of PCR with high throughput platforms played a tremendous role in realizing the Human Genome Project that documented the entire human genome sequence [24]. The project led to the identification and documentation of genetic variations. These variations in turn become landmarks on the map of the human genome and allow genetic studies to be carried out. Genotyping, the determination of the alleles present in an individual, becomes the aim of many genetic studies. In asthma research, genotyping enables linkage studies to detect chromosomal regions housing asthma or asthma-trait–related genes (e.g., 5q31–33, 6p21, 12q13–q24, and 17q12–q21) [25] and genetic association studies (both genome-wide or candidate genes) to identify asthma or asthma-trait–related genes (e.g., *ADAM33*, *ADRB2*, *CD14*, *GSTP1*, *HLA-DRB1*, *HLA-DQB1*, *IL4*, *IL4R*, *IL10*, *IL13*, *LTA*, *MS4A2*, *STAT6*, and *TNFA*) (PMID:18301422). It can be insightful to group disease-associated genes into classes according to biological functions. For example, the grouping of 65 asthma-associated genes revealed that more than half of the genes (54%) have an immune response function and 18% of the genes are involved in tissue remodeling. Finally, 17 genes (28%) fall into the "other" category suggesting that diverse biological pathways are also involved in asthma pathogenesis (Figure 3.7) [26]. More research is needed to identify and understand how these biological pathways underlie asthma pathogenesis.

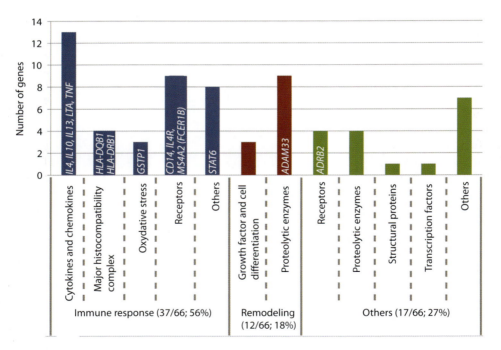

Figure 3.7 Classification of 66 major asthma genes. This figure presents the grouping of 66 genes according to their biological functions (each gene has been reported to associate with asthma in at least five studies). The genes can be grouped into three main categories: immune response (blue bars), tissue remodeling (red), and others (green). (This diagram is an excerpt from an article by Madore, A. M., and Laprise, C., *J Asthma Allergy*, 3, 107–121, 2010 and has been modified to include new publications since January 2010–July 2016 [site PubMed of NCBI: http://www.ncbi.nlm.nih.gov/gene]. The classification was made using the Panther Classification System [http://www.pantherdb.org/]. Genes that were not recognized by this tool were classified using the information from the Entrez gene web site by NCBI.

## Multiplex PCR

Several technical derivations of the original PCR have been developed, including multiplex PCR and real-time/quantitative PCR. Multiplex PCR allows multiple targeted sequences to be amplified through the use of an assembly of primers that are specific to each target (e.g., variant). An example of a multiplex PCR technology is the Sequenom iPLEX technology (www.sequenom.com). It is designed specifically to genotype, that is, a total of 34 single-nucleotide polymorphisms (SNPs). A SNP is a single-nucleotide change at a genomic location; hence creating two alleles (A1, A2) at the site. Genotyping is possible by combining PCR and matrix-assisted laser desorption/ionization time-of-flight (MALDI-TOF) mass spectrometry. Briefly, PCR primers are designed to end at one base upstream of a targeted SNP. The extension of a single base generates a different mass depending on the nucleotide incorporated and products can be separated using mass spectrometry [27]. Sequenom iPLEX platform has been used to identify asthma-associated genes [28,29]. Another example of a multiplex PCR technology is the Illumina array (or chip) technology (www.illumina.com). Depending on the array, the number of SNPs to be genotyped in parallel ranges from 384 to 1536 SNPs. Briefly, an allele-specific extension reaction is followed by amplification using PCR. The amplified products are then hybridized on a network of beads to which certain types of primers are attached (up to 1536 different primers). Each SNP (or primer) is represented numerous times to increase precision. Multiplex PCR is extremely useful in investigating candidate genes because it genotypes numerous SNPs simultaneously in a single PCR reaction, thus reducing the amount of time, sample, and cost considerably. In addition to the realization of the Human Genome Project, extremely high throughput multiplex PCR technology enables the feasibility of conducting genome-wide association studies (GWAS) by genotyping +4,000,000 SNPs [30,31]. A novel asthma locus *ZPBP2/GSDMB/ORMDL3* was identified by GWAS [32].

Gene sequencing, the task of determining the nucleotide order of a gene, is analogous to the spelling of a word and is made possible with PCR. Briefly, gene sequencing begins with the hybridization of a primer complementary to the fragment to be sequenced. The addition of deoxyribonucleotides (dATP, dCTP, dGTP, and dTTP) terminates the elongation process and reveals the last incorporated nucleotide. By comparing the sequence of a gene of interest between the affected and nonaffected subjects, differences can be subsequently investigated for causality. If the mutation occurs in exons, it could potentially modify the structure and function of the translated protein. Alternatively, a mutation in the regulatory regions of a gene (e.g., 3′untranslated region [UTR], 5′UTR or promoter) could affect protein expression. High throughput sequencing technologies have also been developed to reduce sequencing effort by targeting specific genetic elements in the genome for sequencing. While exome sequencing focuses on sequencing the coding portions, next-generation sequencing (NGS) targets exomes and regulatory regions. For example, by using whole-exome sequencing in one pedigree with asthma, researchers have identified 10 novel nonsynonymous variants found only in affected individuals in the pedigree [33]. These technologies and available platforms have been described schematically and comprehensively elsewhere [34].

Gene sequencing with high throughput PCR platforms also facilitates the study of methylation in disease pathogenesis. Methylation is one of the epigenetic mechanisms that alters the transcription process of a gene without changing the gene sequence. While hypermethylation is generally associated with transcriptional repression, hypomethylation is with transcriptional activation [35]. Epigenetic mechanisms are, in most cases, essential for cell development and cell activities during the life of an individual. Importantly, these alterations are reversible. Hence, the ability to measure epigenetics such as DNA methylation is invaluable. DNA methylation in humans occurs on a cytosine residue that is followed by a guanine residue, denoted as CpG where p stands for phosphate. These CpGs are uniformly distributed in the human genome and are enriched in the promoter regions. One of the most commonly used techniques to measure DNA methylation is bisulfite pyrosequencing [36]. Briefly, isolated DNA first undergoes a bisulfite treatment to convert all cytosine residues into uracil residues (Figure 3.8). For a methylated cytosine residue (i.e., methylcytosine), no conversion occurs. Each amplified product undergoes pyrosequencing to determine its sequence. Pyrosequencing is a PCR-based platform with the *Taq* polymerase presented

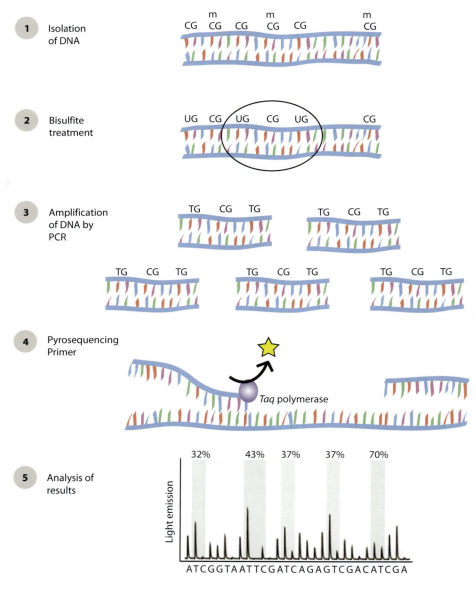

Figure 3.8 Detection of methylations using pyrosequencing. Step 1: DNA sample is isolated from biological specimen (e.g., blood or saliva). Step 2: DNA sample is treated with bisulfite to convert nonmethylated cytosine (C) residues to uracil (U) residues whereas methylated cytosine (Cm) residues remained as Cm. Step 3: The targeted DNA region, usually a promoter region containing several guanine residues preceded by a cytosine residue, called CpG islands, is amplified by PCR. The cytosine-converted uracil residues on the template strand are amplified with its complementary adenosine (A) residues on complementary strand. The A residues on the newly generated template are then amplified with the complementary thymine (T) residues. Step 4: PCR products are sequenced by pyrosequencing. In pyrosequencing, each nucleotide is added by Taq polymerase one at a time during elongation. The incorporation of a new nucleotide released a pyrophosphate accompanied by a light output. Step 5: By corresponding the light output with the sequence in which the nucleotides are added, the sequence of the target is decoded. Methylated cytosine residue can be seen with a mixed-based C:T signal.

with the four nucleotides, one at a time. The incorporation of the correct nucleotide releases a pyrophosphate molecule and subsequently generates a light output. By detecting which nucleotide gives off the light output the identity of the incorporated nucleotide at that location is known. However, the decoded sequence needs to distinguish a TG dinucleotide from a "true" TG or a CG dinucleotide (which converted to UG then TG during the bisulfite treatment). By identifying genomic locations where there are mixed base (T:C) signals, the extent of methylation can be estimated. The various high throughput pyrosequencing platforms used for measuring methylation levels of an entire genome have been compressively reviewed elsewhere [37]. Using bisulfite pyrosequencing methylation assays, polymorphisms at the promoter regions of interleukin 1 receptor type II (*IIL1R2*), solute carrier family 22 (organic 3 cation/carnitine transporter) member 5 (*SLC22A5*), zona pellucida binding protein 2 (*ZPBP2*), and gasdermin A (*GSDMA*) were found to influence the methylation level at its gene's promoter region [38]. The data also suggested interactions between the methylation level of *ZPBP2*, *GSDMA* and asthma in female asthmatic subjects and *SLC22A5* in male asthmatic subjects [38]. The study illustrated the intricate relationship between genotypes, methylation levels, and disease status.

## Multiplex real-time PCR

Real-time PCR measures the amount of DNA amplified at each cycle and it is carried out in a specific type of thermocycler. Similar to Northern blot, real-time PCR can quantify DNA expression products (i.e., mRNA) [39,40] (Figure 3.9). Although the genome is identical in every single cell of an organism, genes are expressed differently according to development (developmental stage specific), space (cell, tissue, or organic type specific), and physiological state (normal, pathologic, or in response to a particular stimulus). The expression level of a transcript can therefore be assessed between affected and nonaffected subjects or between treated and untreated subjects.

High throughput multiplex real-time PCR measures thousands of gene expressions simultaneously per sample. It integrates various disciplines including microelectronics, nucleic acid chemistry, image analysis, and computational biology. Generally, an array is synthesized with single-stranded oligonucelotides immobilized on a solid matrix. The oligonucleotides are complementary DNA (cDNA) or RNA sequences specific to targeted genes. Two main types of real-time PCR array are commonly used in research. The first is DNA microarrays/chips by Affymetrix (www.affymetrix.com). Each array, known as GeneChip, is slide-based with thousands of probes synthesized directly onto a chip using the proprietary photolithography technology. The protocol to measure gene expression begins with isolated mRNA being converted to the more stable cDNA and labeled with fluorophore. After cDNA—oligonucleotide hybridization, a fluorescence signal is given and detected using confocal microscopy. A positive signal indicated the targeted gene was expressed in the sample. To reduce genes being falsely identified as expressed, each targeted gene is represented by a set of oligonucleotides corresponding to the various locations of the gene. To account for nonspecific binding between cDNA and an oligonucleotide, each oligonucleotide is synthesized and immobilized with a witness, an oliogonucleotide with identical sequence except one base change in the middle. The relative level of expression is thus the means of the differences between the oligonucleotide and its witness. DNA microarrays are also often used to compare two samples such as samples from two different tissues or same tissues exposed to different treatment. In this case, the RNA or cDNA are labeled with distinct fluorophores (e.g., Cy-3 [green] and Cy-5 [red]). The level of expression is assessed using the fluorescence emission ratio of each fluorophore at a different wavelength [41]. In one study, the entire transcriptome was measured in the white blood cells of severe asthmatic, controlled asthmatic, and healthy nonasthmatic children by using affymetrix arrays [42]. Of the 1378 genes differentially expressed between asthmatic and healthy children, the transcription levels of various taste receptor genes (*TAS2R13*, *TAS2R14*, and *TAS2R19*) were found to be elevated in severe asthmatic children and correlated with disease severity in both children and adults.

In addition to affymetrix, microarrays by Illumina (www.illumina.com) are also available for high throughput real-time PCR. Unlike the *in situ* synthesis of oligonucleotides onto a chip by Affymetrix, Illumina uses magnetic beads to anchor the oligonucleotides. The array is assembled when the beads are distributed onto a chip and each bead randomly falls into a well on a chip. Each bead is attached with hundreds of thousands of copies of one specific oligonucleotide for subsequent cDNA hybridization. To identify which bead is located in each well, each bead is synthesized with a 23mer address sequence followed by a 50mer probe. Their detection requires the reading system designed by Illumina and the decoding is performed at the company facility. By using the Illumina arrays in CD4+ T cells of asthmatic and nonasthmatic subjects, IL-17RB transcription level is found to correlate with the variation in immunoglobulin E levels in male asthmatic subjects only [43], implicating a sex-specific effect underlying the mechanism of IgE production via IL-17RB.

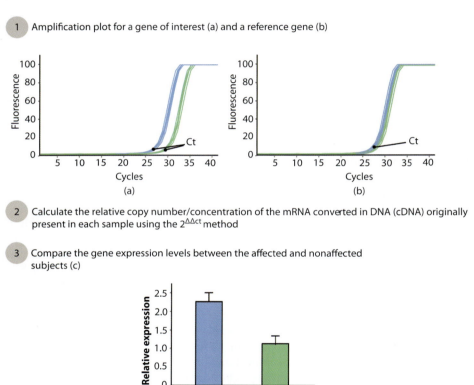

Figure 3.9 Measuring relative gene expression levels using real-time PCR to determine if a gene of interest is differentially expressed in affected individuals as compared to nonaffected individuals. Step 1: An amplification plot is generated for each mRNA (reverse transcribed to cDNA) sample and a threshold line is set. It is set where the precision and predictability of the data are the greatest, usually where the curves are vertically parallel (i.e., exponential phase) to each other. The intersecting point between the curve and the threshold line is the cycle threshold (Ct). A smaller Ct indicates fewer cycles are needed to start the exponential phase of the PCR. (a and b) The amplification plots for affected (blue) and nonaffected (green) samples for gene A and gene B, respectively. Step 2: The relative amount of cDNA in each sample is calculated using the $2^{\Delta\Delta Ct}$ method (compared the Ct value of one gene against a reference gene). Step 3: The relative cDNA quantity of affected and nonaffected samples are evaluated for statistical differences.

## Molecular cloning

Molecular cloning is another commonly used technique to amplify a targeted sequence. The cloning technique, as illustrated in Figure 3.10, requires two components: a sequence of interest known as an insert and a cloning vector. An insert can be either isolated from living cells or synthesized; a vector is a DNA sequence that can be combined with foreign DNA and can replicate within an organism such as a bacterium

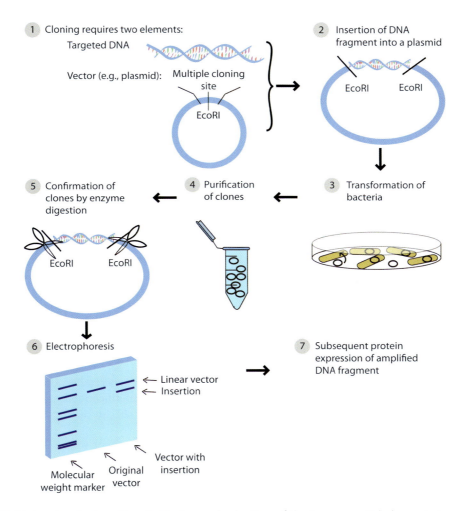

Figure 3.10 Molecular cloning. Step 1: Design and selection of the two essential elements in molecular cloning: a DNA fragment of interest (the recombinant) and a vector. Step 2: The recombinant is inserted into the multicloning site (MCS) of the vector with cleavage by one or more restriction enzymes. Step 3: The newly inserted vectors are being taken up by bacteria, in which the vectors replicated. As the bacteria proliferated, clones are created. Step 4: Vectors are isolated from the bacterial hosts and purified. Step 5: Enzymatic digestion is used to confirm the vectors contained the recombinant. Vectors from each clone are digested using the enzyme that first allowed insertion of the recombinant. Linear fragments of the vector and inserted fragment are obtained. Step 6: It will now be possible to distinguish the original vector from the recombinant plasmid by comparing the size of the DNA fragments on an electrophoresis gel using a molecular weight marker. Step 7: Positive clones (i.e., successful insertion) are to be stored and used for research purposes. The clones can be expressed as proteins subsequently in expression vectors.

or yeast [44,45]. Some commonly used vectors are plasmid, phage, cosmids, bacterial artificial chromosomes (BAC), and yeast artificial chromosomes (YAC). Vectors have three major sites: an origin of replication (ORI), a multicloning site (MCS), and a selectable marker. Briefly, an insert is created from the donor DNA with a restriction enzyme (e.g., EcoRI) and the vector is also cut with the same restriction enzyme. The insert is placed into the vector at the cut site. The newly created recombinant DNA is taken up by the replicating organism in a process called transformation. The vector replicates within the organism and the amplification of the insert becomes exponential as the organism proliferates. Various selection schemes are used to identify the transformed organisms with recombinant vectors from those that are nontransformed or transformed with nonrecombinant vectors. The targeted DNA sequences are then excised and isolated from the recombinant vectors for analysis [46].

Although both are DNA amplifying techniques, molecular cloning can amplify longer sequences (up to 1 mega basepairs) as compared to PCR; hence, cloning is used when the targeted DNA sequence is long (e.g., the entire coding sequence of a gene). Molecular and expression cloning have enabled the molecular characterization of a vast number of proteins associated with asthma pathogenesis [47–49].

## Clustered regularly interspaced short palindromic repeats-associated proteins (CRISPR-Cas9) system

Clustered regularly interspaced short palindromic repeats (CRISPR) refers to the natural occurrence of a DNA repeating sequence separated by a nonrepeating sequence, called spacer, in the prokaryotic genomes [50] (Figure 3.11). It is a defense mechanism used by prokaryotes to fight off viral infection [51,52]. Briefly, a spacer corresponding to a previously exposed viral sequence is kept between repeating DNA sequences so that it can be used to recognize the same virus in the future. To recognize and defend against a viral infection, the prokaryote transcribes the sequence into an RNA strand and together with a *Cas* enzyme, the complex drifts around inside the cell. Once a viral sequence matches the RNA sequence, the *Cas* enzyme snips the viral DNA and prevents the virus from replicating. Of the various *Cas* enzymes, *Cas*9 is the best known and it comes from *Streptococcus pyogenes* [53]. The derived gene-editing system is thus known as the CRISPR-Cas9 system. Briefly, this gene-editing method begins with a Cas9 enzyme guided to a specific DNA site with the help of a customized 17–20-nucleotide long guide RNA (gRNA). Cas9 snips the targeted DNA at the precise location generating a double-strand break (DSB) [54]. The cleaved DSB can be repaired by an error prone nonhomologous end joining (NHEJ) mechanism and generates random microinsertion or microdeletion (INDEL) mutations, or it can be replaced with a gene modification by homology-directed repair (HDR) in the presence of donor template [55]. Hence, NHEJ and HDR can be adapted to either silence a gene or replace a gene, respectively [56].

The specific and flexible CRISPR-Cas9 system becomes a major breakthrough in gene editing in eukaryotic cells [57–59]. Most of the derived genome editing applications have been carried out successfully in cell culture systems and even adapted for *in vivo* use [56–60]. One advantage of the CRISPR-Cas9 system over the conventional gene editing techniques is time. Transgenic animals with the desired genetic changes can be generated in one generation, allowing the causal link between a genetic mutation and a trait to be rapidly identified [61,62]. High throughput gene knockout in a cellular system can be done rapidly to establish the relationship between genes, pathways, networks, and a trait [63]. Furthermore, CRISPR-Cas9 system can be adapted to elicit transcriptional activation, repression, or epigenetic modification of multiple genes for functional studies [64–67]. Genome-wide CRISPR-Cas9 screen has been performed to identify genes whose loss of function promotes tumor growth and metastasis in a mouse model of cancer [68].

One of the most exciting applications of the CRISPR-Cas9 system is the possibility of treating genetic disorders by replacing faulty genes. Proof of concept in cellular or animal models has been established for facioscapulohumeral muscular dystrophy [69], retinitis pigmentosa [70], Duchenne muscular dystrophy

Polymerase chain reaction 47

① Recognition of the cleavage site by Cas9 using the guide RNA and double-strand break

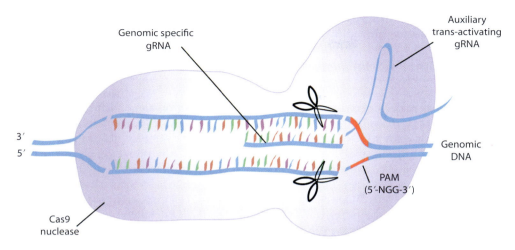

② DNA repair by nonhomologous end joining (NHEJ) or homology-directed repair (HDR)

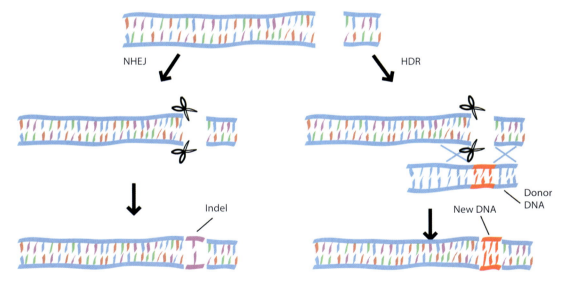

Figure 3.11 CRISPR-Cas9 system as a gene-editing tool. In the CRISPR-Cas9 system, the guide RNA (gRNA) is composed of two parts: the genomic specific sequence of 17–20 nucleotides long that is specific to the target sequence and the auxiliary trans-activating sequence. The CRISPR-CAS9 system is mainly consisted of two steps. Step 1: The Cas9 enzyme is guided by the gRNA to the cleavage site immediately downstream of the three nucleotides (NGG) protospacer-adjacent motif (PAM) sequence. After its binding to the target sequence, Cas9 induces a double-strand break of the genomic DNA. Step 2: The DNA repair can be done by two different mechanisms: (i) nonhomologous end joining (NHEJ) mechanism that often provokes insertion or deletion during the repair process to the native sequence and (ii) homology-directed repair (HDR) mechanism that uses a donor DNA sequence to add a specific sequence into the double-strand break site.

[71–74], and Meesmann's epithelial corneal dystrophy [75]. Given the complexity of the genetic contribution to asthma development, the CRISPR-Cas9 system proves to be more useful in eliciting the role of the encoded protein in disease pathogenesis. For example, using the CRISPR-Cas9 system, the pro-inflammatory role of MUC18 was determined after the gene was knocked out in airway epithelial cells [76].

## Cellular and animal model systems

Cellular models are useful for studying the physiopathology of respiratory diseases and they are described in great detail in Chapter 5. Both commercially available systems of cellular and animal model or in-house cell lines are used in research. Among popular commercially available cell lines are the HeLa cells. They are immortal cells originally isolated from Henrietta Lacks' tumor samples, hence the name of the cells. Because HeLa cells proliferate rapidly, they shorten the study time. Alternatively, cells can be isolated from tissue samples, cultured and become "primary" cell lines. Unlike immortalized cell lines, primary cells are mortal and undergo an aging process. Primary cell lines can be immortalized by transforming cells with an oncogenic agent so that the cells divide perpetually. However, the cell immortalization process modifies the cell phenotype and may no longer be relevant to *in vivo* application. Generally, research in asthma either uses in-house primary cell lines or purchase commercially available primary cell lines.

To study a disease that occurs in humans, modeling it in other animals is a logical step. In asthma, murine models are used the most because they offer several advantages. First, mouse models are relatively inexpensive. Second, the overall murine immune system is well documented; hence, any effects of environmental or therapeutic exposures can be quickly detected based on the abnormalities. Given that mice do not develop asthma naturally, various models have been developed to induce asthma-like reactions in these animals [77]. In asthma, mouse models are commonly used to investigate the role of a targeted protein in disease pathogenesis. Briefly, the ortholog of the targeted protein is identified in mice, then its gene can be silenced or altered, conventionally by homologous recombination, and its effect in the animals can be assessed. These mice are called knock-out mice. Contrarily, a gene with a mutation associated with asthma can be introduced into the orthologic gene in mice and its functional effect can be assessed; these mice are termed "knock-in" mice. These genetically altered mice are called transgenic mice [78]. A recent article reviews the use of animal models in biotechnology research [79]. With the development of CRISPR-Cas9 gene-editing system, more transgenic animals other than mice are expected to be used for modeling diseases in the future.

## Perspectives: Precision Medicine - from phenotypes to endotypes

The last few decades have seen considerable efforts by research scientists to characterize the "omics" of chronic respiratory diseases such as asthma. Our understanding and knowledge of these diseases have expanded tremendously largely attributed by the development of methodological and analytical tools. The adoption of cellular systems to model disease pathogeneses and the development of analytical tools to integrate data across different experiments are particularly powerful in understanding diseases. A complex disease such as asthma can now be characterized with more precision. In the past a patient's asthma could be categorized based on the nature of inflammation (e.g. eosinophilic versus neutrophilic) and treatment response (e.g. steroid responsive versus steroid resistant). Nowadays the availability of "omics" data provides a glimpse of the underlying molecular mechanisms, thus allowing for a more precise characterization of a disease.

The term endophenotyping or endotyping refers to the classification of a trait based on its molecular mechanisms or treatment responses (80). While the term endotype was first coined in 1966, asthma endotypes have only been proposed recently, largely because of the technological and analytical advances (81). Lötvall *et al.* recognized that asthma is a syndrome with phenotypic (observable) characteristics including physiologies, triggers, and inflammatory parameters and they reported six endotypes of asthma: aspirin sensitive, allergic bronchopulmonary mycosis, asthma-predictive indices-positive preschool wheezer, adult allergic, severe late-onset hypereosinophilic, and asthma in cross-country skiers (82). For severe asthma,

Wenzel proposed five endotypes: early onset allergic, persistent eosinophilia, allergic bronchopulmonary mycosis, obese-female, and neutrophilic (83). Furthermore, Poon et al., proposed to endotype severe asthma based on cytokine signaling pathways: IL-4/IL-13, IL-5/IL-33, IL-17, and IL-18/IFN- (84).

It is only perceivable that precision medicine is within reach as more data are available and integrated; endotypes will only become more precise and prognoses more accurate. Disease preventions, interventions, and treatments tailored to one's biology will soon become a reality.

## Conclusion

This chapter briefly describes some of the techniques commonly used in the physiopathology research of respiratory diseases and specific examples are given for asthma. Asthma, being a complex trait, requires investigational techniques which examine the disease mechanisms from all angles. While some of the techniques have been developed decades ago, by adapting new technology such as the CRISPR-Cas9 gene-editing system in established cellular and animal models and coupled with high throughput platforms, the rate of discovery will be unprecedented. Ultimately, these discoveries will lead to more effective treatments to improve the quality of life of those who are affected and those who care for them.

## References

1. Loftus P. A. and Wise S. K. 2016. Epidemiology of asthma. *Curr Opin Otolaryngol Head Neck Surg.* 24:245–249.
2. Masoli M., Fabian D., Holt S., and Beasley R. 2004. The global burden of asthma: Executive summary of the GINA Dissemination Committee report. *Allergy.* 59:469–478.
3. Young B. and Heath J. W. *Weather's Functional Histology. A Text and color Atlas.* 6th edition. London, UK: Elsevier Churchill Linvingstone.
4. Oduola T., Bello I., Adeosun G., Ademosun A. W., Raheem G., and Avwioro G. 2010. Hepatotoxicity and nephrotoxicity evaluation in Wistar albino rats exposed to Morinda lucida leaf extract. *N Am J Med Sci.* 2:230–233.
5. Song-Tao A., Yan-Yan Q., and Li-Xia W. 2010. The severity of coronary artery disease evaluated by central systolic pressure and fractional diastolic pressure. *N Am J Med Sci.* 2:218–220.
6. Taha R., Hamid Q., Cameron L., and Olivenstein R. 2003. T helper type 2 cytokine receptors and associated transcription factors GATA-3, c-MAF, and signal transducer and activator of transcription factor-6 in induced sputum of atopic asthmatic patients. *Chest.* 123:2074–2082.
7. Prefontaine D., Lajoie-Kadoch S., Foley S., Audusseau S., Olivenstein R., Halayko A. J., Lemiere C., Martin J. G., and Hamid Q. 2009. Increased expression of IL-33 in severe asthma: Evidence of expression by airway smooth muscle cells. *J Immunol.* 183:5094–5103.
8. Kay A. B., Ying S., and Durham S. R. 1995. Phenotype of cells positive for interleukin-4 and interleukin-5 mRNA in allergic tissue reactions. *Int Arch Allergy Immunol.* 107:208–210.
9. Engvall E. and Perlmann P. 1971. Enzyme-linked immunosorbent assay (ELISA). Quantitative assay of immunoglobulin G. *Immunochemistry.* 8:871–874.
10. Liao S. C., Cheng Y. C., Wang Y. C., Wang C. W., Yang S. M., Yu C. K., Shieh C. C., Cheng K. C., Lee M. F., Chiang S. R., Shieh J. M., and Chang M. S. 2004. IL-19 induced Th2 cytokines and was up-regulated in asthma patients. *J Immunol.* 173:6712–6718.
11. Komai-Koma M., McKay A., Thomson L., McSharry C., Chalmers G. W., Liew F. Y., and Thomson N. C. 2001. Immuno-regulatory cytokines in asthma: IL-15 and IL-13 in induced sputum. *Clin Exp Allergy.* 31:1441–1448.
12. Bottcher M. F., Bjurstrom J., Mai X. M., Nilsson L., and Jenmalm M. C. 2003. Allergen-induced cytokine secretion in atopic and non-atopic asthmatic children. *Pediatr Allergy Immunol.* 14:345–350.

13. Southern E. M. 1975. Detection of specific sequences among DNA fragments separated by gel electrophoresis. *J Mol Biol.* 98:503–517.
14. Southern E. 2006. Southern blotting. *Nat Protoc.* 1:518–525.
15. Ohe M., Munakata M., Hizawa N., Itoh A., Doi I., Yamaguchi E., Homma Y., and Kawakami Y. 1995. Beta 2 adrenergic receptor gene restriction fragment length polymorphism and bronchial asthma. *Thorax.* 50:353–359.
16. Trayhurn P. 1996. Northern blotting. *Proc Nutr Soc.* 55:583–589.
17. Cromwell O., Hamid Q., Corrigan C. J., Barkans J., Meng Q., Collins P. D., and Kay A. B. 1992. Expression and generation of interleukin-8, IL-6 and granulocyte-macrophage colony-stimulating factor by bronchial epithelial cells and enhancement by IL-1 beta and tumour necrosis factor-alpha. *Immunology.* 77:330–337.
18. Burnette W. N. 1981. "Western blotting": Electrophoretic transfer of proteins from sodium dodecyl sulfate–polyacrylamide gels to unmodified nitrocellulose and radiographic detection with antibody and radioiodinated protein A. *Anal Biochem.* 112:195–203.
19. Sugarbaker E. V., Thornthwaite J. T., Temple W. T., and Ketcham A. S. 1979. Flow cytometry: General principles and applications to selected studies in tumor biology. *Int Adv Surg Oncol.* 2:125–153.
20. Schwartz A. and Fernandez-Repollet E. 2001. Quantitative flow cytometry. *Clin Lab Med.* 21:743–761.
21. Sklar Larry A. (Editor) 2005. *Flow Cytometry for Biotechnology.* Oxford: Oxford University Press.
22. Vazquez-Tello A., Halwani R., Li R., Nadigel J., Bar-Or A., Mazer B. D., Eidelman D. H., Al-Muhsen S., and Hamid Q. 2012. IL-17A and IL-17F expression in B lymphocytes. *Int Arch Allergy Immunol.* 157:406–416.
23. Mullis K., Faloona F., Scharf S., Saiki R., Horn G., and Erlich H. 1986. Specific enzymatic amplification of DNA in vitro: The polymerase chain reaction. *Cold Spring Harb Symp Quant Biol.* 51(Pt 1):263–273.
24. International Human Genome Sequencing Consortium. 2004. Finishing the euchromatic sequence of the human genome. *Nature.* 431:931–945.
25. Ober C. and Yao T. C. 2011. The genetics of asthma and allergic disease: A 21st century perspective. *Immunol Rev.* 242:10–30.
26. Madore A. M. and Laprise C. 2010. Immunological and genetic aspects of asthma and allergy. *J Asthma Allergy.* 3:107–121.
27. Gabriel S., Ziaugra L., and Tabbaa D. 2009. SNP genotyping using the Sequenom MassARRAY iPLEX platform. *Curr Protoc Hum Genet.* Chapter 2: Unit 2 12.
28. Li F. X., Tan J. Y., Yang X. X., Wu Y. S., Wu D., and Li M. 2012. Genetic variants on 17q21 are associated with asthma in a Han Chinese population. *Genet Mol Res.* 11:340–347.
29. Iordanidou M., Paraskakis E., Giannakopoulou E., Tavridou A., Gentile G., Borro M., Simmaco M., Chatzimichael A., Bush A., and Manolopoulos V. G. 2014. Vitamin D receptor ApaI a allele is associated with better childhood asthma control and improvement in ability for daily activities. *OMICS.* 18:673–681.
30. Himes B. E., Hunninghake G. M., Baurley J. W., Rafaels N. M., Sleiman P., Strachan D. P., Wilk J. B., Willis-Owen S. A., Klanderman B., Lasky-Su J., Lazarus R., Murphy A. J., Soto-Quiros M. E., Avila L., Beaty T., Mathias R. A., Ruczinski I., Barnes K. C., Celedon J. C., Cookson W. O., Gauderman W. J., Gilliland F. D., Hakonarson H., Lange C., Moffatt M. F., O'Connor G. T., Raby B. A., Silverman E. K., and Weiss S. T. 2009. Genome-wide association analysis identifies PDE4D as an asthma-susceptibility gene. *Am J Hum Genet.* 84:581–593.
31. Li X., Howard T. D., Zheng S. L., Haselkorn T., Peters S. P., Meyers D. A., and Bleecker E. R. 2010. Genome-wide association study of asthma identifies RAD50-IL13 and HLA-DR/DQ regions. *J Allergy Clin Immunol.* 125:328–335 e311.
32. Moffatt M. F., Kabesch M., Liang L., Dixon A. L., Strachan D., Heath S., Depner M., von Berg A., Bufe A., Rietschel E., Heinzmann A., Simma B., Frischer T., Willis-Owen S. A., Wong K. C., Illig T., Vogelberg C., Weiland S. K., von Mutius E., Abecasis G. R., Farrall M., Gut I. G., Lathrop G. M., and Cookson W. O. 2007. Genetic variants regulating ORMDL3 expression contribute to the risk of childhood asthma. *Nature.* 448:470–473.

33. DeWan A. T., Egan K. B., Hellenbrand K., Sorrentino K., Pizzoferrato N., Walsh K. M., and Bracken M. B. 2012. Whole-exome sequencing of a pedigree segregating asthma. *BMC Med Genet.* 13:95.
34. Bick D. and Dimmock D. 2011. Whole exome and whole genome sequencing. *Curr Opin Pediatr.* 23:594–600.
35. Barnes P. J. 2009. Targeting the epigenome in the treatment of asthma and chronic obstructive pulmonary disease. *Proc Am Thorac Soc.* 6:693–696.
36. Tost J. and Gut I. G. 2007. DNA methylation analysis by pyrosequencing. *Nat Protoc.* 2:2265–2275.
37. Dedeurwaerder S., Defrance M., Calonne E., Denis H., Sotiriou C., and Fuks F. 2011. Evaluation of the infinium methylation 450K technology. *Epigenomics.* 3:771–784.
38. Al Tuwaijri A., Gagne-Ouellet V., Madore A. M., Laprise C., and Naumova A. K. 2016. Local genotype influences DNA methylation at two asthma-associated regions, 5q31 and 17q21, in a founder effect population. *J Med Genet.* 53:232–241.
39. Chang J. T., Chen I. H., Liao C. T., Wang H. M., Hsu Y. M., Hung K. F., Lin C. J., Hsieh L. L., and Cheng A. J. 2002. A reverse transcription comparative real-time PCR method for quantitative detection of angiogenic growth factors in head and neck cancer patients. *Clin Biochem.* 35:591–596.
40. Aarskog N. K. and Vedeler C. A. 2000. Real-time quantitative polymerase chain reaction. A new method that detects both the peripheral myelin protein 22 duplication in Charcot-Marie-Tooth type 1A disease and the peripheral myelin protein 22 deletion in hereditary neuropathy with liability to pressure palsies. *Hum Genet.* 107:494–498.
41. Lee P. and Hudson T. J. 2000. Les puces à ADN en médecine et en sciences. *Médecine Sci.* 16:43–49.
42. Orsmark-Pietras C., James A., Konradsen J. R., Nordlund B., Soderhall C., Pulkkinen V., Pedroletti C., Daham K., Kupczyk M., Dahlen B., Kere J., Dahlen S. E., Hedlin G., and Melen E. 2013. Transcriptome analysis reveals upregulation of bitter taste receptors in severe asthmatics. *Eur Respir J.* 42:65–78.
43. Hunninghake G. M., Chu J. H., Sharma S. S., Cho M. H., Himes B. E., Rogers A. J., Murphy A., Carey V. J., and Raby B. A. 2011. The CD4+ T-cell transcriptome and serum IgE in asthma: IL17RB and the role of sex. *BMC Pulm Med.* 11:17.
44. Timmis K., Cabello F., and Cohen S. N. 1975. Cloning, isolation, and characterization of replication regions of complex plasmid genomes. *Proc Natl Acad Sci U S A.* 72:2242–2246.
45. Hershfield V., Boyer H. W., Yanofsky C., Lovett M. A., and Helinski D. R. 1974. Plasmid ColEl as a molecular vehicle for cloning and amplification of DNA. *Proc Natl Acad Sci U S A.* 71:3455–3459.
46. Dale J. W. and von Schantz M. 2007. *From Genes to Genomes: Concepts and Applications of DNA Technology*, 2nd edition. Chichester, UK: John Wiley & Sons.
47. Welsch D. J., Creely D. P., Hauser S. D., Mathis K. J., Krivi G. G., and Isakson P. C. 1994. Molecular cloning and expression of human leukotriene-C4 synthase. *Proc Natl Acad Sci U S A.* 91:9745–9749.
48. Penrose J. F. 1999. LTC4 synthase. Enzymology, biochemistry, and molecular characterization. *Clin Rev Allergy Immunol.* 17:133–152.
49. Lynch K. R., O'Neill G. P., Liu Q., Im D. S., Sawyer N., Metters K. M., Coulombe N., Abramovitz M., Figueroa D. J., Zeng Z., Connolly B. M., Bai C., Austin C. P., Chateauneuf A., Stocco R., Greig G. M., Kargman S., Hooks S. B., Hosfield E., Williams D. L., Jr., Ford-Hutchinson A. W., Caskey C. T., and Evans J. F. 1999. Characterization of the human cysteinyl leukotriene CysLT1 receptor. *Nature.* 399:789–793.
50. Haft D. H., Selengut J., Mongodin E. F., and Nelson K. E. 2005. A guild of 45 CRISPR-associated (Cas) protein families and multiple CRISPR/Cas subtypes exist in prokaryotic genomes. *PLoS Comput Biol.* 1:e60.
51. Mojica F. J., Diez-Villasenor C., Garcia-Martinez J., and Almendros C. 2009. Short motif sequences determine the targets of the prokaryotic CRISPR defence system. *Microbiology.* 155:733–740.
52. Wright A. V., Nunez J. K., and Doudna J. A. 2016. Biology and applications of CRISPR systems: Harnessing nature's toolbox for genome engineering. *Cell.* 164:29–44.

53. Marraffini L. A. 2016. The CRISPR-Cas system of *Streptococcus pyogenes*: Function and applications. In *Streptococcus pyogenes: Basic Biology to Clinical Manifestations*. J. J. Ferretti, D. L. Stevens, and V. A. Fischetti, editors. Oklahoma City, OK: The University of Oklahoma Health Sciences Center.
54. Mali P., Yang L., Esvelt K. M., Aach J., Guell M., DiCarlo J. E., Norville J. E., and Church G. M. 2013. RNA-guided human genome engineering via Cas9. *Science*. 339:823–826.
55. Ran F. A., Hsu P. D., Wright J., Agarwala V., Scott D. A., and Zhang F. 2013. Genome engineering using the CRISPR-Cas9 system. *Nat Protoc*. 8:2281–2308.
56. Kaminski R., Chen Y., Fischer T., Tedaldi E., Napoli A., Zhang Y., Karn J., Hu W., and Khalili K. 2016. Elimination of HIV-1 genomes from human T-lymphoid cells by CRISPR/Cas9 gene editing. *Sci Rep*. 6:22555.
57. Cong L., Ran F. A., Cox D., Lin S., Barretto R., Habib N., Hsu P. D., Wu X., Jiang W., Marraffini L. A., and Zhang F. 2013. Multiplex genome engineering using CRISPR/Cas systems. *Science*. 339:819–823.
58. Fu Y., Sander J. D., Reyon D., Cascio V. M., and Joung J. K. 2014. Improving CRISPR-Cas nuclease specificity using truncated guide RNAs. *Nat Biotechnol*. 32:279–284.
59. Xue H., Wu J., Li S., Rao M. S., and Liu Y. 2016. Genetic modification in human pluripotent stem cells by homologous recombination and CRISPR/Cas9 System. *Methods Mol Biol*. 1307:173–190.
60. Kalebic N., Taverna E., Tavano S., Wong F. K., Suchold D., Winkler S., Huttner W. B., and Sarov M. 2016. CRISPR/Cas9-induced disruption of gene expression in mouse embryonic brain and single neural stem cells in vivo. *EMBO Rep*. 17:338–348.
61. Low B. E., Kutny P. M., and Wiles M. V. 2016. Simple, efficient CRISPR-Cas9-mediated gene editing in mice: Strategies and methods. *Methods Mol Biol*. 1438:19–53.
62. Ran F. A., Hsu P. D., Lin C. Y., Gootenberg J. S., Konermann S., Trevino A. E., Scott D. A., Inoue A., Matoba S., Zhang Y., and Zhang F. 2013. Double nicking by RNA-guided CRISPR Cas9 for enhanced genome editing specificity. *Cell*. 154:1380–1389.
63. Shalem O., Sanjana N. E., Hartenian E., Shi X., Scott D. A., Mikkelsen T. S., Heckl D., Ebert B. L., Root D. E., Doench J. G., and Zhang F. 2014. Genome-scale CRISPR-Cas9 knockout screening in human cells. *Science*. 343:84–87.
64. Chen Y. S., Hsieh G. W., Chen S. P., Tseng P. Y., and Wang C. W. 2015. Zinc oxide nanowire-poly(methyl methacrylate) dielectric layers for polymer capacitive pressure sensors. *ACS Appl Mater Interfaces*. 7:45–50.
65. Qi L. S., Larson M. H., Gilbert L. A., Doudna J. A., Weissman J. S., Arkin A. P., and Lim W. A. 2013. Repurposing CRISPR as an RNA-guided platform for sequence-specific control of gene expression. *Cell*. 152:1173–1183.
66. Thakore P. I., D'Ippolito A. M., Song L., Safi A., Shivakumar N. K., Kabadi A. M., Reddy T. E., Crawford G. E., and Gersbach C. A. 2015. Highly specific epigenome editing by CRISPR-Cas9 repressors for silencing of distal regulatory elements. *Nat Methods*. 12:1143–1149.
67. Thakore P. I., Black J. B., Hilton I. B., and Gersbach C. A. 2016. Editing the epigenome: Technologies for programmable transcription and epigenetic modulation. *Nat Methods*. 13:127–137.
68. Chen S., Sanjana N. E., Zheng K., Shalem O., Lee K., Shi X., Scott D. A., Song J., Pan J. Q., Weissleder R., Lee H., Zhang F., and Sharp P. A. 2015. Genome-wide CRISPR screen in a mouse model of tumor growth and metastasis. *Cell*. 160:1246–1260.
69. Himeda C. L., Jones T. I., and Jones P. L. 2016. CRISPR/dCas9-mediated transcriptional inhibition ameliorates the epigenetic dysregulation at D4Z4 and represses DUX4-fl in FSH muscular dystrophy. *Mol Ther*. 24:527–535.
70. Bassuk A. G., Zheng A., Li Y., Tsang S. H., and Mahajan V. B. 2016. Precision medicine: Genetic repair of retinitis pigmentosa in patient-derived stem cells. *Sci Rep*. 6:19969.

71. Nelson C. E., Hakim C. H., Ousterout D. G., Thakore P. I., Moreb E. A., Castellanos Rivera R. M., Madhavan S., Pan X., Ran F. A., Yan W. X., Asokan A., Zhang F., Duan D., and Gersbach C. A. 2016. In vivo genome editing improves muscle function in a mouse model of Duchenne muscular dystrophy. *Science*. 351:403–407.
72. Iyombe-Engembe J. P., Ouellet D. L., Barbeau X., Rousseau J., Chapdelaine P., Lague P., and Tremblay J. P. 2016. Efficient restoration of the dystrophin gene reading frame and protein structure in DMD myoblasts using the cinDel method. *Mol Ther Nucleic Acids*. 5:e283.
73. Long C., Amoasii L., Mireault A. A., McAnally J. R., Li H., Sanchez-Ortiz E., Bhattacharyya S., Shelton J. M., Bassel-Duby R., and Olson E. N. 2016. Postnatal genome editing partially restores dystrophin expression in a mouse model of muscular dystrophy. *Science*. 351:400–403.
74. Tabebordbar M., Zhu K., Cheng J. K., Chew W. L., Widrick J. J., Yan W. X., Maesner C., Wu E. Y., Xiao R., Ran F. A., Cong L., Zhang F., Vandenberghe L. H., Church G. M., and Wagers A. J. 2016. In vivo gene editing in dystrophic mouse muscle and muscle stem cells. *Science*. 351:407–411.
75. Courtney D. G., Moore J. E., Atkinson S. D., Maurizi E., Allen E. H., Pedrioli D. M., McLean W. H., Nesbit M. A., and Moore C. B. 2016. CRISPR/Cas9 DNA cleavage at SNP-derived PAM enables both in vitro and in vivo KRT12 mutation-specific targeting. *Gene Ther*. 23:108–112.
76. Chu H. W., Rios C., Huang C., Wesolowska-Andersen A., Burchard E. G., O'Connor B. P., Fingerlin T. E., Nichols D., Reynolds S. D., and Seibold M. A. 2015. CRISPR-Cas9-mediated gene knockout in primary human airway epithelial cells reveals a proinflammatory role for MUC18. *Gene Ther*. 22:822–829.
77. Nials A. T. and Uddin S. 2008. Mouse models of allergic asthma: Acute and chronic allergen challenge. *Dis Model Mech*. 1:213–220.
78. Cho A., Haruyama N., and Kulkarni A. B. 2009. Generation of transgenic mice. *Curr Protoc Cell Biol*. Chapter 19:Unit 19 11.
79. Tew K., Constantine S., and Lew W. Y. 2011. Intraosseous hemangioma of the rib mimicking an aggressive chest wall tumor. *Diagn Interv Radiol*. 17:118–121.
80. John B and Lewis KR. Chromosome variability and geographic distribution in insects. *Science* 1966; 152:711–21
81. Bønnelykke K and Ober C. Leveraging gene-environment interactions and endotypes for asthma gene discovery. *J Allergy Clin Immunol* 2016;137:667–79.
82. Lötvall J *et al.*, Asthma endotypes: a new approach to classification of disease entities within the asthma syndrome. *Allergy Clin Immunol* 2011;127:355–60
83. Wenzel S. Severe asthma: from characteristics to phenotypes to endotypes *Clin Exp Allergy* 2012; 42:650–8
84. Poon AH *et al.*, Pathogenesis of severe asthma. *Clin Exp Allergy* 2012; 42:625–37

# 4

# Acute respiratory insufficiency

MATHIEU SIMON

| | |
|---|---|
| Introduction | 55 |
| Respiratory insufficiency | 56 |
| Upper airways obstruction | 56 |
| Hypoxemic, hypercapnic, and mixed respiratory insufficiencies | 57 |
|     Hypoxemic respiratory insufficiency | 57 |
|         Shunt | 57 |
|         $\dot{V}/\dot{Q}$ Abnormalities | 58 |
|         Alveolar hypoventilation | 58 |
|     Clinical translation | 59 |
|     Hypercapnic respiratory insufficiency | 60 |
|     Alveolar hypoventilation | 60 |
|     Dead space | 60 |
|     Mixed respiratory insufficiency | 60 |
|     Therapeutic approach | 62 |
| Treatment of hypoxemia | 62 |
|     Oxygen therapy | 62 |
|     Mechanical ventilation | 62 |
|     Hypoxemia versus hypoxia | 63 |
| Hypercapnia treatment | 64 |
|     Oxygen therapy | 64 |
|     Mechanical ventilation | 64 |
| Conclusion | 64 |
| References | 64 |

## Introduction

Breathing requires, in humans, the integrity of five highly integrated functions:

- Rhythmicity of central nervous system in charge of respiration
- Integrity of the effect of respiratory apparatus
- Airways permeability

- Ventilation
- Oxygenation

The nervous centers responsible for breathing are located in the midbrain. They coordinate the various afferent nerve inputs mainly from central and peripheral chemoreceptors that monitor blood pH, $pCO_2$, and $pO_2$ [1]. From these variables, the $pCO_2$ is the most important. Other afferent inputs come from mechanoreceptors disseminated throughout the lung parenchyma and from cortical centers integrating the various voluntary and emotional components of breathing. Central coordination of these different afferents allows adaptation of breathing to the needs of the organism.

The effector respiratory apparatus includes various nervous efferents and the respiratory muscles control provided by these last. The phrenic nerve stimulates the diaphragm and is the main effector muscle of breathing. At rest, the phrenic nerve–diaphragm couple ensures the quasi-totality of the work of breathing. The increase in respiratory load following an effort or following a pathologic condition brings the recruitment of accessory muscles of breathing: the main ones are the scalene, sternocleidomastoid, and intercostal muscles [2].

Penetration of air in the lung is passive, resulting from the depressurization of pleural spaces then alveolar, secondary to the action of respiratory muscles that increase the thoracic cage volume. Air entry in the lung requires therefore that the airways are open from the nose to the respiratory bronchioles.

Ventilation refers to the elimination by the respiratory system of $CO_2$ produced by the cellular metabolism. Ventilation depends upon the volume of fresh gas penetrating the alveolar space with each inspiration and from respiratory frequency. Oxygenation is a function almost independent of ventilation. It is essentially under the dependence of the $O_2$ partial pressure in the gas mixture inhaled and from the integrity of the alveolar–capillary interface (see Chapter 2).

## Respiratory insufficiency

Respiratory insufficiency represents the final common pathway of pathologies that brings disequilibrium between respiratory needs of the organism and performance of the respiratory apparatus. The clinical translation will depend on the specific pathology and its rapidity of onset.

To orient the diagnostic and therapeutic steps, we generally distinguish four types of acute respiratory insufficiency:

- Related to upper airways obstruction
- Hypoxemic
- Hypercapnic
- Mixed

The etiology, physiopathology, and diagnostic and therapeutic approaches of these conditions are specified with each entity (Table 4.1).

## Upper airways obstruction

Obstruction from extrinsic compression (e.g., goitre, thymoma, cervical hematoma, and angioedema) or endoluminal injury (e.g., foreign body, blood clot, tumor, and vocal cord paralysis) of the pharynx, larynx, glottis, trachea, or major bronchi can cause a respiratory distress that will manifest clinically by an increase in the work of breathing and a perception of breathlessness (dyspnea). More distal obstruction will not generally cause respiratory insufficiency in the healthy subject. In the presence of respiratory insufficiency, the patient usually looks anxious, uses respiratory accessory muscles, and breathing can be noisy for example, in the form of a stridor. At a more advanced stage, respiratory fatigue begins with the development of paradoxical

Table 4.1 Hypercapnic respiratory insufficiencies—alveolar hypoventilation (type 2)

| Site of lesion | Examples |
| --- | --- |
| **Ventilatory disorders of rhythmicity** | |
| Central nervous system | Intoxication (opioids, alcohol) |
|  | Head trauma |
|  | Cerebral hypoperfusion (stroke, schock) |
| **Insufficiency of effector ventilatory apparatus** | |
| Peripheral nervous system | Diaphragm paralysis |
|  | Quadriplegia from lesion of the spinal cord at a high level |
| Myoneural neuromuscular junction | Myasthenia gravis |
|  | Neuromuscular blockers |
| Muscle | Muscular dystrophy |
| Lung parenchyma | Pneumonia |
|  | Pulmonary edema |
|  | Acute respiratory distress syndrome |

abdominal respiration, movements of the thorax and abdomen being in opposition; the pCO$_2$ increases and the patient moves from an agitated state to a state of sleepiness. Hypoxemia is only a late manifestation of this type of respiratory insufficiency.

The treatment of upper airway obstruction depends on its etiology. A foreign body can be removed by an energetic external compression of the diaphragm such as the one performed during the Hemlich maneuver. It could, similar to a lesion causing a partial obstruction, be extracted by bronchial endoscopy or during open surgery [3]. Extrinsic bronchial compressions, according to their etiology and the time available for the intervention, will be treated with bronchial dilatation, insertion of a tutor, or surgical intervention. Endoluminal or extrinsic neoplastic lesions affecting the airways subacutely or chronically may also benefit, according to the case, from radiotherapy or chemotherapy.

# Hypoxemic, hypercapnic, and mixed respiratory insufficiencies

## Hypoxemic respiratory insufficiency

The acute hypoxemia encountered in clinical settings is most often a manifestation of one of the three following phenomena, either isolated or associated [4]:

- Shunt
- Ventilation/perfusion ($\dot{V}/\dot{Q}$) mismatch
- Alveolar hypoventilation

### Shunt

The term "shunt" describes the return of the nonoxygenated venous blood into the systemic circulation. Intracardiac shunt results from a process that allows direct communication between the right and left heart chambers. It is unusual to find this last as the only cause acute hypoxemia as it supposes pulmonary hypertension making possible blood flow from the right to the left heart. Hypoxemia originating from the lung following an associated reflex vasoconstriction can, however, cause an increase in the pulmonary arterial pressure and force the opening of foramen ovale, otherwise not permeable. The intracardiac shunt in these circumstances contributes to the worsening of hypoxemia.

An intrapulmonary shunt appears when the venous blood flow crosses the pulmonary circulation without being arterialized at the contact of the alveolar–capillary membrane exchange site. Here, the shunt is most often secondary to the absence of ventilation in the alveoli that are normally perfused (Figure 4.1). This occurs following atelectasis of the alveolar beds in a postoperatory period, for example, or when the alveolar are filled with fluid which could be blood, pus, or edema fluid. The pure intrapulmonary shunt rarely contributes markedly to hypoxemia as low $PaO_2$ in the nonventilated alveoli causes a vasoconstriction of the associated capillary beds. We call this phenomenon hypoxemic vasoconstriction [5]. The venous blood is then redirected to alveolar units with more elevated $PaO_2$ and then the shunt is corrected.

### V/Q Mismatch

$\dot{V}/\dot{Q}$ ratio abnormalities represent the main cause of hypoxemia. They describe the inhomogeneity of perfusion and ventilation in the lung parenchyma. So, certain alveolar units will have quasi-normal perfusion which will produce a partial shunt. Other well-ventilated and poorly perfused units will become close to the definition of a dead space. Only the former will contribute to hypoxemia (Figure 4.1). Contrary to the hypoxemia resulting from a true shunt, the secondary hypoxemia following $\dot{V}/\dot{Q}$ abnormalities will be corrected in increasing the $FiO_2$. Pneumonia, bronchospasm, pulmonary embolism, and chronic pulmonary obstructive disease (COPD) are clinical situations where the $\dot{V}/\dot{Q}$ abnormalities will represent the main mechanism leading to hypoxemia (Figure 4.2).

### Alveolar hypoventilation

The main role of alveolar ventilation is not oxygenation but elimination of $CO_2$. When ventilation is reduced from a fatigue of the ventilatory apparatus or the depression of ventilatory centers, the $PaCO_2$ will increase progressively. In the extreme cases, elevation of $PaCO_2$ can lead to hypoxemia. How is that possible? Let's consider the alveolar gas equation described in Chapter 2:

$$PAO_2 = \left(P_{Atm} - P_{H_2O}\right) \times F_iO_2 - \frac{PaCO_2}{R}.$$

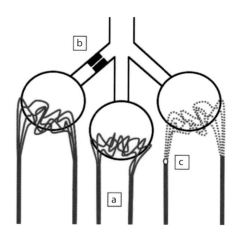

Figure 4.1 Alveolar capillary exchange zones. Schematic representation of the three zones of interaction between ventilation and perfusion. In **(a)**, an alveolus normally ventilated and perfused at $\dot{V}/\dot{Q}$ ratio equal to 1. Exchanges between inhaled air and the blood are optimized. The shunt zones **(b)** and dead space effect **(c)** represent respectively low and high $\dot{V}/\dot{Q}$ ratio. It results respectively in a reduction of the $PaO_2$ and an increase in the $PaCO_2$.

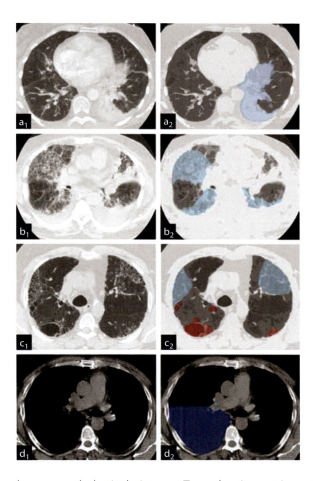

Figure 4.2 Shunt and dead space: pathological pictures. Tomodensitometric sections of lung pathologies. In (**a₁** and **a₂**), pneumonia; (**b₁** and **b₂**), acute respiratory distress syndrome (ARDS); (**c₁** and **c₂**), idiopathic pulmonary fibrosis; (**d₁** and **d₂**), proximal pulmonary embolism. The images on the left are real while the ones on the right represent the same sections enhanced to show zones of a shunt in blue and dead space in red. Note that the pulmonary embolism illustrated in (**d₁** and **d₂**) brings both dead spaces and shunt.

According to this equation, if $PaCO_2$ is normal (40 mmHg), the $PAO_2$ will be at 100 mmHg. However, if $PaCO_2$ doubles (80 mmHg), the $PAO_2$ will be reduced at 50 mmHg. Even if we assume that there is no alveolo–arterial gradient, the $PaO_2$ will be well under the threshold of hypoxemia (60 mmHg). Therefore, when we are facing a hypoxemic patient, the first reflex should be to measure the $PaCO_2$, which is close to the $PaCO_2$.

## Clinical translation

Hypoxemia will present initially with few specific clinical manifestations. The first physiological reaction that can be noted is a tachypnea which is sometimes felt by the patient as dyspnea. The resulting increase in ventilation will allow reduction of $PaCO_2$ and increase of the $PaO_2$ as the alveolar gas equation shows. Bradycardia and anxiety are also the manifestations of severe hypoxemia. Later on, confusion, psychomotor impairment, euphoria, and loss of consciousness will precede arrhythmias and ischemic heart disease leading to death.

## Hypercapnic respiratory insufficiency

Hypercapnic respiratory insufficiency in the patient hospitalized at the intensive care unit results from an excessive production of $CO_2$ or insufficient performance of the ventilatory apparatus [6]. The first condition is rare and it results in an excessive carbohydrate intake in a patient in a critical state in regard to his metabolism, when the ventilatory response is limited. The disorders of the ventilator apparatus are more common. They cause hypercapnia from alveolar hypoventilation or in increasing dead space.

## Alveolar hypoventilation

Two main types of ventilatory apparatus defects produce alveolar hypoventilation and cause a retention of $CO_2$ (Table 4.1): disorders of ventilatory rhythm and effector ventilatory apparatus insufficiency. These conditions result in a reduction in the capacity of excretion of $CO_2$, an increase in $PaCO_2$ and secondarily in $PaCO_2$.

As described previously, an increase in $PaCO_2$ can bring, according to the alveolar gas equation, a reduction in $PAO_2$ and then of $PaCO_2$. This condition is qualified mixed respiratory insufficiency (see "Mixed Respiratory Insufficiency" section).

## Dead space

While hypoxemia results from zones of inhomogeneity with a low $\dot{V}/\dot{Q}$ ratio (poorly ventilated but well perfused) similar to shunt, the inhomogeneity zones with a high $\dot{V}/\dot{Q}$ ratio (well ventilated but poorly perfused) result in dead space conditions leading to hypercapnia (Figure 4.1). Here, the $PaCO_2$ is normal or low but cannot equilibrate with $PaCO_2$. This type of $\dot{V}/\dot{Q}$ abnormalities may be the result of a destruction of the lung parenchyma (e.g., emphysema, acute respiratory distress syndrome [ARDS]) or the creation of West zone 1 where the alveolar pressure is superior to the pulmonary capillary pressure (e.g., shock, ventilation at high volumes, and pulmonary embolism; Figure 4.2).

## Mixed respiratory insufficiency

As we saw before, $\dot{V}/\dot{Q}$ ratio inhomogeneities are responsible for a large majority of abnormalities of arterial gasometry at the intensive care unit. A specific pathology can generate many zones which will favor hypoxemia while others will predispose to hypercapnia (Figure 4.2). Furthermore, a chronic respiratory condition can be complicated with an acute affection that will allow the simultaneous presence of a low $PaO_2$ and high $PaCO_2$. The $PaO_2$ is linked to $PaCO_2$ by the alveolar gas equation, which shows that an increase in $PaCO_2$ secondary to an elevation of the $PaCO_2$ will produce a hypoxemia. These various clinical situations cause a respiratory insufficiency that we can qualify as mixed with associated hypoxemia and hypercapnia. The therapeutic approach will have to take into account the coexistence of these two problems [7].

Most often, the majority of respiratory insufficiencies are mixed (Table 4.2), the underlying pathologies generating both a shunt and a dead space. However, due to the facility of equilibration of $CO_2$ on both sides of the alveolar capillary membrane, dead space is more easily compensated by the residual parenchyma while the shunt is difficult to correct by a redistribution to healthy alveolar spaces. Hypercapnia, if it does not depend on ventilatory rhythmicity problems, indicates therefore that the lung pathology is both diffuse and severe. Pulmonary embolism is an example of such concept. Resulting in a vascular obstruction without

Table 4.2 Frequent pulmonary pathologies and mechanisms of alteration of gas exchanges

| | Shunt | Dead space | Hypoxemia | Hypercapnia | Usual clinical presentation |
|---|---|---|---|---|---|
| **Hypoxemic respiratory insufficiency** | | | | | |
| Pneumonia | ++ | + | +++ mixed? | + | • Hyperthermia<br>• Purulent phlegm<br>• Localized infiltrate on radiograph |
| Pulmonary edema | ++++ | 0 | ++++ | 0 | • Angina or or silent myocardial ischemia<br>• Signs of systemic overload<br>• electrocardiographic modifications<br>• Symetric infiltrates on radiograph |
| Interauricular communication | ++++ | 0 | ++++ | 0 | • Cyanosis<br>• Clubbing<br>• Signs of pulmonary hypertension<br>• Widening of cardiac silhouette |
| Pulmonary embolism | +++ | + | +++ mixed? | + | • Acute dyspnea<br>• Pleuritic pain<br>• Signs of thrombophlebitis<br>• No specific translation on radiograph (regular chest x-rays) |
| **Hypercapnic respiratory insufficiency** | | | | | |
| Status asthmaticus | + | +++ | + mixed? | +++ | • Anxiety<br>• Wheezing<br>• Respiratory fatigue (tachypnea?)<br>• Hyperinflation on radiograph |
| Muscular dystrophy | ++ | ++++ | + mixed? | ++++ | • Slowly progressive condition<br>• Diffuse muscular atrophy<br>• Secondary deformations of thoracic cage |
| Cyphoscoliosis | ++ | +++ | + mixed? | +++ | • Slowly progressive condition<br>• Primary deformations of thoracic cage<br>• Pulmonary asymmetry |
| **Mixed respiratory insufficiency** | | | | | |
| ARDS | ++++ | +++ | ++++ | ++ | • Severe underlying pathology, pulmonary or extrapulmonary<br>• Often associated with a multiorganic dysfunction<br>• High mortality rate |
| COPD exacerbation | ++ | +++ | ++ | +++ | • Underlying COPD<br>• Exacerbation usually from infectious origin<br>• Very frequent lung disease |

ARDS, acute respiratory distress syndrome; COPD, chronic pulmonary obstructive disease.

alveolar defect, this essentially results in the formation of a dead space. However, in clinic, it is quite rare that pulmonary embolism will manifest as hypercapnia. Hypoxemia is more prevalent. This last will be the result of the formation of shunt zones $\dot{V}/\dot{Q}$, due to the bronchoconstriction adjacent to the embolism zone in the parenchyma still perfused. Many humoral mediators including endothelin, histamine, and serotonin are involved in the physiopathology of this phenomenon [7].

## Therapeutic approach

We have to distinguish, here, a specific treatment of the pathology from the support treatment which only aims at correcting the oxygenation and ventilation abnormalities. So, the specific treatment could include antibiotics for pneumonia, diuretics for pulmonary edema, or anticoagulants for pulmonary embolism. In patients in critical state, blood gas abnormalities can be such that they will need a non-specific support treatment, at least one that is transitory, while waiting for the therapeutic effect of the treatment initiated for a specific etiology. The intensive care units have been developed in the second half of the twentieth century to do so.

## Treatment of hypoxemia

### Oxygen therapy

The first intervention to offer to the hypoxemic patient will be oxygen supplementation according to the mode of administration and the flow of oxygen chosen. It will be possible to increase the $FiO_2$ at levels varying from 25% to 100%. The nasal prongs are the first line of intervention in a patient suffering from a mild to moderate hypoxemia. It will be minimally insufficient in a patient with a high breathing flow or presenting essentially an oral respiration. A venturi mask will generally allow oxygen to be brought more effectively to these patients. Some of these masks have a reservoir that allows accumulating oxygen during the expiratory phase, to make it more readily available during the next inspiration. They offer the best $FiO_2$.

### Mechanical ventilation

It represents a general term describing all forms of mechanical assistance to the oxygenation and ventilation functions of the lung. In the treatment of severe hypoxemia, its effects are combined with oxygen therapy. The mechanical ventilation contributes to correcting the hypoxemia essentially by reducing respiratory work and in doing so, the total consumption of $O_2$ by the patient (reduction of $VO_2$), the recruitment of collapsed alveolar beds kept open by the application of a positive ventilatory pressure and a reduction of $PaCO_2$ in the case of severe hypercapnia.

A mechanical ventilator supports spontaneous ventilation at different levels. It can substitute entirely for breathing if the clinical condition requires.

In the presence of a mild to moderate hypoxemia and a quickly reversible pathology, the clinician will privilege noninvasive interface with a silicon mask in a format adapted to the facial anatomy of the patient. This interface will avoid the need for a profound sedation and will allow preservation of the oral feeding and communication with the patient. In addition to being more comfortable, it will avoid the risks of procedures and infections associated with the endotracheal intubation (Figure 4.3) [8].

The invasive interface is so called because it introduces an artificial airway or an artificial access to the airways, most often using an endotracheal tube is inserted in the airways (Figure 4.3b). It allows a protection against aspiration of gastric content, and, in the profoundly hypoxemic patient, use of increased ventilatory pressure ensures better oxygenation. This technique is, however, uncomfortable as it requires profound sedation both at the insertion of the tube and during its maintenance [9,10]. Bypassing the usual airway

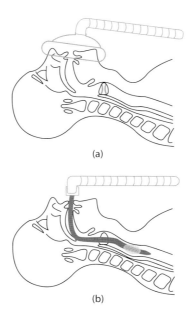

Figure 4.3 Ventilation interfaces. **(a)** Noninvasive ventilation with a mask covering both the nose and mouth. The mask is maintained in place by elastic bands (not shown). **(b)** Invasive ventilation with flexible endotracheal tube introduced by the mouth to the glottis. The sealing of the interface is provided by a balloon inflated below the vocal cords.

defense mechanisms, endotracheal intubation is a significant source of bacterial contamination which often results in nosocomial pneumonia.

## Hypoxemia versus hypoxia

The correction of $PaO_2$ is not the main objective of the hypoxemic treatment. More than gasometrical values, we will try to optimize the tissue oxygenation of which $PaO_2$ is only a minor determinant. In fact, the arterial $O_2$ blood saturation and its hemoglobin content and cardiac flow are more important functions of the cardiovascular apparatus to deliver oxygen to the tissue ($DO_2$).

$$DO_2 = DC \times (1.3 \times Hb \times SatO_2) = 0.003 \times PaO_2$$

where

$DC$ = cardiac flow (L/min)

$Hb$ = serum hemoglobin (g/L)

$SatO_2$ = arterial $O_2$ saturation (0–100)

$PaCO_2$ = arterial partial pressure of $CO_2$ (mmHg)

1.34 = hemoglobin $O_2$ transport capacity (mL/g)

1.34 = plasma $O_2$ transport capacity (mL/mmHg)

## Hypercapnia treatment

### Oxygen therapy

Supplementary oxygen is not useful in the treatment of isolated hypercapnia. In fact, in some patients suffering from COPD we see an increase in the respiratory acidosis following the initiation of oxygen therapy. This phenomenon derives from three mechanisms: (1) the release of $CO_2$ by the hemoglobin molecule when $O_2$ is fixed on this last (Haldane effect); (2) a redistribution of the pulmonary blood flow toward units with a low $\dot{V}/\dot{Q}$ ratio in releasing hypoxic bronchoconstriction; there is, then, a steal of blood flow at the expense of the units relatively better ventilated resulting in an increase of the physiological dead space; and (3) a reduction of the hypoxemic ventilatory stimulation.

Oxygen therapy is useful to support the profoundly hypercapnic patients in whom a normal $FiO_2$ is insufficient to ensure adequate oxygenation according to the alveolar gas equation. Although supplementary oxygen can worsen hypercapnia by the mechanisms mentioned earlier, once it is installed, the withdrawal of oxygen therapy is not usually welcome as it can lead to a profound hypoxemia.

### Mechanical ventilation

The treatment of hypercapnia is usually an increase in alveolar ventilation. This can be accomplished by one of the two following mechanisms: increasing tidal volume or increasing ventilatory frequency.

The product of those two variables is called *minute ventilation*. This last can be increased by mechanical ventilation either invasive or not. Contrary to alveolar recruitment, which needs an elevated ventilatory pressure, an increase in minute ventilation usually requires only modest working pressures that allow non-invasive interface to be the best option in the majority of clinical cases. However, if the hypercapnia results from a depression of the sensorium or if it has been caused by depressive effects, the invasive interface will be favored to allow the protection of the airways.

## Conclusion

Acute respiratory insufficiency is a frequent condition and its physiopathology often depends on the participation of many mechanisms. The shunt and the dead space are the main components as their sources are hypoxemia and hypercapnia, respectively. Once the causal pathology is treated, the shunt will be treated essentially by supplementary oxygen and the alveolar recruitment by pressurization of alveolar spaces while hypercapnia will be corrected by increasing alveolar ventilation. Very often, and in almost all severe cases, hypoxemia and hypercapnia occur simultaneously and require a combined therapeutic approach.

## References

1. Loeschcke HH. Respiratory chemosensitivity in the medulla oblongata. *Acta Neurobiologiae Experimentalis* 1973;33:97–112.
2. Kubin L, Alheid GF, Zuperku EJ, McCrimmon DR. Central pathways of pulmonary and lower airway vagal afferents. *Journal of Applied Physiology* (1985) 2006;101:618–27.
3. Murgu SD, Colt HG. Interventional bronchoscopy from bench to bedside: New techniques for central and peripheral airway obstruction. *Clinics in Chest Medicine* 2010;31:101–15.
4. Henig NR, Pierson DJ. Mechanisms of hypoxemia. *Respiratory Care Clinics of North America* 2000;6:501–21.

5. Mark Evans A, Ward JP. Hypoxic pulmonary vasoconstriction—Invited article. *Advances in Experimental Medicine and Biology* 2009;648:351–60.
6. Epstein SK, Singh N. Respiratory acidosis. *Respiratory Care* 2001;46:366–83.
7. El Solh AA, Ramadan FH. Overview of respiratory failure in older adults. *Journal of Intensive Care Medicine* 2006;21:345–51.
8. Barreiro TJ, Gemmel DJ. Noninvasive ventilation. *Critical Care Clinics* 2007;23:201–22, ix.
9. Kabrhel C, Thomsen TW, Setnik GS, Walls RM. Videos in clinical medicine. Orotracheal intubation. *New England Journal of Medicine* 2007;356:e15.
10. Walz JM, Zayaruzny M, Heard SO. Airway management in critical illness. *Chest* 2007;131:608–20.

# 5

# Pathophysiology of asthma

LOUIS-PHILIPPE BOULET

| Introduction: definition and characteristics of asthma | 68 |
| Epidemiology and prevalence | 68 |
|     Risk factors of asthma | 70 |
| Consequences | 71 |
| Etiologic factors and asthma phenotypes | 71 |
|     Phenotypes/endotypes of asthma | 71 |
|     Mechanisms of development of asthma | 73 |
| Genetic factors | 73 |
| The role of airway inflammation | 74 |
|     Development of allergic asthma | 74 |
|     Pathogenesis of asthma | 75 |
|     Airway inflammation: a description of its main components | 75 |
|     Description of the main inflammatory cells playing a role in asthma | 77 |
|         Mast cells and basophils | 77 |
|         Eosinophils | 77 |
|         Neutrophils | 77 |
|         Monocytes and macrophages | 77 |
|         T- and B-lymphocytes | 78 |
|         Innate lymphoid cells | 78 |
|         Dendritic cells | 79 |
|         Epithelial cells | 79 |
|     Airway structural changes: airway remodeling | 80 |
|     Neurogenic mechanisms | 83 |
|     The "model" of allergic asthma | 84 |
|     Nonallergic asthma | 85 |
|     Exercise-induced asthma | 86 |
|     Aspirin-induced asthma | 86 |
| Asthma and respiratory infections | 86 |
|     Asthma exacerbations | 86 |
|     Severe asthma | 86 |
|     Asthma–COPD Overlap (ACO) | 88 |
|     Clinical expression of asthma | 88 |

| | |
|---|---|
| Physiologic Changes in Asthma | 88 |
|     Airway obstruction | 88 |
|     Airway hyperresponsiveness | 89 |
| How can knowledge of asthma physiopathology help the clinician in the evaluation and treatment of asthma? | 90 |
| Prevention of asthma | 90 |
| Therapeutic targets | 90 |
| Conclusion: Future developments | 92 |
| References | 92 |

# Introduction: definition and characteristics of asthma

The 2017 Global Initiative for Asthma (GINA) report defines asthma as "a heterogeneous disease, usually characterized by chronic airway inflammation. It is defined by the history of respiratory symptoms such as wheeze, shortness of breath, chest tightness, and cough that vary over time and in intensity, together with variable expiratory airflow limitation [1]. These variations are often triggered by factors such as exercise, allergen or irritant exposure, change in weather, or viral respiratory infections."

Asthma is therefore a chronic disease of the airways in which airway inflammation is considered to play a major role in its development in the majority of asthma sufferers [2]. Many cells such as mast cells, eosinophils, basophils, T-lymphocytes, macrophages, neutrophils, and epithelial cells are involved in this process. Asthmatic lower airways are characterized by an increased responsiveness to stimuli, contracting more intensely or more easily either spontaneously or following various triggers. This may then result, combined with other effects such as airway inflammation and structural changes, in airway obstruction. This reduction in airway lumen size, which varies from one patient to another, may be due to the inflammatory process, including airway wall edema, mucus hypersecretion, and/or airway smooth muscle contraction. Classically, this generalized airway obstruction is changing in intensity over time or following treatment with bronchodilators and/or corticosteroids (Table 5.1). The type and severity of asthma symptoms can also vary from an individual to another. For example, some will only have a cough (called cough variant of asthma), although an isolated cough is often due to upper airway cough syndrome (UACS) or gastroesophageal reflux disease (GERD), or only report effort intolerance while others have many symptoms as mentioned above [1,3].

For diagnostic purposes, the variability of airway obstruction (then inducing airflow limitation) is considered as significant if there is an increase in 12% or more of the forced expiratory volume in 1 second ($FEV_1$) after administration of a fast-acting bronchodilator or a change of 20% or more of $FEV_1$ or peak expiratory flow (PEF) spontaneously with time [4] (Table 5.1, Figure 5.1).

# Epidemiology and prevalence

The prevalence of asthma varies from a country to another (from 1% to 18%) [1]. It is the most common chronic disease of the child [7]. The World Health Organization estimates that there are currently over 300 million individuals suffering from asthma worldwide and that this number will increase significantly in the following decades [8]. Asthma can begin at any age and there is currently no cure for this disease. However, it can be controlled, with no or minimal symptoms, allowing a normal life. The GINA report suggests that asthma is well controlled when asthma symptoms do not occur more than twice/week, when there is no night awakening due to asthma, no need for "reliever" therapy (fast-acting bronchodilator) more than twice/week, and no limitation of activities due to asthma. Furthermore, the patient should not be at risk of adverse asthma outcomes such as exacerbations or fixed airflow limitation and have no side effects of medication [1].

Table 5.1 Main characteristics of asthma

| | |
|---|---|
| Symptoms | Cough, dyspnea, chest tightness, wheezing, and phlegm production, which vary over time and in intensity |
| | Can predominantly occur at night and be aggravated by exercise, respiratory irritants, laughter, cold air exposure, relevant allergens, and viral respiratory infections |
| Variable airway obstruction | Airway obstruction at least documented once as $FEV_1/FVC$ lower than normal—it is >0.75–0.80 in adults, although it can be lower in elderly patients, and >0.90 in children. This obstruction is considered variable if $FEV_1$ increases >12% of postbronchodilator (at least 200 mL in adults) or if $FEV_1$ or PEF increases >12% (more convincingly if 20%) spontaneously or after 4 weeks of bronchial anti-inflammatory treatment. Such variability may be absent in some patients, for example, if asthma is mild, or if it is markedly uncontrolled) [1] |
| Airway hyperresponsiveness | Provocative concentration of methacholine inducing a 20% fall in $FEV_1$ ($PC_{20}$)[a] <16 mg/mL on methacholine test[b] or significant fall in $FEV_1$ after other types of bronchoprovocation (e.g., ≥10% after eucapnic voluntary hyperpnea (EVH) test or exercise or ≥15% after mannitol) [5,6] |
| Bronchial inflammation | Often eosinophilic, but sometimes neutrophilic, mixed, or paucigranulocytic (with few or no inflammatory cells) |
| Structural changes (remodeling) | Subepithelial fibrosis, increase in airway smooth muscle, deposition of proteoglycans in the bronchial wall, angiogenesis, and others.... |

[a] Concentration of methacholine causing a fall of 20% of $FEV_1$ on bronchoprovocation test [5].
[b] There is a "gray zone" between 4 and 16 mg/mL where responsiveness is considered to be "borderline" [6]. Airway responsiveness can increase after allergen exposure and decrease with corticosteroid treatment.

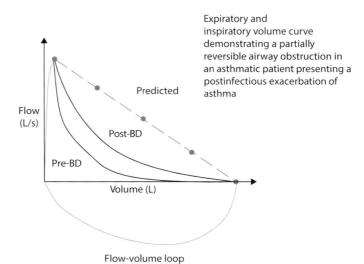

Figure 5.1 Forced expiratory volume curve. Post-BD, post-bronchodilator; pre-BD, pre-bronchodilator.

Asthma most often begins in childhood and is associated with atopy, following sensitization to common allergens. Almost all children developing asthma after the age of 6 are atopic. However, asthma can also develop in the absence of underlying allergy, usually in the mid-late adult age. In these latter ages, asthma is more severe and corticosteroid resistant. In early childhood, asthma is more common in boys than girls but this changes at puberty. Between a third and a half of asthmatic children become asymptomatic at adolescence but remissions at the adult age are rare [9]. Asthma varies in severity, from mild, seasonal, intermittent, or occurring only during physical exercise, to severe, requiring heavy daily medication including high doses of inhaled corticosteroids (ICS) and even sometimes, in addition to bronchodilators, other medications such as oral corticosteroids, anticytokines, or anti-immunoglobulin (Ig)E monoclonal antibodies.

## Risk factors of asthma

There are many risk factors of asthma [10]. Table 5.2 summarizes some of the risk factors that could contribute to the development of asthma. The prevalence of asthma has increased in the last decades. This increase is probably multifactorial. Many hypotheses have been proposed to help explain this phenomenon. The "hygiene hypothesis" attributes this increase in prevalence to changes in lifestyle, with a reduced exposure to infectious agents or endotoxins inducing a change in the immune system that favors the proliferation of T helper type 2 (Th2)-type lymphocytes involved in allergy to the detriment of Th1 mechanisms, which are classically involved in defense against infectious agents [11]. Early-life exposures to environments with a high microbial content and endotoxins (e.g., farms, daycare centers) have indeed been associated with a lower prevalence of asthma. A recent study comparing Amish and Hutterite schoolchildren revealed marked differences in the prevalence of asthma despite similar genetic ancestries and lifestyles, probably related to the protective effect of sustained exposure to microbes that activate innate pathways, related to traditional farming methods in the former, influencing immune response [12].

In the first 2 years of life, children are often infected with respiratory syncytial virus (RSV) and rhinoviruses and these could contribute to the development of asthma, although a developmental defect of the respiratory and/or immune system making them more susceptible to develop asthma may also be involved. Other factors have also been suggested, such as obesity, dietary factors such as a reduction of antioxidant intake, vitamin D

Table 5.2 Risk factors involved in the development of asthma

- Genetic factors (having a close relative with asthma)[a]
- Having another allergic disease than asthma
- Viral infections in childhood
- Low socioeconomic status and stress
- Prematurity/low birthweight/cesarean section
- Duration of breastfeeding or use of antibiotics in early childhood
- Environmental exposures:
  - Allergens
  - Sensitizing agents at workplace
  - Cigarette smoke (particularly maternal smoking)
  - Urban habitat
- Modern lifestyle (western lifestyle)
- Obesity (including obesity of the mother during pregnancy)
- Diet (low levels of antioxidants, high salt intake)
- Possibly acetaminophen/paracetamol intake during childhood**

[a] See the various genes associated with asthma in Chapter 3.
** Possibly confounded by its use during respiratory infections.

deficiency, increased contact with domestic allergens, or various indoors or outdoors pollutants, in addition to an increased recognition of the disease and overdiagnosis [13,14]. There has been an increasing interest about the possible role of the airway microbiome and response to microorganisms on the development of asthma. For example, a delayed increase in IgG1 serum titers against bacteria such as *Haemophilus influenzae* and *Streptococcus pneumoniae* has been associated with a risk of atopy and asthma at age 5 [15].

Although the role of sensitization to allergens and some occupational agents (e.g., isocyanates), and respiratory infections, as asthma "inducers" is quite obvious, it is less so for others such as exposure to air pollutants such as ozone, nitrogen dioxide ($NO_2$), volatile organic compounds (VOCs), and particulate matter (PM). Increased exposure to these can, however, be responsible for exacerbations of the disease and they may also play a role as promoters of allergen sensitization. For tobacco smoke, it is now considered an independent risk factor for asthma. Maternal smoking (and even grandmaternal smoking) during pregnancy is associated with an increased risk of asthma in the child.

Obesity is associated with an increased incidence and severity of asthma but how it influences asthma development is uncertain [16]. It is probably multifactorial, involving respiratory mechanical changes resulting in breathing at very low lung volumes, in addition to low-grade inflammation and hormonal and metabolic changes.

## Consequences

The mortality associated with asthma increased in the 1970s and 1980s, at least in part due to delay in consulting during exacerbations, overuse of β2 agonists, and insufficient use of anti-inflammatory agents such as ICS. Although currently asthma is still responsible for major morbidity, it is now quite less often associated with asthma death [17]. When not controlled properly, however, asthma can affect quality of life, cause troublesome symptoms, and reduce tolerance to environmental irritants and exercise, in addition to be associated with frequent needs for healthcare, particularly emergency care, therefore resulting in increased healthcare costs [18,19].

## Etiologic factors and asthma phenotypes

The cause of asthma is still unknown, although we know that, in those suffering from asthma, there is an abnormal response of the immune and respiratory systems to various stimuli [20]. The physiological manifestations of asthma such as airway hyperresponsiveness (AHR), variable airway obstruction, mucus hypersecretion, and airway remodeling seem to result from the activation of innate and adaptive immune systems and their interaction with epithelial cells. As mentioned previously, factors contributing to the development of asthma include allergen or industrial substance exposure in sensitized subjects, acute or chronic exposure to toxic substances, and respiratory infections (Table 5.3).

Indoor allergens are even more commonly associated with asthma than those found outdoors [21] and allergens originating from house dust mites, cockroaches, fungi, and animals show enzymatic properties, facilitating their penetration through the airway epithelium to interact with antigen-presenting dendritic cells. Various stimuli can however trigger asthma symptoms in inducing a bronchoconstriction of variable intensity, depending on the degree of baseline airway responsiveness, but without influencing significantly the severity of asthma. The mode of presentation of asthma varies, therefore, according to the etiologic factors involved and the type of symptoms experienced by the individual (Table 5.4).

## Phenotypes/endotypes of asthma

Although there have been suggestions not to use the terms "asthma" or "chronic obstructive pulmonary disease (COPD)" to categorize obstructive airways diseases and to mainly call them according to their

Table 5.3 Asthma triggers and inducers (examples)

**INDUCERS**

Which can induce the development of asthma
Allergens:
- House dust mites
- Animal danders
- Pollens (trees, grasses, and ragweed)
- Feathers, molds, etc.

Industrial substances:
- Sensitizing agents of animal origin (laboratory animals, fisheries, etc.)
- Chemical or biological agents (isocyanates, platinum salts, nickel, phthalic anhydride, etc.)
- Exposure to high levels of toxic agents (ammonia, $SO_2$, chlorine, etc.)

Respiratory infectious agents (mainly viruses)

**TRIGGERS**

Which can induce symptoms and/or increase or change the type of airway inflammation:
- Airborne pollutants
- Cigarette smoke

Which can cause a marked bronchoconstriction if they are ingested (usually with other nonrespiratory symptoms that can be predominant):
- Aspirin and nonsteroidal anti-inflammatory agents
- Some food additives (sulfites, benzoates, and monosodium glutamate)

Which can cause a bronchoconstriction but usually without significant influence on airway inflammation:
- Exercise (apart from high-level athletes—see later) and cold air
- Emotion and stress
- Weather changes
- Low levels of various respiratory irritants

Table 5.4 Some characteristics of the main categories of asthma

**Allergic asthma**
- Young patients
- Often associated with a rhinoconjunctivitis, eczema, or atopic dermatitis
- Positive allergy skin tests, presence of specific IgE
- Intermittent symptoms, sometimes seasonal
- Sputum eosinophilia
- Favorable prognosis

**Nonatopic asthma (intrinsic asthma)**
- Mostly adults (late onset)
- Absence of allergic manifestations
- More severe with continuous dyspnea
- Can evolve toward corticosteroid dependence

(*Continued*)

Table 5.4 (*Continued*) Some characteristics of the main categories of asthma

**Occupational asthma**
(A) *Classical presentation*: Asthma induced by a substance at work from a sensitizing process
(B) *Irritant-induced asthma*: Asthma induced by the inhalation of high/toxic concentrations of a respiratory irritant (occupational asthma without latency period)
Note: A transient increase in asthma symptoms in a patient with a previously diagnosed asthma, caused by exposure at work to an allergen or a respiratory irritant, is usually not considered to be occupational asthma but only "work-exacerbated asthma"

**Exercise-induced asthma**
This is usually a mild form of asthma that may occur only during physical exertion, although most asthmatics can experience a bronchoconstriction if they perform exercises, particularly if they are not well controlled

**Aspirin-induced asthma (ASA triad)**
- Intolerance to aspirin and nonsteroidal anti-inflammatory agents (e.g., for arthritis)
- Polypoid rhinitis
- Asthma (often severe)

**Chronic cough**
Asthma can also manifest as an isolated persistent cough, particularly in the child
(also called "cough variant of asthma")

characteristics (e.g., chronic eosinophilic bronchitis associated with partly reversible airway obstruction), this type of description is not widely accepted yet [22]. However, in the last decade, as for other diseases such as cancer and arthritis, asthma has been increasingly considered as an "umbrella-like" term that includes various groups with specific phenotypes or endotypes, influenced by genetic and environmental factors among others [23]. A "phenotype" is defined as any observable characteristic of a disease, such as morphology, development, biochemical or physiological properties, or behavior, while an "endotype" refers to the endogenous mechanisms of development/maintenance of a specific condition [24].

During the last few years, there has been an attempt to better characterize the various phenotypes/endotypes of asthma and see how they compare in regard to the various features of the disease. These phenotypes can be categorized as clinical, physiological, and inflammatory or even molecular [25] (Table 5.5). They often overlap, however, and they can change with time (e.g., asthma in a smoker becomes more neutrophilic, occupational asthma can resolve when exposure to the offending agent is stopped, obesity-associated asthma can improve or resolve following bariatric surgery). Many of these phenotypes and their effects on clinical outcomes or on treatment remain to be characterized.

## Mechanisms of development of asthma

Asthma usually develops following environmental exposures in genetically predisposed individuals. This particularly occurs in atopic subjects sensitized to common airborne allergens (Figure 5.2).

## Genetic factors

Many genetic variants can identify the predilection to developing asthma if a parent is predisposed to the development of atopy, AHR, and asthma [26]. There is therefore a hereditary component to asthma and it has been said that a child with both parents suffering from asthma has a probability of about 75%–80% to develop asthma, while it is approximately 40%–50% if only one has asthma, depending on environmental

Table 5.5 Phenotypes of asthma[a]

**According to etiologic factors or triggers in addition to comorbid conditions**
- Allergic
- Nonallergic
- Occupational (induced by occupational allergens or irritants)
- Aspirin and nonsteroidal anti-inflammatory drugs (NSAID)-induced asthma (ASA triad)**
- Asthma in the smoker
- Asthma in the obese
- Exercise-induced asthma and sports-induced asthma in the high-level athlete
- Asthma influenced by hormonal changes (e.g., premenstrual asthma)
- Asthma associated with Allergic Bronchopulmonary Aspergillosis (see p. 274)

**According to some clinical manifestations**
- Mild, moderate, or severe (defined according to severity)
- Exacerbation prone
- Early or late onset
- Labile (brittle asthma)
- With frequent exacerbations
- Treatment resistant, steroid insensitive

**According to physiological factors**
- With or without a fixed component of airway obstruction
- With a marked component of air trapping

**According to the bronchial inflammatory profile**
- Eosinophilic (allergic, occupational, corticosteroid weaning, etc.)
- Neutrophilic (infection, cigarette, pollutants, obesity, occupational, etc.)
- Mixed (see previous both categories)
- Paucigranulocytic (steroid-resistant, high doses of corticosteroids)

**Molecular phenotypes**
- TH2-type asthma
- Non-TH2-type asthma

[a] Many of these phenotypes may overlap and/or remain to be better documented.
** The triad incudes asthma, NSAID intolerance and nasal polyps

exposures, however. Not only can somebody be genetically predisposed to develop asthma but also there can be genetic factors that will influence response to medications used to treat this condition [27].

## The role of airway inflammation

Asthma can develop following an intense or repeated airway inflammatory process. The latter involves many effector cells and inflammatory mediators and it seems to be responsible for changes in the airway structure and function observed in asthma [20]. The bronchial epithelial damage induced by the inflammatory process can also contribute to the development of AHR [28].

## Development of allergic asthma

The majority of children and at least half of affected adults have allergic asthma, developing from sensitization to various allergens against which they produce immunoglobulin E (IgE). Most often, atopic eczema and/or a rhinitis will develop and later, following what is called "the allergic march," asthma may develop [29]. The concept "united airways disease" has been proposed, suggesting that allergic rhinitis and asthma are manifestations of the same underlying disease that may influence each other [30].

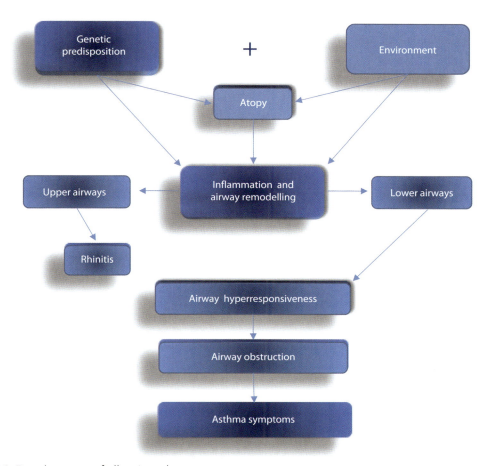

Figure 5.2 Development of allergic asthma.

## Pathogenesis of asthma

Airway inflammation, a major feature of asthma, is of Th2 (or T2) type in more than 80% of children and in a majority of adults who become sensitized to common allergens [31]. Asthma is indeed considered a typical Th2 airways disease, commonly associated with eosinophilic-type airway inflammation, sometimes controlled by type 2 innate lymphoid cells (ILC2) acting with basophils. However, asthma can also exist as a Th2-low disease, in which there is an increase in neutrophils in the sputum but eosinophil counts are normal under the influence of a Th17 subset of helper T cells. Airway inflammation can be of a mixed type, both eosinophilic and neutrophilic, and occasionally, it can present without obvious inflammation (pauci-granulocytic phenotype).

## Airway inflammation: a description of its main components

As mentioned, in most asthmatic patients, airway inflammation involves Th2 lymphocytes, particularly in allergic asthma (Figure 5.3). Asthma and AHR are therefore associated with an inflammatory process in which eosinophils, mast cells, and lymphocytes (mainly CD4+) classically play an important role [20]. These

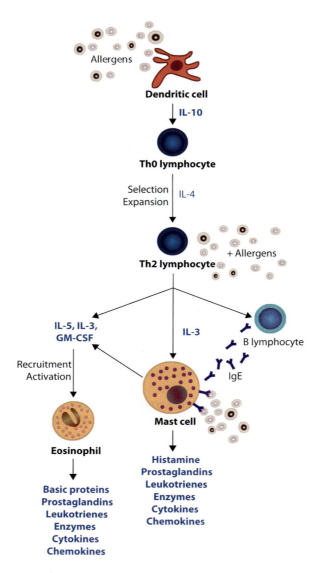

Figure 5.3 Asthmatic reaction of allergic origin.

cells are not only present in increased numbers in the airways of asthmatic subjects, but they are also activated and release various pro-inflammatory substances. Asthma is likely the result of the persistence of this inflammatory process and its consequences on the various structural bronchial elements (remodeling) [32]. This inflammatory process has been mostly described in conducting airways, but also involves peripheral airways, probably to different degrees in different individuals [33].

A variable relationship has been found between the degree of inflammation and the severity of asthma, probably due to the involvement of various other phenomena, such as airway remodeling. However, exacerbations of asthma are classically associated with an increase in airway inflammation, often eosinophilic and/or neutrophilic. The frequency of these exacerbations has been associated with an increased decline in the lung function in the asthmatic patients [34].

## Description of the main inflammatory cells playing a role in asthma

### Mast cells and basophils

These cells, also called metachromatic cells, are located in the bronchial mucosa and the peribronchovascular space and are involved in the process of sensitization to the allergens during the type 1 allergic response. They have high-affinity receptors for IgE (FcεRI) and can produce and release various inflammatory mediators such as histamine, proteinases, leukotrienes, thromboxane, prostaglandins and interleukins (IL-3, IL-4, IL-5), tumor necrosis factor (TNF), granulocyte macrophage colony-stimulating factor (GM-CSF), and platelet-activating factor (PAF) [35]. In mild to moderate allergic asthma, most mucosal mast cells are from TH2 cell-dependent tryptase type, while in more difficult-to-treat asthma, they contain both tryptase and chymase.

### Eosinophils

Eosinophils are considered key cells in asthma. Airway eosinophilia is mainly driven by IL-5, which promotes the production of eosinophils in the bone marrow and contributes to the recruitment of eosinophils through the influence of chemokines such as eotaxins 1, 2, and 3 (CCL11, CCL24, and CCL26, respectively); regulated upon activation, normal T cell expressed and secreted (RANTES); macrophage inflammatory protein (MIP)-1α; and arachidonic acid metabolites including cysteinyl leukotrienes and 5-keto eicosatetraenoic acid [36]. This type of cell increases in the bronchial mucosa after an allergic response. Its pro-inflammatory effects result in the liberation of cytokines, such as IL-3, IL-4, IL-5, and IL-13, various basic proteins, chemokines, growth factors, enzymes, and lipid mediators.

The eosinophil can also activate many other cells such as monocytes, fibroblasts, and B-lymphocytes, and its products, such as eosinophil peroxidase, can increase airway responsiveness from the activation of adaptive immunity through effects on dendritic cells directly. It has also been suggested that eosinophils could promote airway remodeling features, such as subepithelial membrane collagen deposition through the release of transforming growth factor-β (TGF-β). In allergic asthma, eosinophilic airway inflammation is driven by adaptive Th2 cells under the influence of dendritic cells, to produce IL-5, IL-13, and IL-4, these last promoting IgE synthesis [37] (Figures 5.4 through 5.6). In nonatopic asthma, eosinophilia can be due to the effect of ILC2 cells, which do not produce significant IL-4 and therefore are not associated with an IgE response from B cells. A recent publication reported the presence of two population of eosinophils: (1) IL-5-dependent cells classically recruited and (2) IL-5-independent tissue eosinophils that may play a beneficial role in some innate homeostatic functions [38].

### Neutrophils

Neutrophils play an important role in antibacterial defense and are found in large numbers in the bronchial mucosa of patients suffering from COPD, in severe asthma and in the smoking asthmatic as well as in elderly asthmatic patients [39]. They can produce various proteinases, oxidants, and numerous mediators such as TNF, IL-1α, IL-6, IL-8, and leukotriene $B_4$. Many mediators are involved in neutrophilic inflammation, such as IL-8, IL-17, and IL-23.

### Monocytes and macrophages

Alveolar macrophages are the most abundant cells in the bronchial lumen and they play a major role in the lung defense mechanisms, particularly the phagocytosis of inhaled particles and the elimination of infectious agents [40]. Alveolar macrophages are an important source of pro- and anti-inflammatory factors. They produce and release leukotrienes, prostaglandins, oxygen-free radicals, and many cytokines including IL-6, IL-8, IL-10, IL-12, IL-13, GM-CSF, TNF, interferon (IFN)-γ, and platelet-derived growth factor (PDGF).

## 78 Pathophysiology of asthma

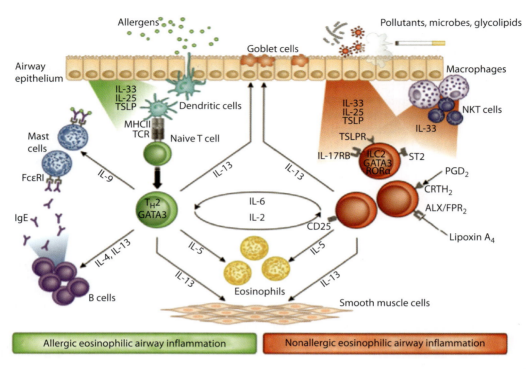

Figure 5.4 Cells and cytokines involved in losing of eosinophilic airway inflammation. (From Brusselle, G.G.I. et al. *Nat Med*, 19, 977–979, 2013.)

### T- and B-lymphocytes

In asthma, the main role of T-lymphocytes seems to be the control of the airway inflammatory process. They show a predominance of Th2 lymphocyte-producing cytokines such as IL-3, IL-4, and GM-CSF. IL-4 triggers the production of immunoglobulin IgE by B-lymphocytes while IL-3, IL-5, and GM-CSF perpetuate the eosinophilic inflammation. Once sensitized, T-lymphocytes migrate in the airways under the influence of various chemokines [41]. These lymphocytes can produce various cytokines of the Th2 type (IL-3, 4, 5, 6, 9, 13, and GM-CSF), predominant in mild to moderate asthma. When the disease becomes more severe, Th1 type as well as T cells of the CD8+ type may become more prevalent with a production of cytokines such as TNF-α and IFN-γ [42]. IL-4, as B cell-activating factor, is essential for B-lymphocytes survival and maturation. Th17 cells are CD4 positive T cells expressing IL17, which play a role in asthma. Finally, T regulatory cells, producing TGF-β and IL-10, are involved in immune responses.

### Innate lymphoid cells

In asthma, these recently described cells developing from common lymphoid progenitors in response to IL-17 and IL-33 were initially classified as non-T, non-B effector cells [43]. They can be activated early after allergen exposure and produce IL-5 and IL-13. They may differentiate into macrophages and granulocytes. Animal models suggest that they have a role in allergic asthma and in the response to respiratory viruses (e.g., influenza, rhinovirus). ILC2s possibly have a major role in patients with severe, nonatopic highly eosinophilic asthma. More research is needed to better define their role in asthma.

The role of airway inflammation 79

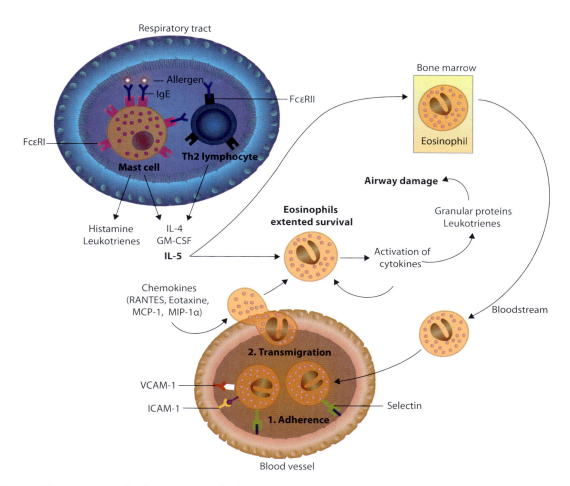

Figure 5.5 Migration of inflammatory cells during the asthmatic response. Many cells, cytokines, and mediators are involved in the asthmatic reaction.

### Dendritic cells

These antigen-presenting cells, which present as various subtypes, play a role in asthma as activators of T cells or ILCs. Animal models have shown that they can induce TH2 and TH17 adaptive immunity to a first contact with inhaled allergens [44].

### Epithelial cells

They are the first-line barrier against the environment [45]. They show cycles of injury and repair and can play a role in airway remodeling, for example, in producing pro-fibroting cytokines and various growth factors, including periostin, PDGF, TGF-β, epithelial growth factor (EGF), neurotrophins (NGFs), and angiogenic mediators including vascular endothelial growth factor (VEGF). They have a role in the development of airway inflammation by activating monocytes and producing chemokines and cytokines that could activate various inflammatory cells such as eosinophils and neutrophils. These cells express various types of pattern recognition receptors for infectious agents or allergens, such as toll-like receptor 4 (TLR4).

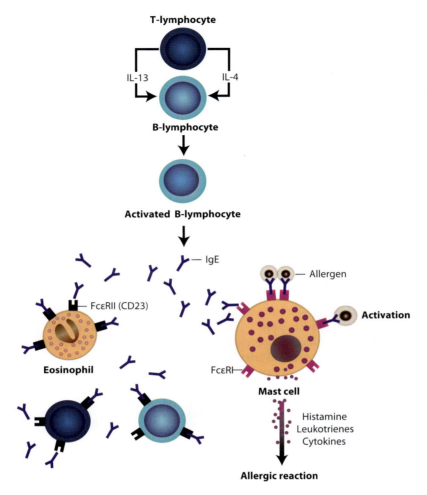

Figure 5.6 Physiopathology of asthma. Activation of lymphocytes plays an important role in the pathogenesis of the asthmatic response.

Lung epithelial cells activated by proteases, viruses, or environmental pollutants produce a triad of cytokines including thymic stromal lymphopoietin (TSLP), IL-33, and IL-25, considered as critical initiators of type 2 eosinophilic inflammatory events in lung, gut, and skin. These cytokines are present in increased levels in airways of asthmatics and correlate with disease severity.

## Airway structural changes: airway remodeling

Airway remodeling (Table 5.6, Figures 5.7 and 5.8) is a process leading to structural changes of the airways, which can be defined as a change in content, type, and quantity of structural elements, secondary to an abnormal repair process following an inflammatory insult or damage of the airway epithelium, although other mechanisms can possibly be involved. Such changes are considered to play a role in the persistence of AHR and in the development of a fixed component of airway obstruction over time in some subjects [46,47]. Mucous hypersecretion can also contribute to air trapping.

The changes that have been most often studied include bronchial epithelial damage (shedding of ciliated epithelial cells) and the development of subepithelial basement membrane thickening from, at least in part,

Table 5.6 Main changes of bronchial structure in asthma (airway remodeling)

- Damage to the airway epithelium with shedding
- Goblet cells metaplasia
- Glandular hyperplasia
- Subepithelial basement membrane thickening with "local" fibrosis
- Angiogenesis/increased number of vessels
- Neuronal proliferation
- Hypertrophy/hyperplasia of smooth muscle
- Changes in the extracellular matrix (deposition of proteoglycans)
- Alteration of bronchial cartilage

extracellular matrix component deposition, including collagen (fibrosis—like a "chronic wound pattern"), as well as the increase in the airway smooth muscle in the airway wall.

We can also find an increased number of blood vessels resulting from increased angiogenesis, under the effects of growth factors such as VEGF and a deposition of proteoglycans in the airway wall, as well as damage to the elastic tissues of the airways and even sometimes of the cartilage, and finally the hyperplasia of bronchial glands and metaplasia of goblet cells (Figure 5.7).

The increase in the airway smooth muscle seems to be mostly due to a hyperplasia of the cells more than a simple hypertrophy, and, particularly in severe asthma, this airway smooth muscle becomes closer to the epithelial basement membrane.

Many observations suggest that inflammation is one of the main mechanisms of development of airway remodeling [46,47]. It could promote structural changes in many ways, including the release of toxic factors by the eosinophils, therefore causing bronchial damage, as well as the synthesis of various chemotactic factors to effector cells and factors involved in the remodeling process. However, the bronchial epithelium itself seems also to have an important role in the development of airway remodeling. For example, under the effect of various mechanical stimuli (e.g., stretching, compression) [48], bronchial epithelial cells can produce factors, such as fibrogenic cytokines and growth factors, involved in these changes. An abnormal airway repair process that could result from an altered communication between epithelial and mesenchymal cells has been proposed as a factor predisposing to airway remodeling (the epithelial-mesenchymal trophic unit) under the influence of genetic determinants [20].

So, the epithelium is not only a physical barrier to the environment but it can also release various substances involved in the repair process and modulate inflammatory responses (Figure 5.7). The bronchial epithelium is altered in asthma and an increase in its permeability can lead to an increased exposure to particles and gases present in the inhaled air. Such epithelial damage can occur not only after respiratory infections but also following contacts with pollutants, probably due to oxidative mechanisms, and from exposure to allergens. Furthermore, in asthma, epithelial cells could be deficient in type I interferon-β and type III interferon-λ, essential cytokines for the elimination of viruses. Epithelial damage could also occur following the activation of *toll-like* receptors. To know more about the epithelial damage in asthma, the reader could consult excellent reviews on this topic such as in Lambrecht and Hammad [43].

We do not know exactly how airway remodeling features such as subepithelial fibrosis influence airway function. These changes may increase airway responsiveness and promote the development of a fixed component of airway obstruction, while it could also be a protective factor against excessive bronchoconstriction. The increase in airway smooth muscle and changes in the function of muscular cells can increase the contractile potential of the airway wall and recent studies on bronchial thermoplasty showing an improvement in airway responsiveness following the reduction of airway smooth muscle support this hypothesis [49]. However, we need more data to better determine the role of these various changes in the clinical expression of asthma. In general, there is a correlation, although quite weak, between the degree of airway responsiveness or remodeling and the severity and duration of asthma. Some individuals may present marked

82 Pathophysiology of asthma

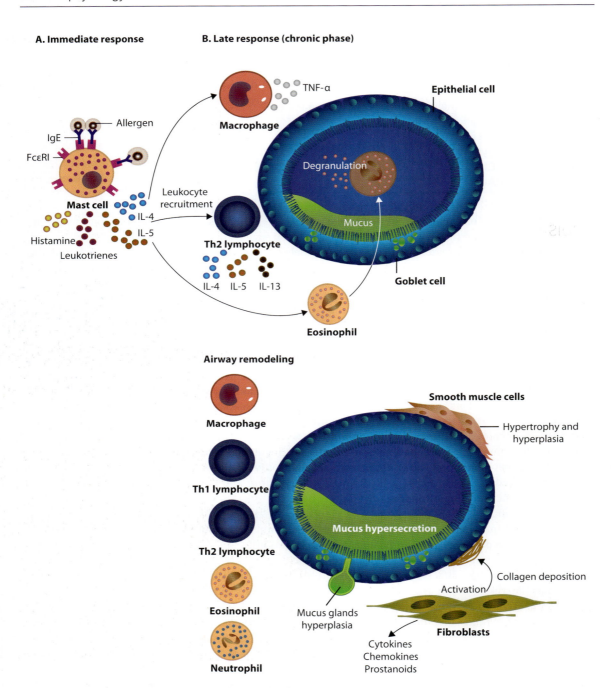

Figure 5.7 Features of airway remodeling and inflammation in asthma and the cells involved.

airway remodeling without any symptoms. This observation can be related to the intensity, type of remodeling, or the absence of an inflammatory component associated with remodeling. The changes observed in airway structure may begin very early in life, although how this process evolves during life remains to be better studied.

The role of airway inflammation 83

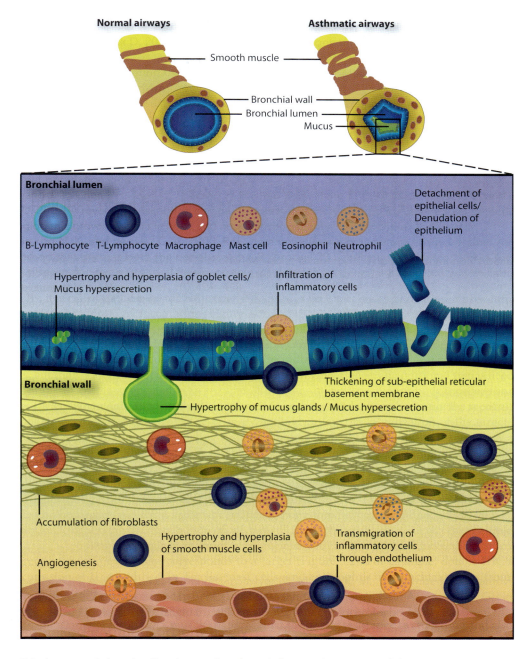

Figure 5.8 Acute and chronic allergic reaction: from inflammation to remodeling.

## Neurogenic mechanisms

Neurogenic mechanisms can influence bronchial tone and contribute to the development of airway inflammation and its modulation [50]. The parasympathetic system, through the vagal nerve, is the main neural influence through its postganglionic fibers, which influence the airway bronchial smooth muscle and bronchial glands. An increase in vagal activity can facilitate bronchoconstriction. Otherwise, adrenergic influences can result from the release of catecholamines, with stimulation of adrenergic receptors, particularly β2 receptors present in various bronchial cells, therefore promoting bronchodilation and mucus production. Even if an increase in vagal tone or a deficiency of the adrenergic system has been evoked to explain AHR in asthma, these influences seem to be mostly limited to a role of modulator of bronchial tone. A third neurogenic influence can be in the form of an involvement of the nonadrenergic, noncholinergic system, which has endings in the epithelium, glands, smooth muscle, and bronchial vessels. This system can promote both bronchodilation and bronchoconstriction. Finally, some neurogenic mediators (tachykinins, neurokinins, etc.) can induce local inflammation. The role of these various influences remains to be determined.

## The "model" of allergic asthma

The model of allergic asthma allowed better characterization of the nature of the asthmatic response [51,52]. Allergic asthma constitutes an "immune type 1 response" involving IgE [53]. When allergic individuals become sensitized to a given substance (e.g., pollens), they acquire specific IgE on the surface of airway inflammatory cells such as mast cells and basophils.

Basic mechanisms involved in the sensitization to allergens involve the uptake and transformation of inhaled allergens by dendritic cells located in the epithelium and bronchial submucosa (Figure 5.3). These cells migrate to the lymphoid tissue under the influence of chemokines, such as ligands for CCR7, where they present selected peptides coming from this antigen to lymphocytes, via HLA (MHC class II) molecules, therefore initiating the immune response to this antigen. The capacity of dendritic cells to produce IL-12 determines the balance between the response of Th1 and Th2 (IL-12 favors Th1-type responses). Once they are sensitized, T-lymphocytes migrate toward the bronchial tree where the numerous cytokines that they are producing can act, particularly in recruiting and activating various cells such as macrophages, basophils, and eosinophils.

Here is the sequence of events occurring in the airways following the inhalation of allergens in the sensitized subjects (Figures 5.3 and 5.9):

1. Allergen penetration into the lower airways.
2. Interaction between allergen and mast cells in the bronchial lumen, with the release of inflammatory mediators and an increase in airway permeability.
3. Release of chemical mediators such as histamine and cysteinyl leukotrienes.
4. These latter induce the airway smooth muscle contraction, mucosal edema, and increased bronchial secretions.
5. These various phenomena cause airway obstruction and asthma symptoms.

The allergic bronchoconstriction usually occurs about 10 minutes after the contact with the allergen (early response) and usually disappears within an hour following this contact (Figures 5.4 and 5.8). However, 2–8 hours after the allergic contact, another asthmatic reaction can occur, even without any further exposure to the allergen. This response is called the "late response" [52].

The immediate response is attributed to the activation and degranulation of mast cells bearing antigen-specific IgE (Figures 5.5, 5.8, and 5.9). The released mediators, such as histamine, cysteinyl leukotrienes, and prostaglandins, lead to a smooth muscle contraction. The mast cell activation also induces the production of cytokines involved in the recruitment and activation of various inflammatory cells. The expression of adhesion molecules at the vascular level is also involved in the mechanism of migration of inflammatory cells from the blood vessels to the airway wall.

The late response is associated with an increase in eosinophils in the bronchoalveolar lavage fluid. Cationic proteins such as the major basic protein (MBP), eosinophil cationic protein (ECP), and eosinophil-derived

# The role of airway inflammation 85

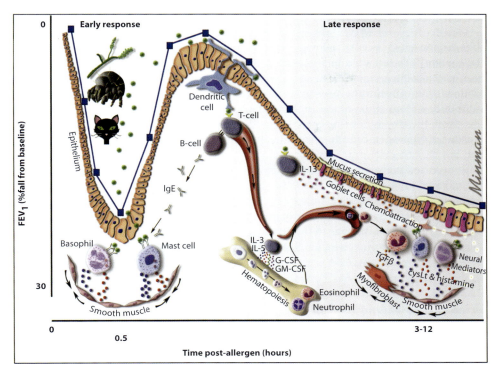

Figure 5.9 Early and late allergen-induced airway responses. Time course and mechanisms of early and late allergic airway responses. (From Diamant, Z. et al., *J Allergy Clin Immunol*, 132, 1045–1055, 2013.)

neurotoxin (EDN) are released. These substances are toxic for the bronchial epithelium and contribute to the inflammatory response in inducing the release of mediators, as well as stimulating other cells. The macrophages and lymphocytes are also involved in the asthmatic response and can also produce various proinflammatory mediators.

Th2 cells expressing the receptor for chemokine CCR4 have been involved in the chronic allergic inflammatory process and the severity of the disease, but the mechanisms involved are also to be determined. Furthermore, with time, inflammation can lead to chronic changes such as collagen/proteoglycan deposition under the subepithelial basement membrane or smooth muscle hypertrophy. Such changes seem to be involved with the chronicity of asthma.

## Nonallergic asthma

Nonallergic (intrinsic) asthma typically develops later in life and is not associated with the typical IgE-related mechanisms. It is often associated with obesity and upper airway diseases such as chronic rhinosinusitis and nasal polyposis, and is more often steroid-dependent and more severe than childhood asthma [54]. The mechanisms of development of nonallergic asthma are still uncertain, probably resulting from a dysregulation of the immune system of unknown etiology. Inflammatory cell activation could be of viral origin or due to the effects of local mechanisms associated to the presence of tissue IgE. This type of asthma may also be of occupational origin, following exposure to chemical agents or other types of toxic substances. We still need to know more about its development, but the type of airway damage observed is similar to allergic asthma.

## Exercise-induced asthma

The asthmatic response that occurs following exercise or inhalation of cold air was initially considered to be due to the cooling of the airways, but it has been shown that it is mostly associated with the drying of the bronchial mucosa, causing an increase in airway lining fluid osmolarity [55]. The latter causes mast cells to release mediators such as histamine, prostaglandins, and cysteinyl leukotrienes [56]. In some patients, exercise can also induce a stimulation of the vagal nerve. A postexercise bronchial vasodilation, following heat and water loss from the airways during exercise (called "rewarming phenomenon"), may possibly modulate response to exercise. Neurogenic mechanisms, involving tachykinins, could also play a role, but this remains to be studied.

There is an increased prevalence of asthma and AHR in high-level endurance athletes. Although it may be related to increased inhalation of allergens in sensitized athletes, following the repeated intense increased ventilation required during exercise, it could be the result of inhalation of air contaminants such as chlorine derivatives (in chlorinated pools), other types of pollutants (e.g., particulate matter, ozone), or cold air exposure (in winter athletes), while damage to the airway epithelial cells from increased breathing efforts (shear stress) and dehydration can be involved [56,57].

## Aspirin-induced asthma

About 5% of individuals suffering from asthma can experience bronchoconstriction, sometimes very severe, after ingesting aspirin or oral anti-inflammatory agents. This response seems to be related to the inhibition of the cyclooxygenase pathway, with the synthesis and release of cysteinyl leukotrienes from their negative regulation by cyclooxygenase products. Cysteinyl leukotrienes have profound effects on the bronchomotor tone [58]. These individuals seem to be more sensitive to the effect of leukotrienes but also produce more leukotrienes compared to non-aspirin-sensitive patients.

## Asthma and respiratory infections

Respiratory virus may cause exacerbations of asthma despite what seems an adequate control of the disease. An increased susceptibility to viruses has been described in asthma and could be due to altered innate antiviral immunity in some individuals, with a defective production of TLR7 or interferons [59].

## Asthma exacerbations

Exacerbations of asthma are a common expression of this disease and there is a phenotype of asthma of "frequent exacerbators" [60]. These episodes of increased symptoms and rapid reduction in lung function over a few minutes/hours or days, sometimes called "asthma attacks," are considered to be the result, in most instances, of an increase in airway inflammation, often in the context of a respiratory infection or allergen exposure.

## Severe asthma

Asthma is considered severe when it requires treatment with a high dose of inhaled corticosteroids (ICS) and a long-acting inhaled β2 agonist (LABA) or another drug such as a leukotriene modifier or theophylline, or systemic corticosteroids for $\geq$50% of the previous year, to prevent it from becoming "uncontrolled," or when it remains "uncontrolled" despite this therapy [61]. When asthma management problems such as nonadherence to therapy or poor inhaler technique are excluded, it seems to affect about 3%–4% of the asthmatic population [62]. Severe asthma is less often associated with atopy than milder forms of asthma [63].

Asthma and respiratory infections 87

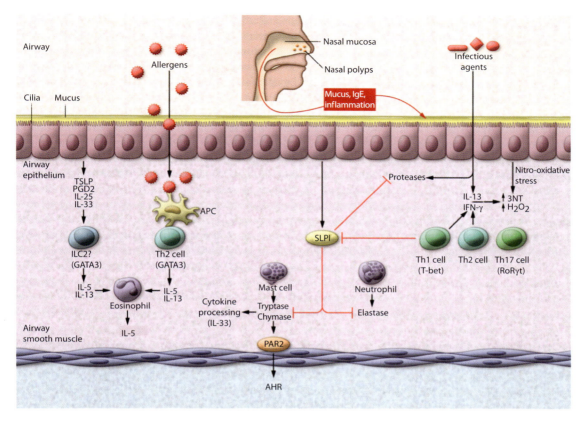

Figure 5.10 Environmental influence on severe asthma and complex relationships among the immune system, airway epithelial cells, and airway smooth muscle cells in the airways of severe asthmatics. (From Ray, A. et al., *J Clin Invest*, 126(7), 2394–2403, 2016.)

Many clinical and molecular phenotypes of severe asthma have been reported. In the atopic individual, severe asthma is associated with high IgE levels, eosinophilia, and early age of onset. In nonatopic individuals, it could as well be associated with TH2 responses, with eosinophilia, and sometimes related to environmental exposures; but it can also be of late onset, non-TH2 type, with eosinophilia, neutrophilia, and even showing poorly formed airway granulomas without vasculitis [64].

Allergens and/or other environmental agents with or without protease activity and different pathogens may elicit severe disease early or late in life (Figure 5.10). Therapies directed against various arms of the type 2 immune response based on the patient's inflammatory response and other characteristics have shown promise in recent clinical trials. While an IFN-γ (Th1/type 1) immune response has been identified in different patient cohorts, no therapy has yet been directed against this arm of the immune response. IFN-γ can inhibit SLPI expression from airway epithelial cells. SLPI is a protease inhibitor secreted by airway epithelial cells that inhibits proteases present in different cell types (mast cells, neutrophils) and infectious agents. Protease-activated PAR2 on airway smooth muscle cells has been implicated in AHR in animal studies. IFN-γ and low levels of the type 2 cytokine IL-13 can synergize to induce nitro-oxidative stress in airway epithelial cells. Future studies will determine the potential role of ILC2s and ILC2-activating cytokines such as IL-33 in severe asthma. Nasal polyps are also encountered in severe asthma, usually in late-onset disease, and crosstalk between the nasal mucosa and the airways may occur due to leakage of cytokines such as IL-5 from the local site (nose) of inflammation.

## Asthma–COPD Overlap (ACO)*

The association of asthma and COPD features in a single patient has been recognized for a long time, but interest about this condition called Asthma–COPD Overlap has increased recently with the reports of an increased morbidity associated with this condition. The 2017 GINA report stresses that: "ACO is not a single disease or phenotype and mentions that ACO is characterized by persistent airflow limitation with several features usually associated with asthma and several features usually associated with COPD. Asthma–COPD overlap is therefore identified in clinical practice by the features that it shares with both asthma and COPD. This is not a definition, but a description for clinical use, as asthma–COPD overlap includes several different clinical phenotypes and there are likely to be several different underlying mechanisms." The pathophysiology of ACO has not been well studied up to now but recent reports suggest various mechanisms potentially involved [65, 66].

## Clinical expression of asthma

Asthma can manifest as typical symptoms of dyspnea, cough, wheezing, chest tightness, and phlegm production. It can sometimes present as an isolated cough or exercise intolerance. Perception and report of symptoms is quite variable from a patient to another and it is considered essential to make the diagnosis of asthma and to perform pulmonary function tests to prove either the presence of variable airway obstruction and/or AHR. In some patients with a poor perception or recognition of symptoms, measures of PEF may help identify loss of control.

In the last two decades, noninvasive measures of airway inflammation such as induced-sputum analysis and exhaled nitric oxide (FeNO) measures have become available in many centers to better phenotype asthma. Sputum-guided treatment has been shown to reduce exacerbations in moderate to severe asthma [67]. Elevated FeNO suggests an underlying Th2-type asthma and in severe asthma, that treatment directed at IgE (if atopic), IL-4/13, and IL5 (severe eosinophilic asthma) could be useful. Other "biomarkers" such as periostin, an extracellular matrix protein induced by IL-4/13 in airway epithelium and lung fibroblasts, have been also suggested as possible predictors of effects of drugs.

## Physiologic Changes in Asthma

### Airway obstruction

The main physiological manifestation of asthma is variable airway obstruction. When asthma is controlled or mild, expiratory flows can be normal. However, according to the degree of bronchial obstruction, the following changes can be observed on the pulmonary function tests (Figure 5.11):

- Reduction in $FEV_1/FVC$ (forced vital capacity) ratio
- Reduction in expiratory flows (e.g., PEF, $FEV_1$) and increase in their circadian variation
- Reduction of mid-expiratory flows (e.g., $FEF_{25\%-27\%}$)*, suggesting small airway obstruction
- Increase in airway resistance
- Occasional reduction in vital capacity, but normal or increased total lung capacity
- Increase in residual volume (RV) and functional residual capacity (FRC), suggestive of air trapping
- Normal lung carbon monoxide diffusion (DLCO)

*Forced expiratory volume between 25% and 75% of forced vital capacity.

---

* Often called ACOS previously, the asthma–COPD overlap "syndrome".

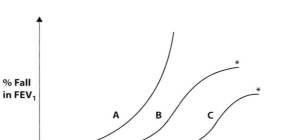

Figure 5.11 Airway responsiveness. In asthma, not only do the airways react to the lower concentrations of methacholine, but we can observe an increase in maximal bronchoconstriction. (A) Moderate asthma. (B) Mild asthma. (C) Normal subject (*Plateau effect observed).

## Airway hyperresponsiveness

The term "airway hyperresponsiveness" is used to describe an increased response of the airways, these last contracting too much or too easily, spontaneously or in response to different stimuli [68]. Such increased response could be found in almost all patients with symptomatic asthma. This responsiveness is usually called "nonallergic"—previously called "nonspecific"—in contrast, for example, to the response to substances such as allergens, which induce a bronchoconstriction only in sensitized patients. The degree of response to external stimuli varies in the general population and asthmatic subjects represent the group showing the more marked airway response, often sufficient to cause respiratory symptoms.

AHR is often quantified using the $PC_{20}$, the provocative concentration—or dose ($PD_{20}$)—of methacholine inducing a 20% fall in $FEV_1$. Methacholine acts on airway smooth muscle muscarinic receptors. Other agents such as histamine have been used but they usually cause more side effects at high doses. AHR is characterized by a shift to the left of the dose-response curve (*sensitivity*), while a steeper slope of this last constitutes an increase in bronchial *reactivity* (Figure 5.11). Furthermore, in asthma, there is a loss of plateau effect of response to agents such as methacholine; the bronchoconstrictive response is indeed normally limited (e.g., between 15 and 50% fall in $FEV_1$, even with higher doses of methacholine) while the asthmatic airways can close completely or near completely (maximal bronchoconstrictor response) [69].

Airway responsiveness has a unimodal distribution in the general population. AHR may remain stable, change over time, increase after contact with sensitizing substances and respiratory infections, and can decrease with treatments such as corticosteroids. The prevalence of AHR may vary from 4% to 40% according to the population studied and the methods used to quantify this responsiveness—it is probably usually around 15% in most countries [68]. It is increased in the atopic population, particularly in the presence of rhinitis, and in endurance athletes. It is asymptomatic in about 50% of hyperresponsive subjects. It can also be found in COPD and rhinitis without thoracic symptoms.

As discussed previously, the specific mechanism of development of AHR is still unknown, but it is probably caused by airway inflammation (variable component) and by structural changes in the airways (a more fixed component). An increase in airway smooth muscle mass and functional changes can contribute to the increase in the bronchial contractility, although other mechanisms are certainly involved.

Another phenomenon observed in asthma is the loss of protective effect of a deep inspiration against induced bronchoconstriction, for example, during a methacholine test [70]. This can be reproduced in the nonasthmatic subjects by avoiding to taking deep inspiration during a period of 20–30 minutes, while normally, deep inspiration can quickly reduce the airway response by a "smooth muscle stretch relaxation" phenomenon [71]. This effect is attributed to a change in the plasticity of airway smooth muscle, causing it to become more responsive. In asthmatic subjects, bronchial structural changes can induce a reduction in the capacity of airways; distension by the elastic forces that the parenchyma exerts on the bronchial wall, which could be responsible for this defect, but this is still controversial [70–72].

## How can knowledge of asthma physiopathology help the clinician in the evaluation and treatment of asthma?

The clinical expression of asthma seems to result from the combined effect of inflammation and specific airway remodeling changes.

### Prevention of asthma

This is still a controversial topic. Allergen avoidance could potentially help prevent asthma in allergic children, but avoidance of exposure may however be difficult. The poor results from allergen strategy avoidance in early childhood (before or after asthma develops—primary or secondary prevention) may be due to the concomitant removal of protective factors such as endotoxins/microbial agents. Multifaceted strategies seem to be more effective [73]. Not being exposed to cigarette smoke, *in utero* or in early childhood, and prevention of obesity may also reduce the risk of asthma. Breastfeeding was considered a possible way to prevent the development of allergy but recent studies do not support this. The role of vitamin D, probiotics, and omega 3 in the prevention and in the treatment of asthma is still uncertain.

### Therapeutic targets

While we cannot cure asthma, the main goal is to control the disease. Recently, a more personalized approach has been suggested, particularly for severe asthma. Key strategies include guided self-management and patient education, environmental control, and use of an asthma action plan for the management of asthma exacerbations. Regular exercise and maintenance of ideal body weight are also suggested. Proper inhaler technique, monitoring of control, and adherence to maintenance medication are essential. Immunotherapy, either subcutaneous or sublingual, has been proposed but is usually only considered for selected cases. They can be more helpful in allergic rhinitis.

Current asthma guidelines suggest that a fast-acting bronchodilator should be introduced as soon as symptoms develop [1] to be used "on demand" at the lowest dose and frequency possible. If symptoms occur more than twice a month, particularly if there are some exacerbations or exercise intolerance, an anti-inflammatory treatment, usually a low-dose ICS, should usually be added. Leukotriene antagonists [74] can be a second choice of controller therapy. If asthma is not perfectly controlled with low doses of ICS (medium doses in the child), after checking therapeutic adherence, inhaler technique, potential contributing environmental factors, smoking or nontreated comorbidities, an add-on treatment with a LABA or leukotriene antagonist (as a second choice) is proposed.

In the evaluation of asthma control, two main aspects should be considered: (1) reduction of symptoms and optimal lung function and (2) the prevention of future untoward events such as exacerbations or a reduction in pulmonary function.

Repeated measurements of AHR are generally not very useful in the follow-up of asthma as, in general, symptoms and expiratory flows as well as frequency of exacerbations and healthcare use are sufficient. More recently, as discussed earlier, the addition of noninvasive measures of airway inflammation by induced sputum or a measurement of the fractional nitric oxide concentration (FeNO) in exhaled breath have been proposed to titrate therapy, particularly in moderate to severe asthma, but these techniques are not yet widely available [75,76].

Table 5.7 Some possible therapeutic targets for future asthma therapies

- Glucocorticosteroid receptors
- Various pro-inflammatory cytokines/interleukins
- Phosphodiesterases
- Nicotinic receptors
- Leukotrienes/5-LO/FLAP
- Migration of inflammatory cells
- IgE-related mechanisms
- Neutrophils migration and function
- Immunomodulation (T-lymphocytes)
- Inhibition/resolution of airway remodeling
- Transcription factors—gene therapy
- Kinase inhibitors
- Endothelin inhibition
- NO inhibition
- Tryptase inhibition
- VLA4
- TSLP, CXCR2, etc.

Table 5.8 Some remaining questions on asthma pathophysiology

- Why does the immune system keep triggering airway inflammation, even without any evidence of persisting environmental factors?
- How can we antagonize the mechanisms responsible for the development or persistence of airway inflammation?
- Can we prevent airway inflammation and structural changes, and consequently prevent the development of AHR and symptomatic asthma?
- Which are the most important pathways leading to asthma?
- How can we predict responses to asthma therapy?

Even if airway remodeling has been described in some individuals before the development of asthma symptoms, such as in rhinitic nonasthmatic patients, it is not recommended to start the anti-inflammatory therapy before asthma symptoms develop, nor in the most trivial form of asthma with rare symptoms. However, as soon as symptoms become more regular, as mentioned above, anti-inflammatory treatment should be prescribed.

ICS are recognized as being efficient to counteract the bronchial inflammatory process in the majority of asthmatic subjects—although some patients seem "resistant" to this treatment (mainly with a non-Th2-type asthma)—but its effects on airway remodeling are still uncertain although they seem modest. Animal studies and studies looking at the effects of high doses of ICS suggest that corticosteroids could block partially the remodeling process before it develops [77]. This has been also demonstrated with leukotriene antagonists [78]. It is however difficult currently to extrapolate these results to humans; more studies are required. There is a reduction in components of airway remodeling such as proteoglycan deposition in the airway or a certain reduction in the subepithelial fibrosis with high doses of ICS but these effects are variable. Other medications that could influence airway remodeling could be beneficial but once again, we need further study, and current treatment should focus on the inflammatory process.

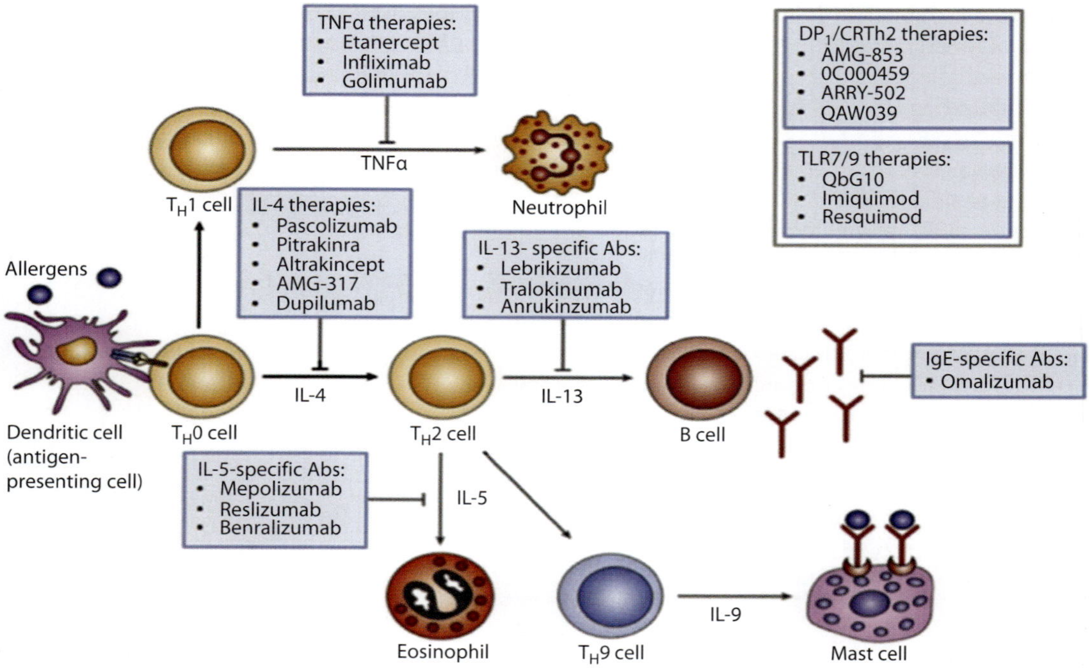

Figure 5.12 Current and potential drugs for asthma according to the targeted site of the inflammatory cascade. (From Bice, J.B. et al., *Ann Allergy Asthma Immunol*, 112, 108, 2014.)

In regard to novel therapies (Table 5.7, Figure 5.12), various drugs targeting the many inflammatory pathways relevant to asthma have been studied [79]. Biologics targeting IgE (e.g., omalizumab) have been used in severe allergic asthma and others targeting IL-5 (e.g., mepolizumab) have become available in many countries for severe eosinophilic asthma. Other drugs target IL-4 and IL-13, TSLP, and other "key cytokines" and may prove useful in some subsets of asthma [79]. Bronchial thermoplasty, the application of radiofrequency energy to the airway wall through endoscopy, aiming to reduce the amount of airway smooth muscle, has shown some benefits, particularly in severe asthma, but more remains to be known about its mechanisms of action [49].

## Conclusion: Future developments

Many questions remain in regard to the development of asthma. Studies of the natural history of the disease and others on immune mechanisms of this condition could help to answer those questions. The potential therapeutic targets useful to treat or prevent asthma are identified in Table 5.7. Many treatments targeting these mechanisms are currently studied.

## References

1. Global Initiative for Asthma. Global strategy for asthma management and prevention 2017. www.ginasthma.org.
2. Hargreave FE, Nair P. The definition and diagnosis of asthma. *Clin Exp Allergy* 2009;39:1652–1658.
3. Dicpinigaitis PV. Cough. 4: Cough in asthma and eosinophilic bronchitis. *Thorax* 2004:59:71–72.

4. Lougheed MD, Lemiere C, Ducharme FM et al. Canadian Thoracic Society Asthma Clinical Assembly. Canadian Thoracic Society 2012 guideline update: Diagnosis and management of asthma in preschoolers, children and adults. *Can Respir J* 2012;19:127–164.
5. Juniper EF, Frith PA, Hargreave FE. Airway responsiveness to histamine and methacholine: Relationship to minimum treatment to control symptoms of asthma. *Thorax* 1981 Aug;36(8):575–579.
6. American Thoracic Society. Guidelines for methacholine and exercise challenge testing–1999. *Am J Respir Crit Care Med* 2000;161:309–329.
7. Lai CKW, Beasley R, Crane J et al. Global variation in the prevalence and severity of asthma symptoms: Phase Three of the International Study of Asthma and Allergies in Childhood (ISAAC). *Thorax* 2009;64:476–483.
8. Lundbäck B, Backman H, Lötvall J, Rönmark E. Is asthma prevalence still increasing? *Expert Rev Respir Med* 2016;10(1):39–51.
9. Vonk JM, Postma DS, Boezen HM et al. Childhood factors associated with asthma remission after 30 year follow up. *Thorax* 2004;59:925–929.
10. Belsky DW, Sears MR. The potential to predict the course of childhood asthma. *Expert Rev Respir Med* 2014 Apr;8(2):137–141.
11. Schaub B, Lauener R, von Mutius E. The many faces of the hygiene hypothesis. *J Allergy Clin Immunol* 2006;117:969–977.
12. Stein MM, Hrusch CL, Gozdz J et al. Innate immunity and asthma risk in Amish and Hutterite farm children. *N Engl J Med* 2016;375:411–421.
13. von Mutius E. The environmental predictors of allergic disease. *J Allergy Clin Immunol* 2000;105:9–19.
14. Aaron SD, Vandemheen KL, Boulet LP et al. Canadian Respiratory Clinical Research Consortium. Overdiagnosis of asthma in obese and nonobese adults. *CMAJ* 2008;179:1121–1131.
15. Hales BJ, Chai LY, Elliot CE et al. Antibacterial antibody responses associated with the development of asthma in house dust mite-sensitised and non-sensitised children. *Thorax* 2012 Apr;67(4):321–327.
16. Boulet LP. Obesity and asthma. *Clin Exp Allergy* 2013;43:8–21.
17. Burney P, Jarvis D, Perez-Padilla R. The global burden of chronic respiratory disease in adults. *Int J Tuberc Lung Dis* 2015;19:10–20.
18. FitzGerald JM, Boulet LP, McIvor RA et al. Asthma control in Canada remains suboptimal: The Reality of Asthma Control (TRAC) study. *Can Respir J* 2006;13:253–259.
19. Beasley R. The global burden of asthma: Executive summary of the GINA Dissemination Committee report. *Allergy* 2004;59:469–478.
20. Holgate ST. Pathogenesis of asthma. *Clinic Exp Allergy* 2008;38:872–897.
21. Boulet LP, Turcotte H, Laprise C et al. Comparative degree and type of sensitization to common indoor and outdoor allergens in subjects with allergic rhinitis and/or asthma. *Clin Exp Allergy* 1997 Jan;27(1):52–59.
22. Sterk PJ. Chronic diseases like asthma and COPD: Do they truly exist? *Eur Respir J* 2016;47:359–361.
23. Wenzel SE. Asthma phenotypes: The evolution from clinical to molecular approaches. *Nat Med* 2012;18:716–725.
24. Anderson GP. Endotyping asthma: New insights into key pathogenic mechanisms in a complex, heterogeneous disease. *Lancet* 2008;372:1107–1119.
25. Wenzel SE. Asthma: Defining of the persistent adult phenotypes. *Lancet* 2006;368:804–813.
26. Ober C. Perspectives on the past decade of asthma genetics. *J Allergy Clin Immunol* 2005;116:274–278.
27. Tantisira K, Weiss S. The pharmacogenetics of asthma treatment. *Curr Allergy Asthma Rep* 2009;9:10–17.

28. Holgate ST. Epithelium dysfunction in asthma. *J Allergy Clin Immunol* 2007;120:1233–1244; quiz 1245–1246.
29. Spergel JM, Paller AS. Atopic dermatitis and the atopic march. *J Allergy Clin Immunol* 2003;112(suppl):S118–S127.
30. Holgate ST, Wenzel S, Postma DS et al. Asthma. *Nat Rev Dis Primers* 2015;1:15025.
31. Busse WW. Mechanisms and advances in allergic diseases. *J Allergy Clin Immunol* 2000;105:S593–S598.
32. Van Hove CL, Maes T, Joos GF, Tournoy KG. Chronic inflammation in asthma: A contest of persistence vs resolution. *Allergy* 2008;63:1095–1109.
33. Kraft M, Martin RJ, Wilson S et al. Lymphocyte and eosinophilic influx into alveolar tissue in nocturnal asthma. *Am J Respir Crit Care J* 1999;159:228–234.
34. Bai TR, Vonk JM, Postma DS, Boezen HM. Severe exacerbations predict excess lung function decline in asthma. *Eur Respir J* 2007;30:452–456.
35. Metcalfe DD, Baram D, Mekori YA. Mast cells. *Physiol Rev* 1997;77:1033–1079.
36. Brusselle GG, Maes T, Bracke KR. Eosinophils in the spotlight: Eosinophilic airway inflammation in nonallergic asthma. *Nat Med* 2013;19:977–979.
37. Weller PF. The immunobiology of eosinophils. *N Engl J Med* 1991;324:1110–1118.
38. Mesnil C, Raulier S, Paulissen G et al. Lung-resident eosinophils represent a distinct regulatory eosinophil subset. *Clin Invest* 2016 Sep 1;126:3279–3295.
39. Cowburn AS, Condliffe AM, Farahi N et al. Advances in neutrophil biology: Clinical implications. *Chest* 2008;134:606–612.
40. Zhang P, Summer WR, Bagby GJ, Nelson S. Innate immunity and pulmonary host defense. *Immunol Rev* 2000;173:39–51.
41. Hamid Q, Tulic M. Immunobiology of asthma. *Annu Rev Physiol* 2009;71:489–507.
42. Truyen E, Coteur L, Dilissen E et al. Evaluation of airway inflammation by quantitative Th1/Th2 cytokine mRNA measurement in sputum of asthma patients. *Thorax* 2006;61:202–208.
43. Lambrecht BN, Hammad H. The immunology of asthma. *Nat Immunol* 2015;16:45–56.
44. van Helden MJ, Lambrecht BN. Dendritic cells in asthma. *Curr Opin Immunol* 2013;25:745–754.
45. Holtzman MJ, Byers DE, Alexander-Brett J, Wang X. The role of airway epithelial cells and innate immune cells in chronic respiratory disease. *Nat Rev Immunol* 2014 Oct;14(10):686–698.
46. Bergeron C, Boulet LP. Structural changes in airway diseases: Characteristics mechanisms, consequences, and pharmacologic modulation. *Chest* 2006;129:1068–1087.
47. Bousquet J, Jeffery PK, Busse WW et al. Asthma. From bronchoconstriction to airways inflammation and remodeling. *Am J Respir Crit Care Med* 2000;161:1720–1745.
48. Tschumperlin DJ, Drazen JM. Chronic effects of mechanical force on airways. *Annu Rev Physiol* 2006;68:563–583.
49. Chakir J, Haj-Salem I, Gras D et al. Effects of bronchial thermoplasty on airway smooth muscle and collagen deposition in asthma. *Ann Am Thorac Soc* 2015;12:1612–1618.
50. Pisi G, Olivieri D, Chetta A. The airway neurogenic inflammation: Clinical and pharmacological implications. *Inflamm Allergy Drug Targets* 2009;8:176–181.
51. Cockcroft DW. Airway responses to inhaled allergens. *Can Respir J* 1998;Suppl A:14A–17A.
52. Diamant Z, Gauvreau GM, Cockcroft DW et al. Inhaled allergen bronchoprovocation tests. *J Allergy Clin Immunol* 2013;132:1045–1055.
53. Kay AB. Allergy and allergic diseases. Second of two parts. *N Engl J Med* 2001;344:109–113.
54. Kim HY, DeKruyff RH, Umetsu DT. The many paths to asthma: Phenotype shaped by innate and adaptive immunity. *Nat Immunol*. 2010;11:577–584.
55. Anderson SD, Kippelen P. Exercise-induced bronchoconstriction: Pathogenesis. *Curr Allergy Asthma Rep* 2005;5:116–122.

56. Kippelen P, Anderson SD. Pathogenesis of exercise-induced bronchoconstriction. *Immunol Allergy Clin North Am* 2013 Aug;33(3):299–312.
57. Boulet LP, O'Byrne PM. Asthma and exercise-induced bronchoconstriction in athletes. *N Engl J Med* 2015 Feb 12;372(7):641–648.
58. Jenneck C, Juergens U, Buecheler M, Novak N. Pathogenesis, diagnosis, and treatment of aspirin intolerance. *Ann Allergy Asthma Immunol* 2007;99:13–21.
59. Kaiko GE, Loh Z, Spann K et al. Toll-like receptor 7 gene deficiency and early-life Pneumovirus infection interact to predispose toward the development of asthma-like pathology in mice. *J Allergy Clin Immunol* 2013 May;131(5):1331–1339.
60. Kupczyk M, ten Brinke A, Sterk PJ et al.; BIOAIR investigators. Frequent exacerbators—A distinct phenotype of severe asthma. *Clin Exp Allergy* 2014 Feb;44(2):212–221.
61. Chung K, Godard P, Adelroth E et al. Difficult/therapy resistant asthma: The need for an integrated approach to define clinical phenotypes, evaluate risk factors, understand pathophysiology and find novel therapies. ERS Task Force on Difficult/Therapy-Resistant Asthma. *Eur Respir J* 1999;13:1198–1208.
62. Hekking PP, Wener RR, Amelink M et al. The prevalence of severe refractory asthma. *J Allergy Clin Immunol* 2015 Apr;135(4):896–902.
63. Ray A, Raundhal M, Oriss TB et al. Current concepts of severe asthma. *J Clin Invest* 2016 Jul 1;126(7):2394–2403.
64. Wenzel SE, Vitari CA, Shende M et al. Asthmatic granulomatosis: A novel disease with asthmatic and granulomatous features. *Am J Respir Crit Care Med* 2012;186(6):501–507.
65. Postma DS, Rabe KF. The asthma–COPD overlap syndrome. *N Engl J Med* 2015;373:1241-1249.
66. Gelb AF, Christenson SA, Nadel JA. Understanding the pathophysiology of the asthma-chronic obstructive pulmonary disease overlap syndrome. *Curr Opin Pulm Med* 2016;22:100-105.
67. Jayaram L, Pizzichini MM, Cook RJ et al. Determining asthma treatment by monitoring sputum cell counts: Effect on exacerbations. *Eur Respir J* 2006 Mar;27(3):483–494.
68. Cockcroft DW, Davis BE. Mechanisms of airway hyperresponsiveness. *J Allergy Clin Immunol* 2006;118(3):551–559.
69. Sterk PJ, Bel EH. Bronchial hyperresponsiveness: The need for a distinction between hypersensitivity and excessive airway narrowing. *Eur Respir J* 1989;2:267–274.
70. Simard B, Turcotte H, Cockcroft DW et al. Deep inspiration avoidance and methacholine response in normal subjects and patients with asthma. *Chest* 2005;127:135–142.
71. Shore SA, Fredberg JJ. Obesity, smooth muscle, and airway hyperresponsiveness. *J Allergy Clin Immunol* 2005;115:925–927.
72. Pyrgos G, Scichilone N, Togias A, Brown RH. Bronchodilation response to deep inspirations in asthma is dependent on airway distensibility and air trapping. *J Appl Physiol* 2011;110:472–479.
73. Scott M, Roberts G, Kurukulaaratchy RJ et al. Multifaceted allergen avoidance during infancy reduces asthma during childhood with the effect persisting until age 18 years. *Thorax* 2012;67:1046–1051.
74. Becker A, Lemière C, Bérubé D et al. Asthma Guidelines Working Group of the Canadian Network for Asthma Care. Summary of recommendations from the Canadian Asthma Consensus guidelines, 2003. *CMAJ* 2005;173:S3–S11.
75. Pin I, Gibson PG, Kolendowicz R et al. Use of induced sputum cell counts to investigate airway inflammation in asthma. *Thorax* 1992;47:25–29.
76. Szefler SJ, Mitchell H, Sorkness CA et al. Management of asthma based on exhaled nitric oxide in addition to guideline-based treatment for inner-city adolescents and young adults: A randomized controlled trial. *Lancet* 2008;372:1065–1072.
77. Chanez P, Bourdin A, Vachier I et al. Effects of inhaled corticosteroids on pathology in asthma and chronic obstructive pulmonary disease. *Proc Am Thorac Soc* 2004;1:184–190.

78. Holgate ST, Peters-Golden M, Panettieri RA, Henderson WR Jr. Roles of cysteinyl leukotrienes in airway inflammation, smooth muscle function, and remodeling. *J Allergy Clin Immunol* 2003;111:S18–S34.
79. Bice JB, Leechawengwongs E, Montanaro A. Biologic targeted therapy in allergic asthma. *Ann Allergy Asthma Immunol* 2014;112:108–115.

# 6

# Chronic obstructive pulmonary disease

JULIE MILOT and MATHIEU MORISSETTE

| | |
|---|---|
| Introduction | 98 |
| Terminology and definitions | 98 |
| Structural changes and remodeling | 98 |
| Repercussions on the normal physiology of respiration | 101 |
|     Repercussions on pulmonary function | 101 |
|     Repercussions on gas exchange | 102 |
| Mechanisms involved in the pathogenesis of COPD | 103 |
|     Effect of cigarette smoking on lung immunity | 103 |
|     Innate immunity: First cause of lung damage? | 103 |
|     Imbalance between protease and antiprotease | 104 |
|     Chronic lung oxidative stress | 104 |
|     Reduction in efferocytosis | 106 |
|     From innate to adaptive immunity: Reaching a point of no return | 106 |
|     Creation of potentially immunogenic neo-molecules | 106 |
|     Adaptive immunity: From back benching to the front line | 107 |
|         B-lymphocytes and autoantibodies | 107 |
|         CD4+ T-lymphocytes | 108 |
|         CD8+ T-lymphocytes | 108 |
|     Increased T-lymphocyte chemotaxis | 109 |
|     Other mechanisms potentially involved in COPD pathogenesis | 109 |
|         Decrease in vascular endothelial growth factor and VEGFR2 receptors levels | 109 |
|         Sensitivity to the ligand TRAIL | 109 |
|         Genetic predispositions | 109 |
| Exacerbation of COPD: Intensification of pulmonary inflammatory response | 110 |
| Effect of pharmacological treatment on pulmonary inflammatory response | 110 |
| Extrapulmonary repercussions of COPD | 111 |
| Conclusions and future perspectives | 111 |
| References | 112 |

## Introduction

Chronic obstructive pulmonary disease (COPD) usually develops after prolonged exposure to inhaled noxious gases [1]. Cigarette smoke is by far the most common of those gases, being involved in more than 90% of COPD cases. Domestic and environmental (industrial, automobiles) pollution, mainly through biomass combustion (cooking oils, coal used for heating), is also responsible for COPD, especially in developing countries. In a smaller proportion of cases (<2%), genetic mutations such as alpha-1 antitrypsin deficiency or a severe viral infection during childhood could be predisposing factors for COPD. If one looks at the whole smokers' population, including former smokers, approximately 15%–20% of them will eventually be diagnosed with a chronic obstructive syndrome. Those numbers may appear modest but they can go up to 40% if we only look at individuals who have been active smokers until they have reached the age of 65.

It is expected that by year 2020, COPD will be the third leading cause of mortality worldwide and the fifth leading source in terms of burden of disease [2]. COPD results in an economic and social burden that is both substantial and increasing worldwide [3–5].

## Terminology and definitions

COPD is defined as a disease state characterized by not fully reversible chronic bronchial obstruction. Bronchial obstruction is usually both progressive and associated with an abnormal inflammatory response. Classically, COPD is divided in two different entities: chronic bronchitis and emphysema.

Chronic bronchitis is a "clinical entity" characterized by chronic cough and increased sputum production secondary to hyperplasia and hypertrophy of submucosal bronchial glands. To make the diagnosis of chronic bronchitis, the productive cough must have been present for at least 3 months in each of two successive years and other causes of chronic cough must have been ruled out. Chronic bronchitis can be found in approximately 50% of smokers while the chronic obstructive syndrome can be found in smokers called "susceptible smokers," meaning that symptoms of chronic bronchitis can be present without being associated to a chronic obstructive syndrome.

In contrast to chronic bronchitis, emphysema is a "pathological entity" characterized by permanent nonreversible destruction of airspaces located distal to the terminal bronchiole. This destruction leads to airspace enlargement and decreased alveolar-capillary contact area. Computed tomography (CT) lung imaging may demonstrate parenchymal changes compatible with the diagnosis of emphysema but the obstructive syndrome must always be present as documented by pulmonary function assessment.

In emphysema, the main symptom is shortness of breath, which is usually progressive and can lead to exercise intolerance. It is important to understand that patients may have clinical symptoms and/or pulmonary function tests (PFTs) compatible with either the diagnosis of chronic bronchitis or emphysema, but we often see patients suffering from both conditions (Figure 6.1).

## Structural changes and remodeling

The bronchial mucosa of patients with emphysema is characterized by epithelial cell metaplasia without thickening of the basal membrane [6] (Figure 6.2). There is also glandular epithelial cells (goblet cells) hyperplasia [7] and hypertrophy of the submucosal glands in large-sized airways [8]. Such alterations are associated with increased mucous production, a key feature of chronic bronchitis.

In addition to these changes, there is also an increased amount of fibrosis and smooth muscle hypertrophy which, in association with the inflammatory reaction, contributes to the thickening of the bronchial wall and narrowing of their lumens [9], mostly seen in small peripheral airways [10]. Finally, there is an increase

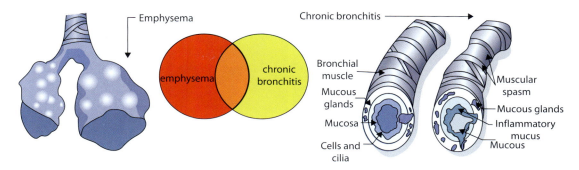

Figure 6.1 Emphysema and chronic bronchitis. Clinical and pathophysiological characteristics of emphysema and chronic bronchitis can be found in the same patient. (From Belleau R, Maltais F., Presses de l'Université Laval, 2008. Reproduced with permission).

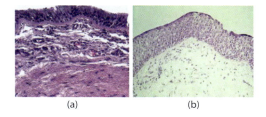

Figure 6.2 Bronchial mucosa. **(a)** Bronchial biopsy specimen from a normal subject **(b)** Bronchial biopsy specimen from an emphysematous smoker ($FEV_1$: 40% of predicted) showing an intact epithelium but presence of some metaplasia. (From Jeffery PK, *Chest*, 117, 251s–260s, 2000. Reproduced with permission).

in the number of goblet cells, which are normally absent in airways with an internal diameter of less than 2 mm (small bronchi and bronchioles) [11–13]. These goblet cells contribute to the formation of mucous plugs, a phenomenon typically observed in the more severe forms of COPD, and that can lead to obstruction [14]. The narrowing and disappearance of terminal bronchioles are the initial events before emphysematous destruction appears and contribute to the increase in peripheral airways resistance observed in COPD [15].

Initially, alveolar wall destruction is only microscopic (Figure 6.3) but as emphysema progresses, macroscopic airspace enlargement occurs with the formation of easily identifiable emphysematous bullae.

Smokers will generally develop proximal acinar or centrilobular emphysema (CLE) characterized by airspace destruction involving the respiratory bronchioles and the central portion of the acini (secondary lobules) surrounded by near normal parenchyma [16]. This type of emphysema is almost exclusively occurring in the upper lobes (Figure 6.4). By contrast, individuals with alpha-1 antitrypsin deficiencies are afflicted by a type of emphysema called panlobular emphysema (PLE), which is mostly observed in lower lobes and is characterized by uniform destruction of the alveolar walls distal to the terminal bronchioles.

Inflammatory and structural changes observed in small airways and lung parenchyma of emphysema patients are the most important contributing factors to airflow obstruction and decline in lung function.

Another typical feature of patients with severe COPD is pulmonary hypertension [17]. Potential explanations for this phenomenon include hypoxic reflex vasoconstriction, destruction of the pulmonary capillary bed, and remodeling of the pulmonary arteries. Pathologically, the most noticeable finding is the thickening of the intima caused by smooth muscle hypertrophy and collagen/elastic matrix deposition [18,19], changes

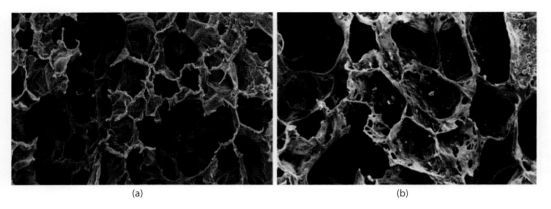

**Figure 6.3** Lung parenchyma. **(a)** Electron microscopy photograph showing normal pulmonary alveoli **(b)** Electron microscopy photograph showing the beginning of alveolar destruction with a typical fenestrated appearance suggesting alveolar wall destruction. (From Jeffery PK, *Chest*, 117, 251s–260s, 2000. Reproduced with permission).

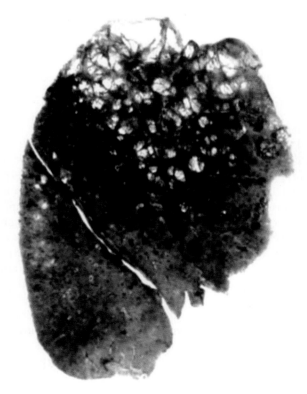

**Figure 6.4** Lung with centrilobular emphysema. Severe centrilobular emphysema with predominant involvement of the upper lobe. (From Jeffery PK, *Am J Respir Crit Care Med*, 164, 28s–38s, 2001. Reproduced with permission).

rarely observed in the media of these arteries [19]. There can also be a lymphocytic infiltration, mostly of CD8+ T-lymphocytes in the adventitia of the pulmonary arteries [10,18]. These structural changes are associated with endothelial dysfunction and an impaired production of endothelium relaxing factors resulting in vasoconstriction [20,21].

## Repercussions on the normal physiology of respiration

### Repercussions on pulmonary function

COPD is defined as a mostly nonreversible expiratory airflow limitation as measured during forced expiration. This airflow limitation relates to an increase in small airway resistance and/or a reduction in pulmonary elastance secondary to parenchymal destruction. This reduction in pulmonary elastance is characterized by loss of elastic recoil, which is essential to maintain patency of small airways.

More than 30 years ago, Fletcher and Peto [22] described the natural history of smokers susceptible to develop COPD and chronic airflow limitation (Figure 6.5). They showed that, depending on age, the maximal forced expiratory volume in 1 second ($FEV_1$) decreases in an accelerated fashion in smokers, while nonsusceptible smokers remain comparable to nonsmokers. The decline in $FEV_1$ was associated with minimal functional and respiratory limitations in nonsmokers and nonsusceptible smokers making them asymptomatic or only mildly symptomatic ($FEV_1$ >80%, $FEV_1$/forced vital capacity [FVC] <70%, Global Initiative for Chronic Obstructive Lung Disease [GOLD]: 0 or 1) (see www.goldcopd.org). On the other hand, susceptible smokers were symptomatic and developed moderately severe ($FEV_1$ 50%–80% of predicted, GOLD 2), severe ($FEV_1$ 30%–50% of predicted, GOLD 3), or very severe ($FEV_1$ <30% of predicted, GOLD 4) emphysema correlating with their smoking history (number of years) and age. The authors also showed that quitting smoking had a beneficial effect by reducing the decline in pulmonary function, regardless of age.

Early airway closure during forced expiration also contributes to increasing total lung capacity (TLC) and residual volume (RV). These changes tend to create pulmonary hyperinflation, which can be further accentuated during exercise due to a shortened duration of expiration creating what is called "dynamic hyperinflation" (Figure 6.6). This greatly contributes to the feeling of discomfort associated with shortness of breath and physical exercise.

When compared to normal individuals, both TLC and RV are increased in emphysema patients due to airflow obstruction and increased compliance. When the emphysema patient is exercising, one can also observe that, as ventilation increases, there is a proportional increase in end-expiratory volumes at

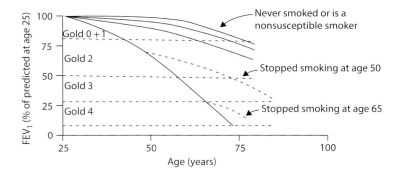

Figure 6.5 Age-dependent decline in $FEV_1$ depending on being a susceptible smoker or not. (From Hogg, J.C., *Lancet*, 364, 709–721, 2004. Reproduced with permission).

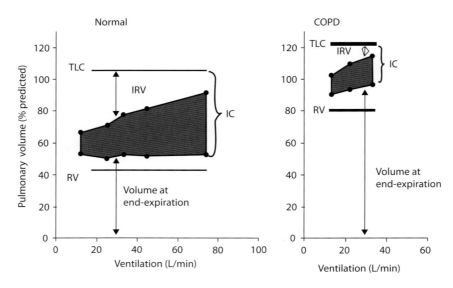

Figure 6.6 Dynamic hyperinflation during exercise.

the expense of the inspiratory reserve volume (IRV). This increase in end-expiratory volume induces a decrease in inspiratory capacity (IC) while IC would remain constant in individuals with normal lung functions.

## Repercussions on gas exchange

The COPD-related changes occurring in airways and lung parenchyma also have significant repercussions on the gas exchange leading to significant ventilation/perfusion ($\dot{V}/\dot{Q}$) mismatch. When the $\dot{V}/\dot{Q}$ ratio is decreased (decreased ventilation with normal perfusion), oxygenation will not be as efficient resulting in systemic hypoxemia. If, on the other hand, the $\dot{V}/\dot{Q}$ ratio is increased (normal ventilation but underperfusion or dead space), respiratory work will increase in order to maintain a normal partial pressure of carbon dioxide ($PaCO_2$). This coping mechanism is effective as long as emphysema is not too severe. Since airway obstruction and lung hyperinflation will eventually lead to respiratory muscles being unable to compensate, the systemic $PaCO_2$ will gradually rise resulting in hypercapnia.

Some individuals suffering from COPD have an increased sensitivity to oxygen. In patients with severe COPD, for instance, attempts to correct hypoxemia by oxygen supplementation may worsen the hypercapnia. In fact, administration of oxygen can inhibit the respiratory drive normally associated with hypoxia, preventing the elimination of carbon dioxide. Another contributing factor to this phenomenon is what is called the "Haldane effect," which results in a decreased blood affinity for $CO_2$ secondary to an elevation of the $PaO_2$. Under these circumstances, oxygen, which has a greater affinity for hemoglobin than $CO_2$, will contribute to the release of $CO_2$ in the circulation and the patient with inadequate ventilation will be unable to compensate for this elevation of the $PaCO_2$. But the factor having the greatest impact on $PaCO_2$ levels is the decreased intensity of the hypoxic pulmonary vasoconstriction reflex succeeding the administration of oxygen. The disappearance of this phenomenon accentuates $\dot{V}/\dot{Q}$ mismatch and leads to increased lung shunting (nonventilated space with normal perfusion).

Hypercapnia and hypoxemia are more common in patients with chronic bronchitis and severe airway obstruction, as blood gases from patients with emphysema tend to remain normal for longer periods of time. Assessment of carbon monoxide diffusing capacity is helpful in estimating the alveolar-capillary exchange surface area and efficiency. Due to parenchymal destruction, the carbon monoxide diffusing capacity is generally decreased in emphysema.

# Mechanisms involved in the pathogenesis of COPD

## Effect of cigarette smoking on lung immunity

One puff of cigarette smoke contains more than 4700 compounds and has more than $10^{15}$ free radicals with high oxidative potential [23]. The host's main defense against this toxic gas includes pulmonary antioxidants, mucous and mucociliary clearance, and the action of inflammatory cells such as macrophages. These mechanisms are mostly involved in damage control through phagocytosis and mucociliary clearance of inhaled particles (Figure 6.7). Unfortunately, tobacco smoke also induces a chronic inflammatory response in the lungs, in addition of causing structural cell damage [24,25].

Tobacco smoke can activate cells involved in innate immunity and also appears to have the potential to activate a pulmonary adaptive response most likely through indirect pathways [25]. The innate immunity is relatively nonspecific but has several powerful antimicrobial mechanisms [26,27] while the adaptive immunity is much more specific, being able to recognize infected cells. The adaptive immunity is also responsible for acquiring and maintaining the "immune memory" toward infectious agents [26]. Most hypotheses that have been put forward to explain the pathogenesis of COPD are based on clinical and preclinical data showing the magnitude of the initial pulmonary damage, the direct or indirect activation of innate immunity, and the progressive appearance of an adaptive immune response.

## Innate immunity: First cause of lung damage?

Pulmonary innate immune cells such as eosinophils, neutrophils, macrophages, and natural killer (NK) cells form the first line of defense against infectious agents. They also contribute to maintaining the integrity of pulmonary structures by eliminating dead cells and repairing tissues. However, when fighting pathogens, these cells can also cause significant lung damage. The percentage of neutrophils in bronchoalveolar

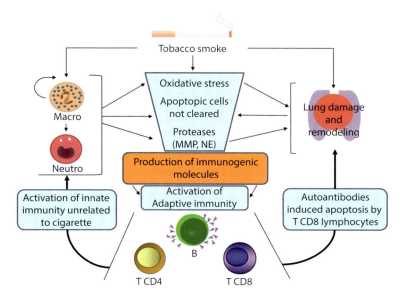

Figure 6.7 Role of immunity in the pathogenesis of chronic obstructive pulmonary disease (COPD). Initiation of an autoimmune reaction through the activation of innate immunity and pulmonary damages caused by tobacco smoke. Macro: macrophage, MMP: matrix metalloproteinase, neutro: polynuclear neutrophils, NE: neutrophil elastase

lavage (BAL) and induced sputum is higher in individuals with emphysema than it is in nonemphysematous smokers and this higher percentage has a positive correlation with the annual decline in $FEV_1$ [28,29]. Similarly, investigators have shown an increase in macrophage numbers in the lungs and BAL of smokers with COPD when compared to non-COPD smokers [30–33]. Finally, there is a positive correlation between the number of macrophages in airways and severity of emphysema [34].

## Imbalance between protease and antiprotease

Proteases are enzymes that degrade various proteins including those forming the extracellular matrix. Constantly secreted and appropriately counterbalanced by antiproteases, proteases are essential to pulmonary homeostasis. Physiologically, they are secreted during cell migration across capillary walls, for instance [35]. These capillary walls are made of endothelial cells and extracellular matrix (collagen, fibronectin), which must be loosened to allow inflammatory cell passage. Proteases are also secreted during infectious episodes where they can destroy the membranes of several pathogens [36], thus limiting their growth and dissemination. Proteases also play an important role in lung tissue repair [37].

Three important observations have lead to the concept of protease/antiprotease imbalance to explain the pathogenesis of COPD: (1) People deficient in alpha-1 antitrypsin, an important antiproteinase present in the lung, can develop an early form of emphysema [38], (2) in animal models (mouse), the instillation of neutrophil elastase (NE), a neutrophil secreted protease, induces, within a few days, the destruction of pulmonary alveoli identical to what is seen in emphysema [39], and (3) when activated, alveolar macrophages and neutrophils are an important source of proteases and both of these inflammatory cells are present in large numbers in emphysematous lungs [28,40].

An important substantial protease release combined with an inability of antiproteases to efficiently inhibit their activity can severely compromise pulmonary homeostasis as maintenance of lung parenchymal integrity largely depends on protein fibers, the prime targets of many proteases. Elastin, which is degraded by NE and matrix metalloproteinase 9 (MMP-9), is responsible for keeping small airways open, allowing them to avoid premature collapse secondary to the reduction in lung volumes occurring during expiration. In addition, the collagen extracellular matrix degraded by collagenases such as matrix metalloproteinase 1 (MMP-1) is essential to maintain the integrity of endothelial and epithelial pulmonary cells. A loss in extracellular matrix integrity can lead to cellular apoptosis and ultimately, and on a larger scale, to an important loss of cellular density contributing to alveolar destruction. An excess of proteases can also lead to local airway and alveolar remodeling. Elevated NE [41], MMP-1, and MMP-9 [42,43] levels are found in the BAL of individuals with emphysema compared to individuals with normal lung functions, levels that are inversely proportional to $FEV_1$ [44,45]. It has also been shown that alveolar macrophages from COPD patients secrete more MMP-9 than healthy smokers [46].

The concept of protease/antiprotease imbalance in the pathogenesis of COPD is mostly attributable to data obtained from observational studies of the BAL. The evidence is, however, not so clear as to whether the population of inflammatory cells found in the BAL is truly representative of what really exists in the lung. Indeed, Finkelstein et al. [30] found that an inversely proportional correlation between severity of lung destruction and number of neutrophils found in BAL exists in individuals with COPD. The same authors have also shown a positive correlation between the presence of T-lymphocytes, severity of parenchymal destruction, and number of alveolar macrophages in BAL. These results suggest that neutrophils are not the only cells involved in the pathogenesis of COPD and that T-lymphocytes and macrophages may play an even more important role (see "Adaptive immunity: From back benching to the front line" on page 107).

## Chronic lung oxidative stress

The oxidative stress is a process during which cells or tissues are exposed to substances called reactive oxygen species (ROS) that can cause lipid, protein, or nucleic acid damage. There are several sources of endogenous or exogenous ROS with a wide range of effects from cell proliferation to cell death. High ROS levels are, however, generally associated to deleterious effects.

COPD is characterized by an increase in oxidative pulmonary stress and it has been shown that the lungs of patients afflicted with COPD have high levels of 4-hydroxy-2-nonenal (4-HNE) [47] and 8-isoprostane [48], two oxidized lipids. The two most important sources of ROS in COPD are tobacco smoke inhalation and the "oxidative burst" of inflammatory phagocytes.

The gaseous part of tobacco smoke contains a large amount of oxidative molecules and free radicals (>10$^{-15}$ molecules per puff) [23], including superoxide and nitric oxide (NO), which interact together to produce a highly reactive composite called peroxynitrite (ONOO–). These substances can also react with unsaturated organic compounds to produce peroxyl radicals (ROO). As far as the tar fraction is concerned, the equilibrium quinone (Q)/semiquinone (Q.)/hydroquinone ($QH_2$) ($Q + QH_2 - 2H^+ + Q$.) is the main source of free radical production. With oxygen, the semiquinone can lead to the production of superoxide ($O_2^-$) ($Q.^- + O \ldots Q + O_2^-$) and then of hydrogen peroxide ($H_2O_2$) ($2O_2 + 2H \ldots O_2 + H_2O_2$). The tar phase is also in contact with iron ions, which are able to catalyze the production of hydroxyl radicals (HO.) from hydrogen peroxide ($H_2O_2$) ($H_2O_2$ + iron$^{++}$…HO. + HO$^-$ + Iron$^{+++}$). Iron recycling (reduction) can be achieved by semiquinones (QH. + Iron$^{+++}$…Q +H$^+$ + Iron$^{+++}$) [49]. This evidence shows that, in addition to containing a very large number of oxidative molecules, constituents of tobacco smoke can keep on generating free radicals for some time after inhalation.

In contrast to what is observed with exposure to tobacco smoke, ROS associated with the respiratory burst are endogenous in origin and relate to a normal and physiological mechanism occurring when phagocytes (neutrophils and alveolar macrophages) become activated. Such activation is generally secondary to the detection of pathogens such as bacteria or to inflammatory mediators such as tumor necrosis factor (TNF) and interferon-gamma (IFN-γ) [48,49]. Within activated phagocytes, NADPH oxidase converts oxygen molecules into superoxide anion ($O_2^-$.) through oxidation of NADPH into NADP+. Superoxide is later transformed to $H_2O_2$ by superoxide dismutase (SOD). The already very reactive $H_2O_2$ will eventually be converted to hypochlorite (OCL$^-$) by myeloperoxidase (MPO). The main purpose of this process is to place the pathogens that have already been submitted to phagocytosis in front of a lethal oxidative burst [50,51].

By direct exposure to tobacco smoke or through inflammatory cell activation, smokers and COPD patients are exposed to chronic lung oxidative stress, which will result in the amplification of the inflammatory response and additional cell damage if not properly counteracted by the antioxidative defense mechanisms.

**Inflammation:** Oxidative stress causes the production of inflammatory mediators such as TNF and interleukin-1 (IL-1), the chemokines monocyte chemoattractant protein-1 (MCP-1) and IL-8, and intracellular adhesion molecule (ICAM)-1 and vascular cell adhesion molecule (VCAM)-1 expressed by structural cells and alveolar macrophages [52]. Stimulation of alveolar macrophages by pro-inflammatory stimuli activates nuclear factor NF-kB and other transcription factors to activate on histone acetyltransferase leading to histone acetylation and transcription of pro-inflammatory genes. Corticosteroids reverse this by binding to glucocorticoid receptors and recruiting histone deacetylase. But inflammatory effects of oxidative stress induce histone acetylase/deacetylase imbalance with reduced levels of histone deacetylase activity. Consequently, the inflammatory response to NF-kB activation is amplified with reduced anti-inflammatory response to corticosteroids [52,53].

**Cellular damage:** An oxidative stress powerful enough can cause a temporary cell cycle arrest, senescence, apoptosis, and even necrosis. DNA damage can lead a cell to stop its cellular cycle, thus allowing for damage repair. This phase is characterized by an increase in the level of cellular cyclin inhibitors such as the p21.

Cellular senescence occurs when oxidative stress induces damage too severe to allow for efficient repair but not severe enough to lead to cell death. A senescent cell has high levels of p16 and B-galactosidase activity. These cells are still metabolically active but can no longer contribute to tissue regeneration. If cellular damage cannot be efficiently repaired, the cell will engage apoptotic pathways involving the transcription factor p53 as well as pro-apoptotic mitochondrial factors Bax, PUMA, and NOXA. These elements will lead the cell toward apoptosis, a "clean" type of cell death with restricted amount of alarmins being released. If cellular damage is very severe, the cell will not have the capacity to engage apoptotic pathways and will become necrotic, releasing alarmins that will trigger and/or amplify the inflammatory response [52,54,55].

Because of its ability to induce an inflammatory response and cause cellular damage, chronic oxidative stress associated with tobacco smoking or ROS release is thus an important player in the initiation of lung destruction and subsequent remodeling.

## Reduction in efferocytosis

Efferocytosis refers to a phenomenon by which cells of the immune system, mainly phagocytes, eliminate apoptotic cells. This apoptotic cell elimination process is common in the lungs and is extremely important for maintaining normal pulmonary homeostasis and tissue regeneration. Apoptotic cells have, on their surface, several molecules including phosphatidylserine (PS) and the ICAM-3, which are recognized by macrophages through a wide spectrum of receptors including receptors for PS, CD14, and CD36 [56].

We have previously mentioned that elevated levels of alveolar apoptosis can be observed in emphysematous patients and in this context, efficient efferocytosis becomes important. However, alveolar macrophages of emphysematous patients have a lowered capacity to phagocytose apoptotic pulmonary epithelial cells [57], which can be reproduced *in vitro* by exposing alveolar macrophages to tobacco smoke [58]. The end result is that apoptotic cells will take longer to be eliminated in smokers and individuals with emphysema.

The significance of efferocytosis goes beyond the simple "tissue cleanliness" since inability to rapidly eliminate apoptotic cells can have serious consequences. When apoptotic cells are phagocytosed, their intracellular content is not released in the surrounding milieu, referred to as a "clean death." If, on the other hand, the apoptotic cells are not rapidly eliminated, their cytoplasmic membrane, whose integrity has been compromised, will no longer be able to hold the intracellular contents and will release it in the surrounding milieu. This can be interpreted by neighboring cells as indicative of danger. This interpretation will be the starting point of an inflammatory response.

## From innate to adaptive immunity: Reaching a point of no return

The role of the innate immunity has always been considered important in the pathogenesis of COPD for its potential destructive power. In a normal situation, during an infection for instance, the neutrophils and macrophages simply die or are deactivated and then eliminated allowing for tissue repair once the initial stimulus is no longer present. However, COPD patients have a persistent lung inflammation despite smoking cessation. In such cases, a most important question to ask is, "What keeps the innate immune system activated under such circumstances?" A possible explanation could have to do with adaptive immunity. In fact, the adaptive immune system is responsible for the specific response to infectious agents as well as for the immune memory. According to some investigators, immunological memory could be controlling the pulmonary destruction mechanisms associated with the chronicity of COPD, despite smoking cessation [59–61].

## Creation of potentially immunogenic neo-molecules

By definition, an immunogenic molecule is able to induce a targeted response from the adaptive immune system. This adaptive immunity can discriminate between host or self-molecules and those from pathogens such as bacteria or virus, also called "non-self molecules." It is those processes that mediate the destruction of a virus-infected cell or cause a bacterium to be opsonized by antibodies that will activate the complement system or inform phagocytes to initiate phagocytosis. Under conditions of homeostasis, the adaptive immune system does not attack host cells or activate the innate immune system. However, cigarette smoke inhalation as well as chronic activation of the innate immune system can lead to the production of immunogenic neo-molecules of nonmicrobial origin that could potentially activate the adaptive immune system (Figure 6.7). Each of the previously discussed hypotheses involving the innate immune system (protease/antiprotease imbalance, chronic oxidative stress, and reduction in efferocytosis) can lead to the emergence of potentially immunogenic molecules.

**Proteases:** Abnormal protease activity can be the source of unusual peptides able to trigger an adaptive immune system response. Bullous pemphigoid skin disease is a good example of an autoimmune reaction set off by elevated cutaneous proteolysis [62].

**Oxidative stress:** In addition to being pro-inflammatory and cytotoxic, oxidants can alter cellular and matrix components (collagen and elastin) and, by doing so, give them an unusual configuration that could ultimately trigger a response from the adaptive immune system. People afflicted with rheumatoid arthritis, for instance, have autoantibodies directed against peptides containing the amino acid citrulline, an oxidative by-product of the amino acid arginine [63].

**Reduction in efferocytosis:** In addition to inducing a local inflammatory reaction, the unusual presence of intracellular material in the extracellular milieu can also initiate a response from the adaptive immune system. Individuals with systemic lupus erythematosus, an autoimmune disorder, produce high levels of antibodies against DNA and nuclear components [64].

In COPD, several factors are in place to promote the generation of autoantigens. Well before the symptoms appear, this autoimmune-like reaction, maintaining the activation of the adaptive immune system, will also support innate immune activation despite smoking cessation.

But do we have the evidence to support the concept that the adaptive immune system is involved in the pathogenesis of COPD?

## Adaptive immunity: From back benching to the front line

### B-lymphocytes and autoantibodies

One of the histological characteristics of the adaptive immune response is the presence of bronchial associated lymphatic tissues (BALTs), which are found in both the lung parenchyma and airway walls of COPD patients [14]. These follicles are made of dividing aggregates of B-lymphocytes and of follicular dendritic cells surrounded by T-lymphocytes (Figure 6.8) [11]. Hogg et al. have shown that there is a significant correlation between an increased number of lymphoid follicles and the progression of COPD severity [14]. They also suggested that the presence of these lymphoid follicles might be a reflection of the adaptive immune system response to repeated infections or microbial colonization, both common in severe COPD.

It has been shown that there are more B-lymphocytes in the lungs of COPD patients and mice exposed to tobacco smoke [14,65]. B-lymphocytes are cells of the adaptive immune system responsible for antibody

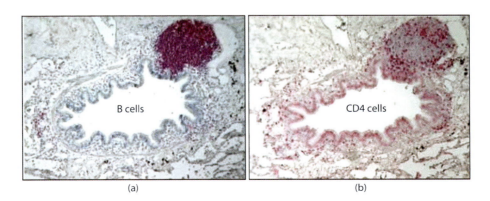

Figure 6.8 Lymphoid follicles. **(a)** Bronchial lymphoid follicle from a patient with severe COPD containing a germinal center whose darker staining is highly positive for B-lymphocytes. **(b)** Same airway stained for CD4+ T-lymphocytes. (From Hogg JC et al., *NEJM*, 350, 2645–2653, 2004. Reproduced with permission).

production. Investigators have also described an antigen-specific oligoclonal reaction in the lymphoid follicle B-lymphocytes [65]. However, the absence of bacterial or viral antigens in the lymphoid follicles may rather suggest a response directed toward an autoimmune pulmonary antigen. Antibodies directed against "self" antigens such as elastin have been found in the blood of COPD patients but not in that of non-COPD individuals [66].

Serum antibodies in COPD patients have *in vitro* cytotoxic effect on epithelial pulmonary cells by activating the complement cascade [67]. This observation, however, seems to be more applicable to emphysema than other types of COPD.

## CD4+ T-lymphocytes

CD4+ T-lymphocytes interact through their T-cell receptor (TCR) with antigen-presenting cells (mature dendritic cells and macrophages) that exhibit a variety of antigens through the major histocompatibility complex (MHC) II. If dendritic cells bear antigens that can powerfully bind the CD4+ T-lymphocyte TCR, the lymphocyte will become activated and enter a proliferative phase (oligoclonal expansion). CD4+ T-lymphocytes are involved in the process of both innate immunity and B-lymphocyte (adaptive immunity) activation [68].

COPD patients have a high proportion of CD4+ T-lymphocytes in their lungs [30,33,69]. In addition to being numerous, the CD4+ T-lymphocytes express more activation markers, specifically high levels of STAT4 and increased secretion of IFN-γ, both correlating with $FEV_1$ decline [70]. One can also find in the lungs of COPD patients, but not in the peripheral blood, CD4+ T-lymphocytes undergoing oligoclonal expansion [71], an observation further supported by the presence of lymphoid follicles. When exposed *in vitro* to elastin fragments, CD4+ T-lymphocytes from the lungs of COPD patients start producing IFN-γ [66], a phenomenon not observed in a normal population or during collagen stimulation. These data suggest that CD4+ T-lymphocytes found in the lungs of COPD individuals have a higher degree of activation, divide as a response to specific antigen stimulation, and can become activated when a specific pulmonary antigen such as elastin is present.

## CD8+ T-lymphocytes

CD8+ T-lymphocytes can be seen as highly specific killer cells. These lymphocytes are, indeed, specialized in fighting intracellular pathogens and can also trigger apoptosis in infected cells expressing viral antigens at their surface. Being activated by antigen-presenting cells similar to what happens with CD4+ T-lymphocytes, CD8+ T-lymphocytes undergo oligoclonal expansion and acquire an effector phenotype. The effector CD8+ T-lymphocytes are recognizable by their high amount of IFN-γ secretion and perforin and granzyme B levels, which play a crucial role by initiating apoptosis in cells targeted by CD8+ T-lymphocytes [68].

As opposed to what is observed in the lungs of normal individuals, the lungs of individuals with COPD contain more CD8+ T-lymphocytes in central airway [72], peripheral airway [10], lung parenchyma [30], and pulmonary arteries [18]. Higher numbers of CD8+ T-lymphocytes in the lung parenchyma correlate positively with the amount of parenchymal destruction, degree of alveolar apoptosis, number of alveolar macrophages, and decline in pulmonary function [67]. In addition, a large proportion of CD8+ T-lymphocytes found in lungs of COPD patients show enhanced cytotoxicity with high levels of perforin and granzyme B expression [73].

Lymphocyte activation is not observed in the systemic circulation of these same individuals [74,75] suggesting that CD8+ T-lymphocytes likely acquire their effector phenotype once recruited in the lungs. In mice exposed to tobacco smoke, CD8+ T-lymphocyte oligoclonal expansion is maintained despite smoking cessation [76]. As documented with CD4+ T-lymphocytes, these data suggest that CD8+ T-lymphocytes divide in response to specific antigen stimulation, in addition to acquiring an effector phenotype in the lungs.

## Increased T-lymphocyte chemotaxis

Chemotaxis is a mechanism by which a ligand has the ability to attract cells harboring a specific receptor. This process is very important for the recruitment of circulating cells to the periphery, including the lungs. Chemokines are classified based on their primary structure but can also be regrouped according to the type of cells that they can attract. Chemokines CXCL9/monokine induced by IFN-γ (MIG) and CXCL10/interferon-inducible protein-10 (IP-10) are highly expressed by pulmonary structural epithelial and endothelial cells. The receptor associated with those chemokines is CXCR3, a receptor well known for its expression by activated CD4+ and CD8+ T-lymphocytes. Indeed, lymphocytes found in the lungs of patients with COPD have a strong expression of the CXCR3 receptor [77] and this level of expression correlates with disease severity. Thus, in addition to local proliferation, T-lymphocytes are specifically recruited to the lungs, illustrating the need of COPD lungs to recruit more new T-lymphocytes.

## Other mechanisms potentially involved in COPD pathogenesis

There is much evidence to suggest that the pathogenesis of COPD is primarily related to alterations in the immune system (Figure 6.7). Other mechanisms have, however, been shown to have a role in the process of lung destruction associated with COPD. Unfortunately, it is unknown where these mechanisms occur in the chronology of disease as well as the full extent of their role.

### Decrease in vascular endothelial growth factor and VEGFR2 receptors levels

The interaction between the vascular endothelial growth factor (VEGF) and its receptor VEGFR2 is responsible for the proliferation, migration, and survival of endothelial cells [78]. A decrease in the levels of VEGF and VEGFR2 expression could compromise the homeostasis of the pulmonary capillary bed to which alveolar epithelial cell survival is closely linked.

VEGF and VEGFR2 expression is reduced in lungs of individuals with COPD compared to normal individuals and correlates negatively with the importance of alveolar apoptosis [79]. In a rat model, animals that received the VEGFR2 inhibitor SU5416 developed a pulmonary phenotype similar to emphysema as well as an increase in alveolar wall apoptosis [80]. This phenomenon was prevented by concomitant administration of an apoptosis inhibitor (Z-Asp-CH2-DCB) [80], suggesting that SU5416-induced emphysema depends on alveolar apoptosis. It has also been shown that tobacco smoke could alter VEGF expression *in vitro* [81]. The exact cause of decreased VEGF and VEGFR2 expression in the emphysematous lung remains unknown although it has been documented that *in vitro* exposure of endothelial cells to tobacco smoke is associated with decreased VEGFR2 expression [81]. In addition, the disappearance of lung epithelial cells could be the main cause of VEGF reduced levels in the lungs of individuals with COPD, as those cells are the main source of VEGF.

### Sensitivity to the ligand TRAIL

The TNF-related apoptosis-inducing ligand (TRAIL) is a member of the family of "tumor necrosis factors," a family that includes TNF and Fas ligand (FasL), and has the ability to initiate cellular apoptosis. The emphysematous lung has a higher sensitivity to TRAIL-mediated apoptosis than normal lungs that show resistance to apoptosis [82]. In fact, the emphysematous lungs shows increased TRAIL-R1, TRAIL-R2, and TRAIL-R3 expression despite cigarette smoking cessation [83]. Elevated levels of the transcription factor p53 and pro-apoptotic factor Bax can also be observed, molecules linked to an increased sensitivity to TRAIL-mediated apoptosis.

### Genetic predispositions

The fact that not all smokers develop COPD suggests a genetic predisposition. The most important genetic factor involved in the pathogenesis of emphysema is the Z alpha-1 antitrypsin allele, an important elastase inhibitor. The presence of this allele translates into a 10%–15% plasma level than the normal M allele [84], as 85% of synthesized Z alpha-1 antitrypsin accumulates in the liver [85]. If individuals who bear the allele Z homozygotes (PI Z) are smokers, their odds of developing emphysema are markedly increased [86]. People with substantial alpha-1 antitrypsin PI Z deficits represent only 1%–2% of the individuals with emphysema and there is also an important variability between smokers and former smokers with a similar genotype PI Z [87]. Such variability suggests that there are probably other genetic-related factors that could predispose to emphysema in PI Z individuals.

Polymorphism in the alpha-1-antichymotrypsin antiproteases and tissue inhibitors of metalloproteinase-2 (TIMP-2) genes could also be responsible for increasing the risks of developing COPD [88,89]. Several investigators have also shown that polymorphisms on genes coding for the antioxidant enzymes heme oxygenase-1 (HO-1), glutathione S-transferase M1 (GSTM1), and GSTP1 were associated with rapid decline in respiratory function in smokers [90–92]. Investigators have also been able to document the presence of emphysema-associated polymorphisms in cytokine-coding genes such as TNF and IL-13 [93,94]. The results of these studies on polymorphism are still debated as these findings could be attributed to ethnic differences. A published meta-analysis has, however, shown the protective role of TGF-beta polymorphisms [95].

## Exacerbation of COPD: Intensification of pulmonary inflammatory response

COPD exacerbations are generally associated with episodes of viral or bacterial bronchial infection and represent a substantial medical and research subject that will not be covered extensively in this chapter. During such episodes, individuals with COPD experience an increase in shortness of breath and sputum production, which becomes more purulent. COPD exacerbations are common, especially in patients with advanced disease. Respiratory infections are important stimuli of pulmonary inflammatory response [96] and this phenomenon contributes to the worsening of the patient's general condition and accelerates the decline in lung function [97,98]. Since 2012, the GOLD has combined spirometry evaluation, symptom severity, and history of exacerbation to improve assessment and management of COPD.

## Effect of pharmacological treatment on pulmonary inflammatory response

Aside smoking cessation, no pharmacological treatment has been shown to slow down disease progression or lower disease-related mortality [22,99]. Most therapies rather aim at relieving symptoms, most notably dyspnea. Inhaled steroids are recommended for the treatment of COPD combined with long-acting β2-agonist bronchodilators (LABA) when $FEV_1$ is less than 50% predicted with history of two or more exacerbations per year. Although, COPD inflammation is less sensitive to steroid for several reasons (neutrophil inflammation, excessive activation of NF-kB, reduced histone deacetylase, and decreased glucocorticoid receptor expression), studies have shown that inhaled corticosteroids can significantly lower the incidence of disease exacerbations [100,101]. The addition of LABA lowers the incidence of exacerbations from 18% (steroid alone) to 25% per year compared to placebo [102]. Few studies have looked at the effect of those therapies on the pulmonary inflammation response. In 2006, Barnes et al. [103] showed that salmeterol/fluticasone propionate decreases the intensity of the inflammatory response in COPD smokers and former smokers by lowering the number of CD4+ and T CD8+ T-lymphocytes, mastocytes, and TNF and IFN-γ expression in bronchial biopsies obtained after 13 weeks of treatment. In 2007, Bourbeau et al. [104] were able to confirm these findings by showing a significant reduction in CD8+ T-lymphocytes and macrophages in bronchial biopsies obtained after 12 weeks of treatment with salmeterol/fluticasone propionate versus fluticasone alone, therefore suggesting a possible anti-inflammatory action of LABA (salmeterol). Other studies are also suggesting that, in addition to their bronchodilator effect, LABA could also accelerate translocation of the glucocorticosteroid/receptor complex nucleus, thus encouraging the transcription and expression of anti-inflammatory factors [105]. Long-acting muscarinic antagonist bronchodilators (LAMA) such as tiotropium have shown anti-inflammatory effects *in vivo* using animal models [106,107]. Recent reports also suggest that tiotropium can inhibit viral activation of inflammation [108,109]. The need for more evidence of the clinical significance of LAMA and LABA anti-inflammatory effects does not prevent them from being effective at relieving dyspnea, increasing exercise tolerance, preventing exacerbations, and improving quality of life [102,110].

Phosphodiesterase-4 (PDE-4) is expressed in most inflammatory and lung cells. Clinical trials with PDE-4 inhibitor showed a significant reduction of 17% (up to 21% with concomitant treatment with LABA) in moderate-to-severe exacerbation rates in patients with COPD [111,112]. *In vivo* studies showed a reduction of neutrophils, eosinophils, and concentration of inflammatory mediators in sputum (IL-8 and NE) and in the serum (TNF-α) [113]. In a bronchial biopsy study, a PDE-4 inhibitor reduced the number of CD8+ T-lymphocytes and macrophages (CD68+ cells) [114].

Macrolides are also used for COPD patients with frequent exacerbation. In addition to their antimicrobial activity, macrolides have significant immunomodulatory/anti-inflammatory properties related to the macrocyclic lactone ring [115]. Macrolides decrease neutrophil activity, oxidant production, and pro-inflammatory mediators such as IL-5, IL-6, IL-8, IL-1β, and IL-10 [116]. Macrolides also inhibit IL-13 and TNF-α production, which have an important role in mucus secretion in the airways [117]. Finally, macrolides interfere with *Pseudomonas aeruginosa* colonization, which is an important airways pathogen in severe COPD, by inhibiting biofilm formation [118]. Clinical studies showed a significant reduction of COPD exacerbations with macrolides. Albert et al. [119] showed a 27% reduction after 1 year using azithromycin 250 mg/day in moderate-to-severe COPD patients. This reduction is up to 43% if recruited COPD patients had history of three or more exacerbations per year [120]. Long-term erythromycin treatment is also associated with decreased COPD exacerbations [121] and this clinical effect may partly be caused by an antiprotease effect [122].

## Extrapulmonary repercussions of COPD

Even if COPD mostly affects the lungs, extrapulmonary repercussions are well documented. COPD patients have an increased incidence of cardiovascular diseases (myocardial infarct, arteriosclerosis), diabetes mellitus, and osteoporosis [123] and are highly susceptible to peripheral muscle atrophy.

In the peripheral blood of stable emphysematous subjects, we can observe an increase in inflammatory mediators such as TNF and IL-6 [73,124–126], acute inflammatory mediators such as C-reactive protein (CRP) and fibrinogen [127,128], as well as the neutrophil chemoattractant CXCL8 [129]. There are also differences between circulating cell types, notably an increase in monocyte chemotactic response [130], an increase in the number of CD8+ T-lymphocytes with Fas-positive expression [131], and a greater proportion of IFN-γ secreting CD4+ T-lymphocytes [132]. The significance of these observations is still under debate with regards to their extrapulmonary impacts.

People afflicted with severe emphysema also have a significant decrease of their peripheral muscle mass [133,134]. This phenomenon can be attributable to malnutrition, systemic inflammation, inactivity, local oxidative stress, use of corticosteroids, and hypoxia. The true mechanisms are, however, not well known nor documented. The loss of peripheral muscle mass is not a negligible issue as it has been shown that, in patients with similar lung function, loss of muscle mass is associated with unfavorable prognosis and increased disease-related mortality [135].

## Conclusions and future perspectives

COPD clinical and basic research performed over the past decades highlights the complexity of the disease. There has been increased and renewed interest in this research from people with all kinds of background including immunologists, geneticists, and specialists in molecular and cell biology. Because of these various contributions, the role of the immune system in the pathogenesis of emphysema-related pulmonary changes is no longer debated. Unfortunately, the exact reasons as to why tobacco smoke triggers in only some smokers, the pathogenic mechanisms of emphysema are still largely unknown and poorly understood. This lack of knowledge with regards to the exact pathogenesis of COPD and pathology limits the development of new drugs that could potentially have a significant impact on COPD progression.

Current research efforts are focusing on a better understanding of the inflammatory response including the exact role of both innate and adaptive immunity triggered by tobacco smoke exposure. Researchers are also trying to understand the differences between smokers without COPD and smokers who developed the disease. Using animal models and refining the methods for cell culture and molecular biology should be helpful in improving our understanding of the consequences of smoking on the lungs and, eventually, helping us understand the pathogenesis of COPD and thus be able to slow down its evolution.

# References

1. Pauwels RA, Buist AS, Calverley PM et al. Global strategy for the diagnosis, management, and prevention of chronic obstructive pulmonary disease. NHLBI/WHO Global Initiative for Chronic Obstructive Lung Disease (GOLD) Workshop summary. *Am J Respir Crit Care Med* 2001; 163: 1256–1276.
2. Anto JM, Vermeire P, Vestbo J, Sunyer J. Epidemiology of chronic obstructive pulmonary disease. *Eur Respir J* 2001; 17: 982–994.
3. Lopez AD, Shibuya K, Rao C et al. Chronic obstructive pulmonary disease: Current burden and future projections. *Eur Respir J* 2006; 27: 397–412.
4. Mathers CD, Loncar D. Projections of global mortality and burden of disease from 2002 to 2030. *PLoS Med* 2006; 3: e442.
5. Belleau R, Maltais F. *Apprendre à vivre avec la bronchite chronique ou l'emphysème. Améliorer votre qualité de vie*. Presses de l`Université Laval, Québec, 2008, 96 pages.
6. Saetta M, Turato G, Maestrelli P et al. Cellular and structural bases of chronic obstructive pulmonary disease. *Am J Respir Crit Care Med* 2001; 163: 1304–1309.
7. Reid LM. Pathology of chronic bronchitis. *Lancet* 1954; 266: 274–278.
8. Dunhill MS, Massarella GR, Anderson JA. A comparison of the quantitative anatomy of the bronchi in normal subjects, in status asthmaticus, in chronic bronchitis, and in emphysema. *Thorax* 1969; 24: 176–179.
9. Jeffery PK. Remodeling in asthma and chronic obstructive lung disease. *Am J Respir Crit Care Med* 2001; 164: S28–S38.
10. Saetta M, Di Stefano A, Turato G et al. CD8+ T-lymphocytes in peripheral airways of smokers with chronic obstructive pulmonary disease. *Am J Respir Crit Care Med* 1998; 157: 822–826.
11. Saetta M, Turato G, Baraldo S et al. Goblet cell hyperplasia and epithelial inflammation in peripheral airways of smokers with both symptoms of chronic bronchitis and chronic airflow limitation. *Am J Respir Crit Care Med* 2000; 161: 1016–1021.
12. Jeffery PK. Comparison of the stucture and inflammatory feature of COPD and asthma. Giles F Filley lecture. *Chest* 2000; 117: 251s–260s.
13. Hogg JC, Macklem PT, Thurlbeck WM. Site and nature of airway obstruction in chronic obstructive lung disease. *N Engl J Med* 1968; 278: 1355–1360.
14. Hogg JC, Chu F, Utokaparch S et al. The nature of small-airway obstruction in chronic obstructive pulmonary disease. *N Engl J Med* 2004; 350: 2645–2653.
15. McDonough JE, Yuan R, Suzuki M et al. Small-airway obstruction and emphysema in chronic obstructive pulmonary disease. *N Engl J Med*; 365: 1567–1575.
16. Kim WD, Eidelman DH, Izquierdo JL et al. Centrilobular and panlobular emphysema in smokers. Two distinct morphologic and functional entities. *Am Rev Resp Dis* 1991; 144: 1385–1390.
17. Kessler R, Faller M, Fourgaut G et al. Predictive factors of hospitalization for acute exacerbation in a series of 64 patients with chronic obstructive pulmonary disease. *Am J Respir Crit Care Med* 1999; 159: 158–164.

18. Peinado VI, Barbera JA, Abate P et al. Inflammatory reaction in pulmonary muscular arteries of patients with mild chronic obstructive pulmonary disease. *Am J Respir Crit Care Med* 1999; 159: 1605–1611.
19. Hale KA, Niewoehner DE, Cosio MG. Morphologic changes in the muscular pulmonary arteries: Relationship to cigarette smoking, airway disease, and emphysema. *Am Rev Resp Dis* 1980; 122: 273–278.
20. Dinh-Xuan AT, Higenbottam TCW, Clelland CA et al. Impairment of endothelium-dependent pulmonary artery relaxation in chronic obstructive lung disease. *N Engl J Med* 1991; 324: 1539–1547.
21. Hogg JC. Pathophysiology of airflow limitation in chronic obstructive pulmonary disease. *Lancet* 2004; 364: 709–721.
22. Fletcher C, Peto R. The natural history of chronic airflow obstruction. *Br Med J* 1977; 1: 1645–1648.
23. Church DF, Pryor WA. Free-radical chemistry of cigarette smoke and its toxicological implications. *Environ Health Perspect* 1985; 64: 111–126.
24. Smith LA, Paszkiewicz GM, Hutson AD, Pauly JL. Inflammatory response of lung macrophages and epithelial cells to tobacco smoke: A literature review of ex vivo investigations. *Immunol Res* 2010; 46: 94–126.
25. D'hulst AI, Vermaelen KY, Brusselle GG et al. Time course of cigarette smoke-induced pulmonary inflammation in mice. *Eur Respir J* 2005; 26: 204–213.
26. Abbas AK, Lichtman AH. *Cellular and Molecular Immunology,* 5th Edition. Philadelphia, PA : Saunders, 2005. 564 pages.
27. Martin TR, Frevert CW. Innate immunity in the lungs. *Proc Am Thorac Soc* 2005; 2: 403–411.
28. Martin TR, Raghu G, Maunder RJ, Springmeyer SC. The effects of chronic bronchitis and chronic airflow obstruction on lung cell populations recovered by bronchoalveolar lavage. *Am Rev Respir Dis* 1985; 132: 254–260.
29. Stanescu D, Sanna A, Veriter C et al. Airways obstruction, chronic expectoration, and rapid decline of FEV1 in smokers are associated with increased levels of sputum neutrophils. *Thorax* 1996; 51: 267–271.
30. Finkelstein R, Fraser RS, Ghezzo H, Cosio MG. Alveolar inflammation and its relation to emphysema in smokers. *Am J Respir Crit Care Med* 1995; 152; 1666–1672.
31. Pesci A, Balbi B, Majori M et al. Inflammatory cells and mediators in bronchial lavage of patients with chronic obstructive pulmonary disease. *Eur Respir J* 1998; 12: 380–386.
32. Keatings VM, Collins PD, Scott DM, Barnes PJ. Differences in interleukin-8 and tumor necrosis factor-alpha in induced sputum from patients with chronic obstructive pulmonary disease or asthma. *Am J Respir Crit Care Med* 1996; 153: 530–534.
33. O'shaughnessy TC, Ansari TW, Barnes NC, Jeffery PK. Inflammation in bronchial biopsies of subjects with chronic bronchitis: Inverse relationship of CD8+ T lymphocytes with FEV1. *Am J Respir Crit Care Med* 1997; 155: 852–857.
34. Di Stefano A, Capelli A, Lusuarsdi M et al. Severity of airflow limitation is associated with severity of airway inflammation in smokers. *Am J Respir Crit Care Med* 1998; 158: 1277–1285.
35. Madri JA, Graesser D. Cell migration in the immune system: The evolving inter-related roles of adhesion molecules and proteinases. *Dev Immunol* 2000; 7: 103–116.
36. Pham CT. Neutrophil serine proteases: Specific regulators of inflammation. *Nat Rev Immunol* 2006; 6: 541–550.
37. Parks WC. Matrix metalloproteinases in lung repair. *Eur Respir J Suppl* 2003; 44: S36–S38.
38. Eriksson S. Pulmonary emphysema and alpha1-antitrypsin deficiency. *Acta Med Scand* 1964; 175: 197–205.
39. Kueppers F, Bearn AG. A possible experimental approach to the association of hereditary alpha-1-antitrypsin deficiency and pulmonary emphysema. *Proc Soc Exp Biol Med* 1966; 121: 1207–1209.

40. Hunninghake GW, Crystal RG. Cigarette smoking and lung destruction. Accumulation of neutrophils in the lungs of cigarette smokers. *Am Rev Resp Dis* 1983; 128: 833–838.
41. Yoshioka A, Betsuyaku T, Nishimura M et al. Excessive neutrophil elastase in bronchoalveolar lavage fluid in subclinical emphysema. *Am J Respir Crit Care Med* 1995; 152: 2127–2132.
42. Betsuyaku T, Nishimura M, Takeyabu K et al. Neutrophil granule proteins in bronchoalveolar lavage fluid from subjects with subclinical emphysema. *Am J Respir Crit Care Med* 1999; 159: 1985–1991.
43. Finlay GA, Russell KJ, McMahon KJ et al. Elevated levels of matrix metalloproteinases in bronchoalveolar lavage fluid of emphysematous patients. *Thorax* 1997; 52: 502–506.
44. Betsuyaku T, Nishimura M, Takeyabu K et al. Evidence for neutrophil involvement in the development of subclinical emphysema. *Chest* 2000; 117: 302s–303s.
45. Kang MJ, Oh YM, Lee JC et al. Lung matrix metalloproteinase-9 correlates with cigarette smoking and obstruction of airflow. *J Korean Med Sci* 2003; 18: 821–827.
46. Russell RE, Culpitt SV, DeMatos C et al. Releases and activity of matrix metalloproteinase-9 and tissue inhibitor of metalloproteinase-1 by alveolar macrophages from patients with chronic obstructive pulmonary disease. *Am J Respir Cell Mol Biol* 2002; 26: 602–609.
47. Rahman I, van Schadewijk AA, Crowther AJ et al. 4-Hydroxy-2-nonenal, a specific lipid peroxidation product, is elevated in lungs of patients with chronic obstructive pulmonary disease. *Am J Respir Crit Care Med* 2002; 166: 490–495.
48. Montuschi P, Collins JV, Ciabattoni G et al. Exhaled 8-isoprostane as an in vivo biomarker of lung oxidative stress in patients with COPD and healthy smokers. *Am J Respir Crit Care Med* 2000; 162: 1175–1177.
49. Pryor WA, Stone K. Oxidants in cigarette smoke. Radicals, hydrogen peroxide, peroxynitrate, and peroxynitrite. *Ann N Y Acad Sci* 1993; 686: 12–27.
50. Dahlgren C, Karlsson A. Respiratory burst in human neutrophils. *J Immunol Methods* 1999; 232: 3–14.
51. Gwinn MR, Vallyathan V. Respiratory burst: Role in signal transduction in alveolar macrophages. *J Toxicol Environ Health B Crit Rev* 2006; 9: 27–39.
52. Martindale JL, Holbrook NJ. Cellular response to oxidative stress: Signaling for suicide and survival. *J Cell Physiol* 2002; 192: 1–15.
53. Barnes PJ, Adcock IM. Glucocorticoid resistance in inflammatory diseases. *Lancet* 2009; 373: 1905–1917.
54. Achanta G, Huang P. Role of p53 in sensing oxidative DNA damage in response to reactive oxygen species-generating agents. *Cancer Res* 2004; 64: 6233–6239.
55. Ryter SW, Kim HP, Hoetzel A et al. Mechanisms of cell death in oxidative stress. *Antioxid Redox Signal* 2007; 9: 49–89.
56. Taylor PR, Martinez-Pomares L, Stacey M et al. Macrophage receptors and immune recognition. *Annu Rev Immunol* 2005; 23: 901–944.
57. Richens TR, Linderman DJ, Horstmann SA et al. Cigarette smoke impairs clearance of apoptotic cells through oxidant-dependent activation of RhoA. *Am J Resp Crit Care Med* 2009; 179: 1011–1021.
58. Hodge S, Hodge G, Scicchitano R et al. Alveolar macrophages from subjects with chronic obstructive pulmonary disease are deficient in their ability to phagocytose apoptotic airway epithelial cells. *Immunol Cell Biol* 2003; 81: 289–296.
59. Cosio MG, Saetta M, Agusti A. Immunologic aspects of chronic obstructive pulmonary disease. *N Engl J Med* 2009; 360: 2445–2454.
60. Morissette MC, Parent J, Milot J. Alveolar epithelial and endothelial cell apoptosis in emphysema: What we know and what we need to know. *Int J Chron Obstruct Pulmon Dis* 2009; 4: 19–31.
61. Duncan SR. What is autoimmunity and why is it likely to be important in chronic lung disease? *Am J Respir Crit Care Med* 2010; 181: 4–5.

62. Liu Z, Li N, Diaz LA et al. Synergy between a plasminogen cascade and MMP-9 in autoimmune disease. *J Clin Invest* 2005; 115: 879–887.
63. Anzilotti C, Pratesi F, Tommasi C, Migliorini P. Peptidylarginine deiminase 4 and citrullination in health and disease. *Autoimmun Rev* 2010; 9: 158–160.
64. Muller S, Dieker J, Tincani A, Meroni PL. Pathogenic anti-nucleosome antibodies. *Lupus* 2008; 17: 431–436.
65. Van der Strate BW, Postma DS, Brandsma CCA, Melgert BN et al. Cigarette smoke-induced emphysema: A role for the B cell? *Am J Respir Crit Care Med* 2006; 173: 751–758.
66. Lee SH, Goswami S, Grudo A et al. Antielastin autoimmunity in tobacco smoking-induced emphysema. *Nat Med* 2007; 13: 567–569.
67. Feghali-Bostwick CA, Gadgil AS, Otterbein LE et al. Antibodies in patients with chronic obstructive pulmonary disease. *Am J Respir Crit Care Med* 2008; 177: 156–163.
68. Janeway CA, Travers P, Walport M, Shlomchik MJ. *Immunobiology: the immune system in health and disease.* 6th Edition. New York. Garland Science, 2005, 823 pages.
69. Majo J, Ghezzo H, Cosio MG. Lymphocyte population and apoptosis in the lungs of smokers and their relation to emphysema. *Eur Respir J* 2001; 17: 946–953.
70. Di Stefano Chrysofakis G, Tzanakis N, Kyriakoy D et al. STAT4 activation in smokers and patients with chronic obstructive pulmonary disease. *Eur Respir J* 2004; 24: 78–85.
71. Sullivan AK, Simonian PL, Falta MT et al. Oligoclonal CD4+ T cells in the lungs of patients with severe emphysema. *Am J Respir Crit Care Med* 2005; 172: 590–596.
72. Lams BE, Sousa AR, Rees PJ, Lee TH. Subepithelial immunopathology of the large airways in smokers with and without chronic obstructive pulmonary disease. *Eur Respir J* 2000; 15: 512–516.
73. Chrysofakis G, Tzanakis N, Kyriakoy D et al. Perforin expression and cytotoxic activity of sputum CD8+ lymphocytes in patients with COPD. *Chest* 2004; 125: 71–76.
74. Morissette MC, Parent J, Milot J. Perforin, granzyme B, and FasL expression by peripheral blood T lymphocytes in emphysema. *Respir Res* 2007; 8: 62.
75. Glader P, von Wachenfeldt K, Lofdahl CG. Systemic CD4+ T-cell activation is correlated with FEV1 in smokers. *Respir Med* 2006; 100: 1088–1093.
76. Motz GT, Eppert BL, Sun G et al. Persistence of lung CD8 T cell oligoclonal expansions upon smoking cessation in a mouse model of cigarette smoke-induced emphysema. *J Immunol* 2008; 181: 8036–8043.
77. Saetta M, Mariani M, Panina-Bordignon P et al. Increased expression of the chemokine receptor CXCR3 and its ligand CXCL10 in peripheral airways of smokers with chronic obstructive pulmonary disease. *Am J Respir Crit Care Med* 2002; 165: 1404–1409.
78. Ferrara N, Gerber HP, LeCouter J. The biology of VEGF and its receptors. *Nat Med* 2003; 9: 669–676.
79. Kasahara Y, Tuder RM, Cool CD et al. Endothelial cell death and decreased expression of vascular endothelial growth factor and vascular endothelial growth receptor 2 in emphysema. *Am J Respir Crit Care Med* 2001; 163; 737–744.
80. Kasahara Y, Tuder RM, Taraseviciene-Stewart L et al. Inhibition of VEGF receptors causes lung cell apoptosis and emphysema. *J Clin Invest* 2000; 106: 1311–1319.
81. Edirisinghe I, Yang SR, Yao H et al. VRGFR-2 inhibition augments cigarette smoke-induced oxidative stress and inflammatory responses leading to endothelial dysfunction. *FASEB J* 2008; 22: 2297–2310.
82. Morissette MC, Parent J, Milot J. Higher sensitivity of the emphysematous lung to TRAIL-mediated apoptosis. Vienna, Austria: European Respiratory Society Congress. 2009.
83. Morissette MC, Vachon-Beaudoin G, Parent J et al. Increased p53 level, Bax/Bcl-x(L) ratio, and TRAIL receptor expression in human emphysema. *Am J Respir Crit Care Med* 2008; 178: 240–247.
84. Eriksson S. Studies in alpha 1-antitrypsin deficiency. *Acta Med Scand Suppl* 1965; 432: 1–85.

85. Lomas DA, Evans DL, Finch JT, Carell RW. The mechanism of Z alpha 1-antitrypsin accumulation in the liver. *Nature* 1992; 357: 605–607.
86. Piitulainen E, Eriksson S. Decline in FEV1 related to smoking status in individuals with severe alpha 1-antitrypsin deficiency (PiZZ). *Eur Resp J* 1999; 13: 247–251.
87. Silverman EK, Province MA, Campbell EJ, Pierce JA, Rao DC. Biochemical intermediates in alpha 1-antitrypsin deficiency: Residual family resemblance for total alpha 1-antitrypsin, oxidized alpha 1-antitrypsin, and immunoglobulin E after adjustment for the effect of the Pi locus. *Genet Epidemiol* 1990; 7: 137–149.
88. Ishii T, Matsuse T, Teramoto S et al. Association between alpha-1-antichymotrypsin polymorphism and susceptibility to chronic obstructive pulmonary disease. *Eur J Clin Invest* 2000; 30: 543–548.
89. Hirano K, Sakamoto T, Uchida Y et al. Tissue inhibitor of metalloproteinases-2 gene polymorphisms in chronic obstructive pulmonary disease. *Eur Respir J* 2001; 18: 748–752.
90. Yamada N, Yamaha M, Okinaga S et al. Microsatellite polymorphism in the heme oxygenase-1 gene promoter is associated with susceptibility to emphysema. *Am J Hum Genet* 2000; 66: 187–195.
91. He JQ, Ruan J, Connett JE et al. Antioxidant gene polymorphisms and susceptibility to a rapid decline in lung function in smokers. *Am J Respir Crit Care Med* 2002: 166: 323–328.
92. Ishii T, Matsuse T, Teramoto S et al. Glutathione D-transferase P1 (GSTP1) polymorphism in patients with chronic obstructive pulmonary disease. *Thorax* 1999; 54: 693–696.
93. Sakao S, Tatsumi K, Igari H et al. Association of tumor necrosis factor alpha gene promoter polymorphism with the presence of chronic obstructive pulmonary disease. *Am J Respir Crit Care Med* 2001; 163: 420–422.
94. Van der Pouw Kraan TC, Kucubaycan M, Bakker AM et al. Chronic obstructive pulmonary disease is associated with the -1055 IL-13 promoter polymorphism. *Genes Immun* 2002; 3: 436–439.
95. Smolonska J, Wijmenga C, Postna DS, Boezen HM. Meta-analyses on suspected chronic obstructive pulmonary disease genes: A summary of 20 years' research. *Am J Respir Crit Care Med* 2009; 180: 618–631.
96. Bhowmik A, Seemungal TCA, Sapsford RJ, Wedzicha JA. Relation of sputum inflammatory markers to symptoms and lung function changes in COPD exacerbations. *Thorax* 2000; 55: 114–120.
97. Donaldson GC, Seemungal TCA, Bhowmik A, Wedzicha JCA. Relationship between exacerbation frequency and lung function decline in chronic obstructive pulmonary disease. *Thorax* 2002; 57: 847–852.
98. Seemungal TA, Donaldson GC, Bhowmik A et al. Time course and recovery of exacerbations in patients with chronic obstructive pulmonary disease. *Am J Respir Crit Care Med* 2000; 161: 1608–1613.
99. Anthonisen NR, Skeans MA, Wise RA et al. The effects of a smoking cessation intervention on 14.5-year mortality: A randomised clinical trial. *Ann Intern Med* 2005; 142: 233–239.
100. Burge PS, Calverley PM, Jones PW et al. Randomised, double blind. Placebo controlled study of fluticasone propionate in patients with moderate to severe chronic obstructive pulmonary disease: The ISOLDE trial. *BMJ* 2000; 320: 1297–1303.
101. Lung Health Study Research Group. Effect of inhaled triamcinolone on the decline in pulmonary function in chronic obstructive pulmonary disease. *N Engl J Med* 2000; 343: 1902–1909.
102. Calverley PM, Anderson JA, Celli B et al. Salmeterol and fluticasone propionate and survival in chronic obstructive pulmonary disease. *N Engl J Med* 2007; 356: 775–789.
103. Barnes NC, Qiu YS, Pavord ID et al. Antiinflammatory effects of salmeterol/fluticasone propionate in chronic obstructive lung disease. *Am J Respir Crit Care Med* 2006; 173: 736–743.
104. Bourbeau J, Christodoulopoulos P, Maltais F et al. Effect of salmaterol/fluticasone propionate on airway inflammation in COPD: A randomised controlled trial. *Thorax* 2007; 62: 938–943.
105. Sin DD, Man SF. Corticosteroids and adrenoceptor agonists: The complements for combination therapy in chronic airways diseases. *Eur J Pharmacol* 2006; 533: 28–35.

106. Wollin L, Pieper MP. Tiotropium bromide exerts anti-inflammatory activity in a cigarette smoke mouse model of COPD. *Pulm Pharmacol Ther* 2010; 4: 345–354.
107. Pera T, Zuidhof A, Valadas J et al. Tiotropium inhibits pulmonary inflammation and remodelling in a guinea pig model of COPD. *Eur Respir J* 2011; 38: 789–796.
108. Bucher H, Duechs MJ, Tilp C et al. Tiotropium attenuates virus-induced pulmonary inflammation in cigarette smoke-exposed mice. *J Pharmacol Exp Ther* 2016; 357: 606–618.
109. Yamaya M, Nishimura H, Hatachi Y et al. Inhibitory effects of tiotropium on rhinovirus infection in human airway epithelial cells. *Eur Respir J* 2012; 40: 122–132.
110. Tashkin DP, Celli B, Senn S et al. A 4-year trial of tiotropium in chronic obstructive pulmonary disease. *N Engl J Med* 2008; 359: 1543–1554.
111. Calverley PM, Rabe KF, Goehring UM et al. Roflumilast in symptomatic chronic obstructive pulmonary disease: Two randomized clinical trials. *Lancet* 2009; 374: 685–694.
112. Fabbri LM, Calverley PM, Izquierdo-Alonso JL et al. Roflumilast in moderate-to-severe chronic obstructive pulmonary disease treated with long acting bronchodilators: Two randomised clinical trials. *Lancet* 2009; 374: 695–703.
113. Grootendorst DC, Gauw SA, Verhoosel RM et al. Reduction in sputum neutrophil and eosinophil by the PDE4 inhibitor roflumilast in patients with COPD. *Thorax* 2007; 62:1081–1087.
114. Gamble E, Grootendorst DC, Brightling CE et al. Anti-inflammatory effects of the phosphodiesterase-4 inhibitor cilomilast (Ariflo) in chronic obstructive pulmonary disease. *Am J Respir Crit Care Med* 2003; 168: 976–982.
115. Rubin BK, Henke MO. Immunomodulatory activity and effectiveness of macrolides in chronic airway disease. *Chest* 2004; 125: 70S–78S.
116. Suresh Babu K, Kastelik J, Morjaria JB. Role of long-term antibiotics in chronic respiratory diseases. *Respir Med* 2013; 107: 800–815.
117. Steel HC, Theron AJ, Cockeran R et al. Pathogen–and host-directed anti-inflammatory activities of macrolide antibiotics. *Mediators Inflamm* 2012; 2012: 584262.
118. Lutz L, Pereira DC, Paiva RM et al. Macrolides decrease the minimal inhibitory concentration of antipseudomonal agents against Pseudomonas aeruginosa from cystic fibrosis patients in biofilm. *BMC Microbiol* 2012; 12: 196.
119. Albert RK, Connett J, Bailey WC et al. Azithromycin for prevention of exacerbations of COPD. *N Engl J Med* 2011; 365: 689–698.
120. Uzun S, Djamin RS, Kluytmans JA. Azithromycin maintenance treatment in patients with frequent exacerbations of chronic obstructive pulmonary disease (COLUMBUS): A randomised, double-blind, placebo-controlled trial. *Lancet Respir Med* 2014; 2: 361–368.
121. Seemungal TA, Wilkinson TM, Hurst JR et al. Long-term erythromycin therapy is associated with decreased chronic obstructive pulmonary disease exacerbations. *Am J Respir Crit Care Med* 2008; 178: 1139–1147.
122. Djekic UV, Gaggar A, Weathington NM. Attacking the multi-tiered proteolytic pathology of COPD: New insights from basic and translational studies. *Pharmacol Ther* 2009; 121: 132–146.
123. Barnes PJ, Celli BR. Systemic manifestations and comorbidities of COPD. *Eur Respir J* 2009; 33: 1165–1185.
124. Di Francia M, Barbier D, Mege JL, Orehek J. Tumor necrosis factor-alpha levels and weight loss in chronic obstructive pulmonary disease. *Am J Respir Crit Care Med* 1994; 150: 1453–1455.
125. Takabatake N, Nakamura H, Abe S et al. The relationship between chronic hypoxemia and activation of the tumor necrosis factor-alpha system in patients with chronic obstructive pulmonary disease. *Am J Respir Crit Care Med* 2000; 161: 1179–1184.
126. Broekhuizen R, Grimble RF, Howell WM et al. Pulmonary cachexia, systemic inflammatory profile, and the interleukin 1 beta-511 single nucleotide polymorphism. *Am J Clin Nutr* 2005; 82: 1059–1064.

127. Dahl M, Vestbo J, Lange P et al. C-reactive protein as a predictor of prognosis in chronic obstructive pulmonary disease. *Am J Respir Crit Care Med* 2007; 175: 250–255.
128. Polatli M, Cakir A, Cildag O et al. Microalbuminuria, von Willebrand factor and fibrinogen levels as markers of the severity in COPD exacerbation. *J Thromb Thrombolysis* 2008; 26: 97–102.
129. Spruitt MA, Gosselink R, Troosters T et al. Muscle force during an acute exacerbation in hospitalised patients with COPD and its relationship with CXCL8 and IGF-I. *Thorax* 2003; 58: 752–756.
130. Aldonyte R, Jansson L, Piitulainen E, Janciauskiene S. Circulating monocytes from healthy individuals and COPD patients. *Respir Res* 2003; 4: 11.
131. Domagala-Kulawik J, Hoser G, Dabrowska M, Chazan R. Increased proportion of Fas positive CD8+ cells in peripheral blood of patients with COPD. *Respir Med* 2007: 101: 1338–1343.
132. Majori M, Corradi M, Caminati A et al. Predominant Th 1 cytokin pattern in peripheral blood from subjects with chronic obstructive pulmonary disease. *J Allergy Clin Immunol* 1999; 103: 458–462.
133. Maltais F. Skeletal muscles in chronic airflow obstruction: Why bother? *Am J Respir Crit Care Med* 2003; 168: 916–917.
134. Caron MA, Debigare R, Dekhuijzen PN, Maltais F. Comparative assessment of the quadriceps and the diaphragm in patients with COPD. *J Appl Physiol* 2009; 107: 952–961.
135. Marquis K, Debigare R, Lacasse Y et al. Midthigh muscle cross-sectional area is a better predictor of mortality than body mass index in patients with chronic obstructive pulmonary disease. *Am J Respir Crit Care Med* 2002; 166: 809–913.

# 7

# Pulmonary vascular diseases

ANNIE C. LAJOIE, VINCENT MAINGUY, SÉBASTIEN BONNET, and STEEVE PROVENCHER

| | |
|---|---|
| Introduction | 120 |
| Overview | 120 |
| Pulmonary hypertension | 120 |
|    Normal pulmonary hemodynamics | 120 |
|    Physiopathology of PH | 122 |
|    Pathogenesis | 124 |
|       Pulmonary arterial hypertension (Group 1) | 124 |
|       PH due to left heart disease (Group 2) | 124 |
|       PH due to lung diseases and/or hypoxia (Group 3) | 124 |
|       Chronic thromboembolic pulmonary hypertension (Group 4) | 127 |
|       PH with unclear and/or multifactorial mechanisms (Group 5) | 127 |
|    Clinical manifestations and diagnosis | 128 |
|    Treatment | 128 |
|    Prognosis | 129 |
| Pulmonary embolism | 131 |
|    Overview | 131 |
|    Pathogenesis | 131 |
|    Pathophysiology | 133 |
|    Clinical manifestations and diagnosis | 133 |
|    Prognosis and treatment | 133 |
| Pulmonary edema | 134 |
|    Overview | 134 |
|       Edema caused by increased capillary hydrostatic pressure | 135 |
|       Edema caused by the increasing capillary permeability | 135 |
|       Other types of pulmonary edema | 135 |
|    Pathophysiology | 136 |
|    Clinical manifestations and treatment | 136 |
| Pulmonary arteriovenous malformations | 137 |

Macroscopic PAVMs 137
    Overview and pathogenesis 137
    Clinical presentation 137
Microscopic arteriovenous malformations 139
    Overview and pathogenesis 139
    Pathophysiology 140
    Clinical presentation 140
Conclusion 141
References 141

## Introduction

The respiratory system receives its blood supply from two distinct circulations, the bronchial and the pulmonary circulation. The bronchial circulation, of systemic origin, supplies the trachea, the bronchi, and the visceral pleura. In presence of a bronchial disorder, these vessels increase in size and number and can be the source of significant hemoptysis. In turn, the pulmonary circulation comes in close contact with the alveoli and plays a key role in gas exchanges between air and blood. This circulation is at the origin of various pulmonary diseases. An overview of the normal pulmonary vascular physiology and the pathophysiology of common pulmonary vascular diseases such as pulmonary hypertension (PH), pulmonary embolism, pulmonary edema, and pulmonary arteriovenous malformations (PAVMs) are discussed in this chapter.

## Overview

The pulmonary arteries divide in parallel with the different bronchial subdivisions. Thus, elastic arteries (>1–2 mm in diameter), muscular arteries (100 μm to <2 mm in diameter), and arterioles (deprived of smooth muscle as they progress) succeed each other. These extra-alveolar blood vessels subsequently give rise to a vast network of capillaries that are in close contact with the alveoli (alveolar vessels). With an alveolocapillary exchange surface of 50–70 m$^2$, the pulmonary circulation accomplishes its essential role of gas exchange between blood and air. Once oxygenated, the blood then travels through the pulmonary veins to join the left atrium.

The pulmonary circulation has many important secondary functions. The small diameter of pulmonary capillaries (<10 μm) allows filtration of particles coming from the venous circulation. It also serves as a blood reservoir between the two ventricles, therefore minimizing fluctuations in pulmonary blood flow. Finally, pulmonary endothelial cells play an impressive metabolic role by inactivating or activating many circulating substances [1]. Vasoactive substances such as angiotensin I, bradykinin, serotonin, and prostaglandin $E_1$, are a few examples of compounds metabolized by the lungs.

## Pulmonary hypertension

### Normal pulmonary hemodynamics

The pulmonary circulation is a low-pressure system. In healthy subjects, the mean pulmonary artery pressure (mPAP) is around 14 ± 3 mmHg [2]. The pulmonary vascular resistance (PVR) and impedance are also low. In relating Ohm's law to fluid flow, the PVR are calculated according to the following equation:

$$PVR = (P_{PA} - P_{LA})/Q$$

where $P_{PA}$ is the mPAP, $P_{LA}$ is the mean left atrium pressure, and $Q$ is the pulmonary (right side) cardiac output. PVR can also be modeled with the *Poiseuille equation*, which describes the parameters influencing the resistance imposed to a constant laminar flow traveling through a rigid tube, according to the following equation:

$$R = (8\eta \cdot l)/(\pi \cdot r^4)$$

where $R$ represents resistance, $\eta$ is fluid viscosity, $l$ and $r$ are respectively length and radius of the tube. Therefore, minimal changes in radius greatly influence resistance. Although these models allow a simple description of the resistive characteristics of the pulmonary arteries, they have major limitations, mainly because the pulmonary arteries are a complex system of distensible branches and because blood is a non-homogenous fluid whose flow is pulsatile (Figure 7.1). Furthermore, PVR only accounts for around 50% of actual right ventricle afterload as it neglects the natural pulsatility of the pulmonary blood flow [3]. The right ventricular afterload can be evaluated by measuring the vascular impedance, which also takes into account the influence of blood flow pulsatility, pulmonary blood vessel elastance, and the reflected wave [4,5].

In the healthy subject, the pulmonary microcirculation accounts for most of PVR. Alveolar hypoxia is the most powerful inducer of arteriolar vasoconstriction [6]. This reaction is potentiated by an increase in plasma $H^+$ concentration or partial pressure of carbon dioxide [7,8]. PVR is also affected by blood viscosity, pleural pressure, and lung volume (Figure 7.2) [9]. PVR decreases with increasing cardiac output due to distension and recruitment of previously less solicited pulmonary vessels.

Finally, many vasoactive mediators are involved in vasoconstriction (e.g., serotonin, endothelin, norepinephrine, thromboxane, angiotensin-II, and histamine) and vasodilation (e.g., nitric oxide, prostaglandin $I_2$ and $E_2$, and bradykinin) of the pulmonary blood vessels [10]. The autonomic nervous system seems to play a limited role in PVR regulation.

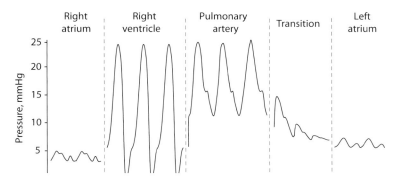

Figure 7.1 Vascular pressure waves measured at the different levels of the pulmonary circulation. The average pressure is generally 2–8, 12–15, and 5–12 mmHg in the right atrium, pulmonary artery, and left atrium, respectively. As compared to right ventricular pressure, the pulmonary artery pressure remains between 5–12 mmHg during diastole because of the pulmonary valve. Inversely, the right ventricular diastolic pressure approaches 0 mmHg. The left atrial pressure can be estimated with the right heart catheterization by measuring the "wedge" or occlusion pressure, which approximates the left atrial pressure in the absence of pathologies affecting venous return. The "real" capillary pressure is intermediate between the diastolic pulmonary artery pressure and the "wedge" or occlusion pressure. Because of the compliance of the elastic pulmonary arteries, the pulsatility of pulmonary blood flow progressively flattens to become a constant flow as it reaches the capillary circulation.

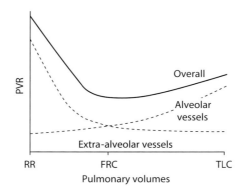

**Figure 7.2** Influence of lung volumes on pulmonary vascular resistance (PVR). PVR increases when lung volumes decrease from functional residual capacity (FRC) to residual volume (RV) as a result of the compression of extra-alveolar blood vessels by positive pleural pressure. A similar increase in PVR is seen with passage from the FRC to total lung capacity (TLC) since alveolar distension then compresses alveolar blood vessels. Thus, PVR is at its lowest value at FRC.

## Physiopathology of PH

The pulmonary artery pressure can be calculated using the following equation [11]:

$$P_{PA} = (Q \times PVR) + PCWP$$

where the pulmonary capillary wedge pressure (PCWP) serves as an estimate of left atrial pressure. It represents a linear ($y = ax + b$) type relation over a physiologic range of cardiac output (Figure 7.3). Thus, PH may result from either an increase in cardiac output, in left atrial pressure or in PVR or a combination of these factors. An isolated increase in cardiac output or left atrial pressure usually has limited effects on pulmonary artery pressure because the pulmonary vascular bed is able to vasodilate and to recruit vessels. Conversely, conditions decreasing the vascular surface result in a disproportionate increase in PVR (Figure 7.4).

PH is defined as a persistent elevation in mPAP of more than 25 mmHg at rest [11]. PH may initially be present only when cardiac output rises, such as during exercise (Figure 7.3). Importantly, PH was also traditionally defined as mPAP of more than 30 mmHg during exercise. This definition was recently abandoned since mPAP during exercise is age related, frequently exceeding 30 mmHg in individuals Changer > 50 years old pour : more than 50 years old. [2]. More recent studies proposed new criteria for exercise-induced PH, which remain to be validated [14,15].

The right ventricle is a thin-walled structure acting mainly as a volume generator. It is very sensitive to any constraints to the expulsion of blood from the right ventricle to the pulmonary circulation (afterload). Therefore, its function can be impaired even when PVR are only marginally increased [16]. The right ventricle partly compensates for this excessive work by increasing its preload. Further stretching of its muscular fibers during diastole will, in turn, result in a greater tension during the subsequent systole. Nevertheless, the initial increase in right ventricular contractility will be insufficient to face the increased afterload, leading to right ventricular–pulmonary artery uncoupling [17]. Eventually, the ejection volume will be reduced and increasing the heart rate eventually becomes the only way to maintain a decent cardiac output, especially during exercise [18,19]. Since both ventricles operate in series, any right heart dysfunction causes a significant decrease in left ventricular preload. The right ventricle's pressure overload eventually causes the interventricular septum to adopt a rectilinear shape or even to present an end-systolic leftward shift [4]. Inside a rather nondistensible pericardium, the right ventricular expansion compromises the left ventricular compliance. These alterations lead to a reduced cardiac output and eventually to a drop in systemic blood pressure which, in turn, will decrease

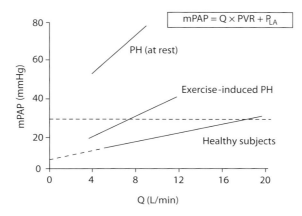

Figure 7.3 Relationship between mean pulmonary artery pressure (mPAP) and cardiac output (Q). The relationship between mPAP and Q is linear within a physiologic range of cardiac output. Their relationship can then be characterized by a linear equation of the $y = ax + b$ type equation. The opening pressure corresponds to the extrapolation of the slope (dotted line) at zero cardiac output. In the supine healthy subject, the opening pressure is comparable to the left atrial pressure. Therefore, any increase in cardiac output, left atrial pressure or PVR engenders elevation of pulmonary artery pressure. However, the healthy subject sees minimal elevation in mPAP during exercise despite *increase in cardiac output* and left atrial pressure as PVR decreases. Significant increases in mPAP are seldom observed in athletes performing intense exercise when they achieve extreme levels of cardiac output. Conversely, up to 50% of healthy elderly patients experience mPAP >30 mmHg during mild-to-moderate exercise, presumably due to significant elevation in left atrial pressure. Patients suffering from pulmonary hypertension (PH) have an abnormally elevated mPAP at rest and show a disproportionate increase in mPAP during exercise. During the preclinical stage of the disease, it is believed that resting mPAP remains within the normal range (<25 mmHg) but significantly increases during exercise, reflecting the loss of the ability to modulate PVR during exertion [12,13].

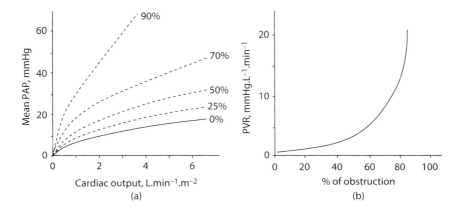

Figure 7.4 **(a)** Relationship between mPAP and cardiac output according to the degree of pulmonary circulation obstruction. **(b)** Relationship between PVR and the degree of pulmonary circulation obstruction. PVR shows little augmentation with vascular obstruction of less than 50%. This is due to recruitment and distension of the residual vascular bed, thus limiting PAP and PVR elevations. The relationship between PVR and obstruction is therefore hyperbolic, as previously described following pulmonary embolism. This relationship is likely applicable physiologically to PH. (From Azarian, R. et al., *J Nucl Med.*, 38, 980–983, 1997; Piazza, G, Goldhaber, SZ., *Circulation.*, 114, e28–e32, 2006).

myocardic perfusion and further decrease cardiac reserve [20]. When the increase in afterload is gradual and sustained, the right ventricle compensates by becoming hypertrophic, a phenomenon that allows it to increase its contractility while reducing its wall tension [21]. Eventually, the rise in right ventricular afterload engenders right heart failure, which becomes symptomatic and eventually leads to death [22]. More recently, however, right ventricular-specific defects have been described, including disorders of angiogenesis [23], metabolism [24], adrenergic signaling, sex hormones [25–27], and genetics and epigenetics [28].

## Pathogenesis

The causes of PH are multiple. Over the years, a new classification was proposed, subdividing them according to the physiopathology, clinical presentation, and therapeutic approach (Table 7.1, Figures 7.5 and 7.6) [29].

### Pulmonary arterial hypertension (Group 1)

Pulmonary arterial hypertension (PAH) is characterized by a progressive increase in resistance to blood flow engendered by the conjugated effects of vasoconstriction, pulmonary blood vessels remodeling, and *in situ* thrombosis (Figure 7.7) [30]. The underlying physiopathology of the disease remains poorly understood. This group of PH includes different entities such as idiopathic pulmonary hypertension (IPAH), hereditary PAH (HPAH), PAH associated with drugs and toxins, as well as associated pulmonary arterial hypertension (APAH) including connective tissue disease, congenital heart diseases, HIV, portopulmonary hypertension, and others. A germline mutation in the gene encoding a type II receptor of the *TGF-β* superfamily (*Bone Morphogenic Protein Receptor II or BMPR2*) is identified in 75% of familial PAH and 10%–30% of "sporadic" PAH [31–34]. These mutations are rarely observed in other forms of PAH. However, BMPR2 expression is reduced even in the absence of mutations [35]. More recently, other mutations associated with HPAH were identified, including activin-like receptor kinase-1 (ALK1), endoglin (ENG), *mothers against decapentaplegic 9 (Smad 9)*, and the potassium channel subfamily K member 3 (KCNK3) [34,36]. Nevertheless, other genes could be involved, possibly from the BMP/*TGF-β* pathway, which plays an important role in regulating pulmonary vasculature. Since the penetrance of the mutations remains low (10%–30%), the development of PAH probably requires a genetic predisposition coupled with certain risk factors. Nongenetic abnormalities are also involved in the progression of disease (Table 7.2) [30].

### PH due to left heart disease (Group 2)

Due to the chronically increased pressure in the left heart cavities, left heart disease can lead to PH (Figure 7.5). The transpulmonary pressure gradient (TPG, i.e., the difference between mPAP and PCWP) is commonly used to distinguish "passive" (TPG <12 mmHg) from "reactive" PH (TPG >12 mm Hg). However, the TPG is influenced by cardiac output, resistance, and the left heart filling pressures [37]. In contrast, diastolic pulmonary artery pressure is less influenced by PAWP than systolic and mPAP, likely explained by a lower sensitivity to vessel distensibility [37,38]. In case of isolated "postcapillary" PH, there is a passive elevation of pulmonary arterial pressure so that PCWP is increased (>15 mmHg) and the diastolic pressure gradient is <7 mmHg. When, in some cases, this chronic PH is complicated by an arteriolar vasculopathy leading to progressive increase in PVR, PH ultimately becomes partly "precapillary," which is generally irreversible, even with normalization in left heart pressures [39,40]. A "combined postcapillary PH and precapillary PH" is defined as a PCWP >15 mmHg and a diastolic pressure gradient is >7 mmHg.

### PH due to lung diseases and/or hypoxia (Group 3)

PH is a common complication of severe chronic respiratory diseases [41,42]. The effect of chronic hypoxia on vascular remodeling is the cornerstone of the disease. However, the intensity of vascular remodeling is variable according to certain genetic polymorphisms [43]. Vascular bed scarcity, as seen in emphysema, and to a lesser extent hypercapnia and blood viscosity also contribute to pathophysiology PH due to lung disease and/or hypoxia [44].

Table 7.1 Clinical classification of pulmonary hypertension

**1. PAH**
- 1.1 Idiopathic (formerly known as primary pulmonary hypertension)
- 1.2 Heritable
  - 1.2.1 Associated with *BMPR2* gene mutation
  - 1.2.2 Associated with *ALK1(ACVRL1)*, *endoglin* (with or without hereditary hemorrhagic telangiectasia), *SMAD9*, *CAV1*, or *KCNK3* gene mutation
  - 1.2.3 Unknown mutation
- 1.3 Drug and toxins induced
- 1.4 Associated with (also known as APAH):
  - 1.4.1 Connective tissue disease
  - 1.4.2 HIV infection
  - 1.4.3 Portal hypertension
  - 1.4.4 Congenital heart disease
  - 1.4.5 Schistosomiasis
- 1′ Pulmonary veno-occlusive disease and/or pulmonary capillary hemangiomatosis
- 1″ PPHN

**2. Pulmonary hypertension due to left heart disease**
- 2.1 Systolic dysfunction
- 2.2 Diastolic dysfunction
- 2.3 Left heart valvular disease
- 2.4 Congenital/acquired left heart inflow/outflow tract obstruction and congenital cardiomyopathy

**3. Pulmonary hypertension due to lung diseases and/or hypoxia**
- 3.1 Chronic obstructive pulmonary disease
- 3.2 Interstitial lung disease
- 3.3 Other pulmonary diseases with mixed restrictive and obstructive pattern
- 3.4 Sleep-disordered breathing
- 3.5 Alveolar hypoventilation disorders
- 3.6 Chronic exposure to high altitude
- 3.7 Developmental lung diseases

**4. Chronic thromboembolic pulmonary hypertension (CTEPH)**

**5. Pulmonary hypertension with unclear and/or multifactorial mechanisms**
- 5.1 Hematological disorders: chronic hemolytic anemia, myeloproliferative disorders, and splenectomy
- 5.2 Systemic disorders: sarcoidosis, pulmonary histiocytosis, and lymphangioleiomyomatosis
- 5.3 Metabolic disorders: glycogen storage disease, Gaucher disease, and thyroid disorders
- 5.4 Others: tumoral obstruction, fibrosing mediastinitis, chronic renal failure, and segmental PH

*Source:* Adapted from Simonneau, G. et al., *J Am Coll Cardiol.*, 62, D34–D41, 2013.
Updated classification of the 4th World Symposium in Dana Point 2008.
APAH, associated pulmonary arterial hypertension; CTEPH, chronic thromboembolic pulmonary hypertension; PAH, pulmonary arterial hypertension; PH, pulmonary hypertension; PPHN, persistent pulmonary hypertension of the newborn.

126 Pulmonary vascular diseases

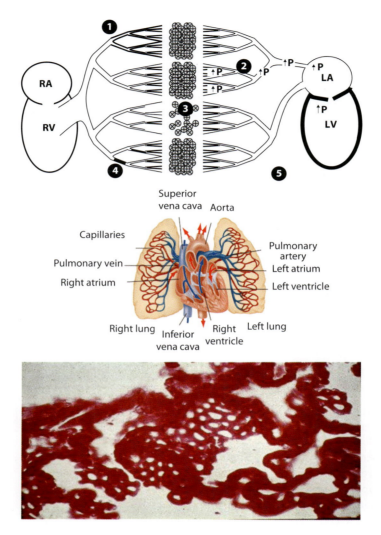

Figure 7.5 Schematic representation of the pulmonary circulation and the different types of PH. Blood ejected during each systole from the right ventricle travels through the pulmonary arteries. The diameter of the arteries progressively diminishes as it reaches the capillaries where blood will ultimately be oxygenated. Blood then accesses the left heart cavities through the pulmonary veins and gains the systemic circulation to eventually repeat the cycle. In pulmonary arterial hypertension (PAH—group 1), the arterioles become progressively narrower, leading to increased PVR. These anomalies are widespread and relatively uniform throughout the lungs. PVR is also increased in PH due to lung diseases or chronic hypoxia (group 3) and chronic thromboembolic disease (group 4). This is largely due to the vascular rarefaction, such as in emphysema, or occlusion of the pulmonary vascular bed by organized thrombi. Although these anomalies are heterogeneous throughout the lungs, diffuse arteriolar remodeling is frequently encountered. PH due to left heart disease (group 2) results from elevated left heart pressures which is, in turn, passively transmitted to the pulmonary venules and eventually the capillaries and pulmonary arteries (i.e., "isolated postcapillary" PH). In some instances, PH ultimately becomes partly "precapillary" (i.e., "combined postcapillary and precapillary PH") due to a reactive process not well understood. Finally, group 5 regroups PH due to multiples or unknown mechanisms. LA: left atrium; LV: left ventricle; P, pressure; RA, Right atrium; RV, right ventricle.

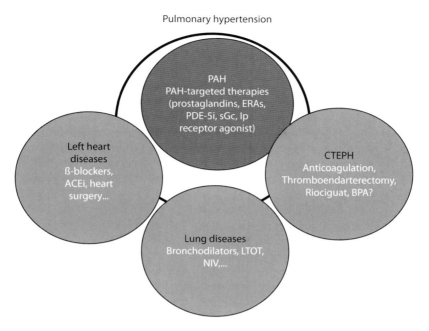

Figure 7.6 Principal categories of PH and their respective treatments. In addition to PAH, a substantial proportion of patients with left heart or chronic respiratory diseases as well as certain patients with previous pulmonary embolism will develop PH. Different therapies that specifically target endothelial dysfunction are used in PAH. Some therapies are aimed at reducing the loss of cyclic adenosine monophosphate (AMP) (such as prostaglandin analogues and selective IP prostacyclin-receptor agonist), some prevent the metabolism of cyclic GMP (phosphodiesterase type 5 inhibitors and soluble guanylate cyclase stimulators) and others block the effects of endothelin-1 (endothelin receptor antagonists). In PH secondary to left heart disease or lung disease, treatment is directed at resolving the underlying cause. In chronic thromboembolic disease, when residual thrombi are proximal, they can be evacuated with thromboendarterectomy. In inoperable cases, vasoactive therapy (Riociguat) should be considered. ACEi, angiotensin-converting-enzyme inhibitors; BPA, balloon pulmonary angioplasty; CTEPH, chronic thromboembolic pulmonary hypertension; ERA, endothelin receptor antagonist; NIV: non invasive ventilation; PAH, pulmonary arterial hypertension; PDE-5i, phosphodiesterase type 5 inhibitors; LTOT, Long-term oxygen therapy; sGc, soluble guanylate cyclase stimulators.

### Chronic thromboembolic pulmonary hypertension (Group 4)

Following a pulmonary embolism, numerous patients have persistent thrombi that eventually become organized and obstruct the part of pulmonary blood vessels [45,46]. In some of these patients, the organized material will be sufficient to be hemodynamically significant. In addition, an arteriolar vasculopathy similar to that of PAH may eventually develop in the nonoccluded blood vessels (Figure 7.7) [47,12]. Consequently, between 0.8% and 3.8% of patients acute pulmonary embolism will develop PH in the years following pulmonary embolism [48,49].

### PH with unclear and/or multifactorial mechanisms (Group 5)

Certain diseases are associated with a direct infringement upon the pulmonary circulation. For example, a granulomatous or histiocytosis cellular infiltration can be seen in the pulmonary arterioles of patients with sarcoidosis or Langerhans cell histiocytosis, respectively.

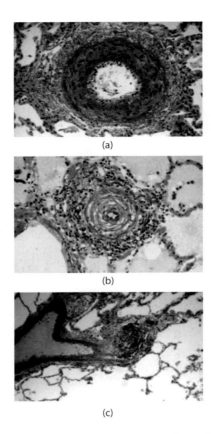

Figure 7.7 The histologic changes seen in PAH. Vascular remodeling affects every layer of the small pulmonary blood vessels. **(a)** Intimal and medial hypertrophy (enlarged X200). **(b)** Concentric lamellar intimal fibrosis (enlarged X200). **(c)** Plexiform lesions. Other changes are sometimes observed and consist of vascular dilatation, *in situ* thrombosis, arteritis, and fibrinoid necrosis.

## Clinical manifestations and diagnosis

PH should be suspected in the presence of dyspnea and/or exercise intolerance, especially when the patient suffers from diseases known to be associated with PH (Table 7.1). An isolated reduction in diffusion capacity of the lung for carbon monoxide (D$_L$CO) is frequently observed on pulmonary function tests. Less frequently, a discrete obstructive and/or restrictive syndrome can be encountered [50]. Symptoms disproportionate to the severity of the underlying cardiac or respiratory disease should also elicit suspicion of secondary PH. Pulmonary arterial pressure can be estimated by cardiac echography. However, the final diagnosis is confirmed by right heart catheterization. A systematic diagnostic approach to PH is detailed in Figure 7.8 [11].

## Treatment

The type of PH will dictate its treatment (Figure 7.6). In patients with PAH (group 1), the treatment will include general and supportive measures, such as diuretics and long-term oxygen therapy for hypoxemic patients. The role of anticoagulation remains controversial. Acute vasoreactivity testing will be initially

Table 7.2 Examples of nongenetic anomalies involved in the pathogenesis and/or progression of pulmonary arterial hypertension

| Anomalies | Consequences |
| --- | --- |
| Endothelial dysfunction | Vasoconstriction and cellular proliferation is favored by deficits in cAMP and cGMP and elevation in endothelin-1 levels. |
| Underexpression of smooth muscle potassium channels | Favors proliferation and contraction of smooth muscle cells. |
| Metabolic shift and cancer-like phenotype of pulmonary artery smooth muscle cells | Pro-proliferative and antiapoptotic phenotype of pulmonary artery smooth muscle cells contributing to pulmonary artery obliteration. |
| Inflammatory anomalies | Elevation of serum IL-1 and IL-6 levels, circulating autoantibodies (in 10%–40% of patients), inflammatory infiltration of plexiform lesions, overexpression of endothelial chemokines. |
| Platelet dysfunction | Activated platelets liberate many factors, such as thromboxane A2, *PDGF*, serotonin, *TGF-ß*, and *VEGF*, therefore predisposing to *in situ* thrombosis, vasoconstriction and cellular proliferation. |

Source: Tuder, R.M. et al., *J Am Coll Cardiol.*, 62, D4–D12, 2013.
cAMP, cyclic adenosine monophosphate; cGMP, cyclic guanosine monophosphate; PDGF, platelet-derived growth factor; TGF-ß, transforming growth factor beta; VEGF, vascular endothelial growth factor.

performed in idiopathic PAH patients to identify the small proportion of patients who may respond to long-term calcium channel blockers. The majority of patients, however, will be nonresponders [51]. Over the last two decades, several drugs targeting the endothelial dysfunction that characterizes PAH were developed and commercialized [52]. A meta-analysis confirmed that PAH-targeted monotherapy reduced short-term mortality as compared to placebo [53]. More recently, a second meta-analysis confirmed that upfront or sequential combination therapy significantly reduced the risk of clinical worsening compared to monotherapy alone, supporting the changing treatment paradigm of PAH [54]. While endothelial dysfunction, pulmonary vascular remodeling, and vasoconstriction are also observed in PH due to left heart (group 2) and lung (group 3) diseases, randomized clinical trials demonstrated that PAH-targeted therapies are either ineffective or even deleterious for these patients [55–60]. In patients with chronic thromboembolic pulmonary hypertension (CTEPH—group 4), pulmonary endarterectomy, a major surgery during which the chronic embolic material is removed from the pulmonary arteries, remains the standard treatment for patients when this material is deemed surgically accessible [45]. In inoperable cases or for patients with persistent PH despite surgery, an oral medication (riociguat) has been shown to improve patients' symptoms and exercise capacity [61]. In the future, balloon pulmonary angioplasty may also prove to be effective in inoperable cases [62,63].

# Prognosis

The occurrence of PH is an independent factor of poor prognosis when it occurs in patients with left heart [64–70] or lung diseases [41,71–75]. Long-term outcomes are also poor for inoperable CTEPH [76,77]. Nonetheless, it is PAH that carries the worst prognosis. Indeed, without PAH-targeted treatments, the median survival in PAH is less than 3 years [22]. Currently available PAH-targeted treatments have significantly improved patients' survival, although long-term outcomes remain limited with a mortality rate of 15% per year for incident idiopathic PAH [78,79].

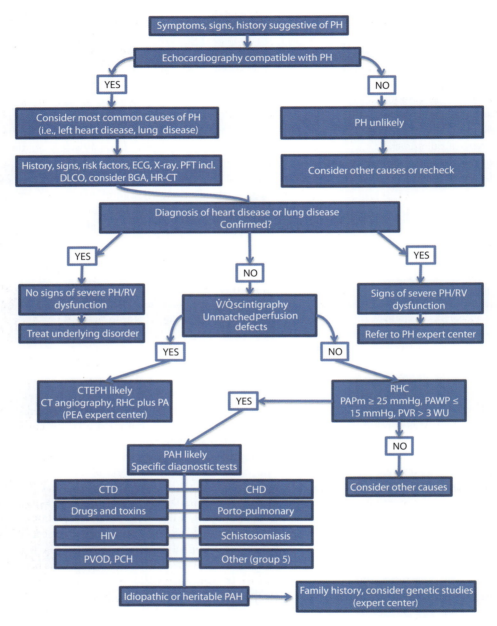

Figure 7.8 Diagnosis of PH. BGA, blood gas analysis; ECG, electrocardiogram; CHD, congenital heart disease; CTD, connective tissue disease; CTEPH, chronic thromboembolic pulmonary hypertension; DLCO, diffusion capacity of the lung for carbon monoxide; HIV, human immunodeficiency virus; HR-CT, high resolution computed tomography; PA, pulmonary angiography; PAH, pulmonary arterial hypertension; mPAP, mean pulmonary artery pressure; PAWP, pulmonary arterial wedge pressure; PCH, pulmonary capillary hemangiomatosis; PFT, pulmonary function tests; PH, pulmonary hypertension; PVOD, pulmonary veno-occlusive disease; PVR, pulmonary vascular resistance; RHC, right heart catheter; RV, right ventricle; V/Q, ventilation/perfusion; WU, woods unit. (Adapted from Hoeper, M.M. et al., *J Am Coll Cardiol.*, 62, D42–D50, 2013.)

# Pulmonary embolism

## Overview

Pulmonary embolism is defined as the sudden obstruction of pulmonary blood flow by material driven by the bloodstream into the pulmonary vessels. There are many types of substances that can result in pulmonary embolism: blood clots, fat, gas, amniotic fluid, tumors, septic, foreign bodies (e.g., contaminants found in intravenous drugs), and parasites (e.g., schistosomiasis). In developed countries, the embolism of blood clots remains the most common.

## Pathogenesis

The vast majority of pulmonary embolism result from the detachment of a thrombus previously formed in the lower extremities following a deep vein thrombosis. Other origins include the pelvic region and less commonly the upper limbs or the right heart chambers. Pulmonary embolism and deep vein thrombosis are two manifestations of thromboembolic disease. Blood stasis, hypercoagulability, and endothelial dysfunction are classic risk factors of deep vein thrombosis and constitute the Virchow triad first described in 1856 [13]. Coagulation is the result of a complex cascade of chain reactions using multiple coagulation factors, most of which are inhibited by anticoagulant factors as illustrated in Figure 7.9 [80,81]. Perturbations in the delicate balance between pro-coagulant and anticoagulant factors lead to hypercoagulability, which can be congenital or acquired as in the context of cancer, congestive heart failure, or pregnancy (Table 7.3).

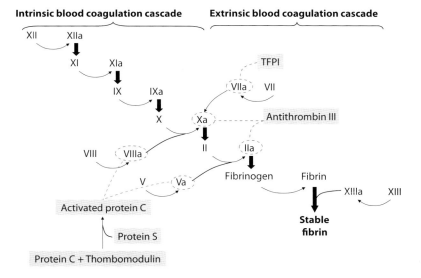

Figure 7.9 Coagulation cascade. Coagulation results from a succession of chained reactions between different coagulation factors. Activated factors then catalyze the subsequent reaction and therefore produce more and more factors as the cascade unveils. Two key coagulation complexes initiate the process of coagulation: the intrinsic and extrinsic blood coagulation cascades. Importantly, coagulation factors are counterbalanced by anticoagulant factors (gray boxes). These factors inhibit specific coagulation factors (dotted line). Tight balance between pro- and anticoagulant factors allows an adequate control of the coagulation system, enabling creation of fibrin clots to prevent further bleeding, while avoiding excessive thrombosis. a, activated factor; TFPI, tissue factor pathway inhibitor. (From Margaglione, M. et al., *Ann Intern Med.*, 129, 89–93, 1998; Koster, T. et al., *Lancet.*, 345, 152–155, 1995.).

Table 7.3 Nonexhaustive list of inherited and acquired thrombophilia predisposing to thromboembolic disease

## Thrombophilia

| Inherited | Prevalence (%)[a] | Risk ratio[a] |
|---|---|---|
| Factor V Leiden mutation | | |
| • Heterozygotes | 3–7 | 7 |
| • Homozygotes | | 80 |
| Prothrombin gene mutation 20210A | 2–2.5 | 2–5 |
| Antithrombin deficiency | 0.02–0.1 | 5–50 |
| Protein C deficiency | 0.2–0.5 | 5–12 |
| Protein S deficiency | 0.1 | 4–11 |
| Hyperhomocysteinemia (*MTHFR* mutation) | | 2.5 |
| Dysfibrinogenemia | low | ? |
| Increase in coagulation factors VIII and XI | | ? |
| Factor XII deficiency | low | ? |
| Heparin cofactor II deficiency | low | ? |
| Fibrinolysis anomalies | low | ? |
| • Plasminogen activator inhibitor (PAI) deficiency | | |
| • α1-antiplasmin deficiency | | |
| • Plasminogen deficiency | | |
| Sticky platelet syndrome | low | ? |

*Acquired*
Age
Solid malignancy
Myeloproliferative or lymphoproliferative syndromes
Hyperviscosity syndromes (e.g., multiple myeloma)
Falciform anemia
Antiphospholipid antibodies
Nephrotic syndrome[b]
Congestive cardiac insufficiency
Hyperhomocysteinemia
Oral contraceptive or hormonotherapy
Pregnancy[c]
Prolonged immobilization
Trauma, surgery, or recent hospitalization
Acute infection
Immobilization (long trips in plane or automobile)
Foreign body/endovascular catheter
Smoking
Obesity

*Source:* Margaglione, M. et al., *Ann Intern Med.*, 129, 89–93, 1998; Koster, T. et al., *Lancet.*, 345, 152–155, 1995.

[a] Prevalence of congenital thrombophilia in the general population. Many epidemiology studies have reported a variable, and sometimes contradictory, prevalence and risk ratio. Therefore, these are approximate values and some prevalence and risk ratio are misunderstood.

[b] The nephrotic syndrome is associated with the loss of plasmatic proteins, such as protein C, protein S, and antithrombin III, in the urine.

[c] Pregnancy is associated with increased venous stasis and numerous coagulation abnormalities, including acquired protein C resistance. There is also modification of factor V, factor VIII, von Willebrand factor, fibrinogen, and protein S. *MTHFR*, methylenetetrahydrofolate reductase enzyme; PAI, plaminogen activator inhibitor.

## Pathophysiology

Pulmonary embolism reduces the pulmonary vascular surface in proportion to the importance of the obstruction caused by the clots (Figure 7.4) [12,82,83]. The consequences of pulmonary embolism on PVR and right ventricular function are similar to those resulting from PH [20,84]. However, acute increase in afterload leaves no time for the right ventricle to compensate with ventricular hypertrophy and therefore limits its ability to propel blood flow into the pulmonary circulation. Indeed, during an acute increase in afterload, the mPAP seldom reaches more than 30 mmHg [20,84]. The severity of pulmonary embolism depends primarily on the degree of pulmonary arterial obstruction and the ability of the heart to overcome such resistance.

Pulmonary embolism is also associated with gas exchange anomalies. The majority of patients have hypoxemia and/or hypocapnia [85]. Hypoxemia results from ventilation–perfusion abnormalities. Poorly ventilated areas will receive better perfusion mainly because of pulmonary blood flow redistribution from obstructed area to intact areas, lowering the $\dot{V}/\dot{Q}$ ratio (physiologic shunt), and also because of a reflex increase in bronchial tone (hypocapnic bronchoconstriction) [86]. This phenomenon is aggravated by inhibition of pulmonary hypoxic vasoconstriction induced by pulmonary embolism [87]. A reduction in cardiac output resulting in a decrease in venous oxygen pressure also contributes to this hypoxemia [88]. Finally, pulmonary embolism may result in cardiac right-to-left shunt through a patent foramen ovale. The mechanisms leading to hypocapnia in pulmonary embolism remain partly unknown.

## Clinical manifestations and diagnosis

The incidence of venous thromboembolism is about one case per 1000 [89]. Pulmonary embolism is largely underdiagnosed, the diagnosis being established postmortem in 70% of patients who died from pulmonary embolism. Small emboli usually lodge in pulmonary arteries of small caliber and lead to pulmonary infarction. Patients are then likely to experience pleuritic chest pain and hemoptysis. Pulmonary embolism occluding larger pulmonary arteries will usually cause isolated acute or subacute dyspnea [90]. Right ventricular dysfunction with distension and hypokinesia of its lateral wall occurs in about 30%–40% of cases [91]. Finally, about 5% of patients will present hypotension or shock. The other possible signs and symptoms include syncope, hyperthermia, tachycardia, pleural rub, jugular vein distension, and symptoms of deep vein thrombosis. Chest radiography is often normal.

In North America and Europe, most cases of pulmonary embolism are now diagnosed using computed tomography pulmonary angiogram (Figure 7.10) [92]. The diagnosis can also be made when there is a mismatch between perfusion (markedly decreased or absent) and ventilation (normal) on ventilation–perfusion lung scan. Conventional pulmonary angiography, previously recognized as the gold standard for the diagnosis of pulmonary embolism, is invasive and now infrequently performed [13,93]. The diagnosis algorithm will be influenced by the clinical presentation, pretest probability, presence of underlying lung disease, relative contraindications to specific tests (e.g., iodine allergy, renal insufficiency), as well as test availability and local expertise.

## Prognosis and treatment

Mortality from pulmonary embolism is low in the absence of right ventricular dysfunction (<3%), compared to patients with cardiac dysfunction (5%–10%) or shock (25%–30%) [91]. Deaths occur mainly in the early hours of the disease. Risk stratification at the time of diagnosis can be assessed using prediction models (e.g., the simplified Pulmonary Embolism Severity Index) and evidence of right ventricular strain or injury on EKG, echocardiography, computed tomography pulmonary angiogram, and serum biomarkers (e.g., troponin, natriuretic peptide) [94].

Treatment was traditionally initiated with unfractionned heparin or low molecular weight heparin, followed by long-term oral anticoagulation with vitamin K antagonists. Nowadays, nonvitamin K antagonist

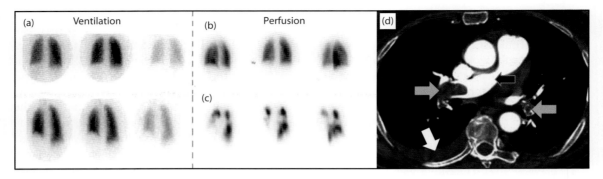

Figure 7.10 Complementary investigation for the diagnosis of pulmonary embolism. During ventilation/perfusion scan, the patient inhales a marked gas (usually Xenon[133]). **(a)** This enables, by observation of the topography of radioactivity, the visualization of the ventilated zones. **(b)** Secondly, albumin aggregates marked with technetium[99m] are injected. Because of their 10–150 μm diameter, the aggregates embolize in the pulmonary capillaries. **(c)** Therefore, this exam can demonstrate well ventilated but non-perfused areas, called a ventilation–perfusion mismatch, which is diagnostic for pulmonary embolism. **(d)** Pulmonary arteries (black arrows) and eventually pulmonary embolism (gray arrows) can be visualized on the contrast enhanced computed tomography pulmonary angiogram. It can also unmask secondary anomalies, such as pleural effusion due to pulmonary embolism (white arrow). Its realization necessitates infusion of contrast product (iodine).

oral anticoagulants (NOAC) including dabigatran, rivaroxaban, apixaban, or edoxaban are now recommended for most patients [95]. The treatment goal is to prevent the progression and formation of new thrombi while endogenous fibrinolysis degrades the clots already formed. Thrombolytic agents are used exclusively in patients with acute hemodynamic instability. Optimal duration of anticoagulation depends on the risk of recurrent disease as well as the risk of bleeding under anticoagulation [95]. In patients with temporary risk factors (e.g., recent surgery, see Table 7.3), 3 months of anticoagulation is generally recommended [95]. In contrast, patients with idiopathic pulmonary embolism, extended anticoagulant therapy (no scheduled stop date) is most commonly recommended in patients at low risk of bleeding, especially those at increased risk of recurrence (e.g., males).

In the days following treatment initiation, there is a rapid degradation of clots. Nevertheless, persistent perfusion defects are observed in 30%–50% of patients after 3–6 months of therapeutic anticoagulation [96,97]. In a minority of patients, these defects will be sufficient to lead to CTEPH [45,46].

## Pulmonary edema

### Overview

Pulmonary edema is defined as the accumulation of fluid in the extravascular tissue of the lung. Hundreds of milliliters of liquid pass through the pulmonary interstitium daily. This fluid movement is a function of hydrostatic and oncotic pressures, as described by the Starling's equation:

$$Q = K_f \left[ (P_c - P_i) - \sigma(\pi_c - \pi_i) \right]$$

where $Q$ represents the net flow of liquid driven out of the capillary, $K_f$ is the filtration coefficient, $P_c$ and $P_i$ are the capillary and interstitial fluid hydrostatic pressure, $\pi_c$ and $\pi_i$ are the capillary and interstitial fluid oncotic pressure, and $\sigma$ is the reflection coefficient, which reflects the ability of the alveolar–capillary membrane to prevent diffusion of proteins. Thus, pulmonary edema occurs when there is a net flow of liquid toward the interstitial space that exceeds its absorption capacity (Table 7.4) [98].

Table 7.4 Pathogenesis of pulmonary edema and potential causes according to mechanisms

| Mechanisms | Potential causes |
| --- | --- |
| Increase in capillary hydrostatic pressure[a] | Myocardial infarction, mitral or aortic stenosis, systolic or diastolic dysfunction of the left ventricle, and volume overload |
| | Rarely, capillary pressure elevation is attributable to specific venous disease such as compression or veno-occlusive disease |
| Increase in capillary permeability[a] | Pulmonary or extrapulmonary infections, pancreatitis, aspiration, toxic fumes inhalation, radiotherapy, pulmonary contusion, hypoperfusion resulting from shock, metabolic disturbances, blood transfusion, medication, and heat stroke |
| Decrease in capillary oncotic pressure[a] | Hypoproteinemia |
| Lymphatic insufficiency[a] | Lymph node invasion |
| Reduction in interstitial hydrostatic pressure[b] | Rapid pulmonary expansion after evacuating pleural effusion or pneumothorax |

Source: Suzuki, S. et al., Chest., 101, 275–276, 1992.
[a] While reduction in capillary oncotic pressure or lymphatic insufficiency predispose to pulmonary edema in presence of elevated hydrostatic pressure, they rarely cause by themselves pulmonary edema.
[b] The physiopathology of reexpansion edema seems to be more complex than the isolated diminution in interstitial hydrostatic pressure. Enhanced capillary permeability resulting from an inflammatory reaction could be superimposed.

### Edema caused by increased capillary hydrostatic pressure

Edema resulting from increased capillary hydrostatic pressure is by far the most common. It results from an increase in pulmonary venous and/or left heart pressures (Table 7.4). It evolves in two stages. Indeed, a peribronchial and perivascular tissue congestion, also called the interstitial stage, is generally followed by the alveolar stage where there is abundant liquid filling the alveoli. The occurrence of pulmonary edema depends on capillary hydrostatic pressure, vessel permeability, and rapidity of these changes (Figure 7.11). Pulmonary edema is prevented by protective mechanisms limiting the pressure gradient between the capillary and interstitium. First, pulmonary lymphatic vessels can increase their capacity to clear excessive interstitial fluid tenfold. Furthermore, fluid accumulation increases hydrostatic pressure and reduces oncotic pressure by diluting proteins within the interstitium [99].

### Edema caused by the increasing capillary permeability

The effect of hydrostatic pressure is potentiated by an increase in capillary membrane permeability (Figure 7.11). Proteins can then cross the vascular wall and reduce the difference in oncotic pressure between either sides of the membrane. This type of edema occurs in a variety of conditions (Table 7.4) and is called, in its most severe form, "acute respiratory distress syndrome" (ARDS). Within the first 7–10 days, an exudative phase takes place. It is marked by histological changes, such as the formation of hyaline membranes composed of precipitated plasma proteins, fibrin, and necrotic debris. This phase is followed by a proliferative phase characterized by extensive alveolar and interstitial remodeling.

### Other types of pulmonary edema

Rarely, pulmonary edema results from a reduction in capillary oncotic pressure, interstitial hydrostatic pressure, or lymphatic drainage (Table 7.4).

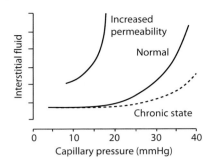

Figure 7.11 Relationship between quantity of interstitial liquid and capillary pressure. In the healthy subject, interstitial fluid starts accumulating when the capillary pressure reaches 18–20 mmHg. At that stage, interstitial fluid accumulation is exponential. In the presence of increased capillary permeability, interstitial fluid may increase despite normal capillary pressure. This phenomenon will be amplified by any increase in capillary pressure. Conversely, some patients suffering from chronic elevation in venous pressure, such as patients with mitral stenosis, can tolerate remarkable capillary pressure elevation without developing significant edema. This is due to lymphatic adaptation and changes in the basal membrane throughout the years. (From Coalson, J.J. et al., *Arch Pathol.*, 83, 377–391, 1967).

## Pathophysiology

The consequences of pulmonary edema resulting from high capillary hydrostatic pressure on gas exchange and respiratory dynamics depend on the severity of the edema. Pulmonary blood volume, including capillary blood volume, is initially increased. This potentiates the diffusing capacity of the lungs. While the impact of interstitial edema on lung compliance remains controversial, a reduction in total lung capacity (TLC) is generally observed in reaction to cardiomegaly and increased pulmonary elastance [100]. Furthermore, swelling of the bronchial walls and subsequent reflex bronchoconstriction can increase airway resistance and induce a bronchospasm, also known as cardiac asthma [101]. Moreover, this phenomenon promotes closure of small airways during expiration, which increases the residual volume (RV). Stimulation of the juxtacapillary (J) receptors, located in the alveolar wall, by the edema causes an increase in minute ventilation. At this stage, patients display slight hypoxemia due to ventilation–perfusion abnormalities. The PVR will be increased due to hypoxic vasoconstriction and possibly due to compression of extra-alveolar pulmonary vessels by the interstitial edema. As the alveoli fill, lung volumes and compliance further decrease significantly and respiratory mechanics are altered [102,103]. Pulmonary edema engenders a reduction in ventilated respiratory units, residual capacity, and pulmonary compliance as well as gas exchange impairment [104,105]. In ARDS, proliferative changes, occurring during the proliferative phase, will cause further deterioration of respiratory dynamics. Other mechanisms of pulmonary edema have similar effects on respiratory dynamics and gas exchanges.

## Clinical manifestations and treatment

Pulmonary edema resulting from increased capillary hydrostatic pressure manifests with rapidly progressive dyspnea, which is exacerbated in the supine position (orthopnea). If the underlying mechanism is cardiac insufficiency due to cardiac ischemia, most patients also experience chest pain. Chest radiography shows interstitial infiltrates, bronchial wall edema and occasionally Kerley B lines representing increased lymphatic drainage (Figure 7.12). Bilateral alveolar infiltrates predominate during the alveolar stage. Pleural effusions are occasionally encountered. Treatment is aimed at improving heart function and lowering the pressure in the left heart cavities with diuretics and systemic vasodilators. Respiratory support is often necessary and can range from oxygen delivery through nasal prongs or face mask to invasive mechanical ventilation.

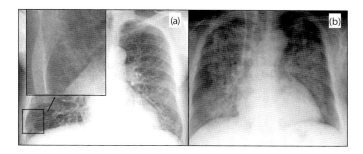

Figure 7.12 Classic radiological images of pulmonary edema. **(a)** At the interstitial edema stage, interstitial infiltration and bronchial wall edema are frequently seen, as well as Kerley lines (see enlargement), reflecting dilated lymphatic vessels compensating with increased drainage. **(b)** At the alveolar stage, infiltrations are more pronounced and adopt an "alveolar" pattern. Infiltrations are generally symmetric and predominate around the hilar portion of the lungs, whereas the subpleural regions are relatively spared.

In ARDS, the noncardiogenic pulmonary edema results in progressive dyspnea, bilateral pulmonary infiltrates, and severe hypoxemia. Treatment consists of respiratory support, most commonly by invasive mechanical ventilation, and treating the underlying cause (Table 7.4). Although the vital prognosis of ARDS remains limited, pulmonary prognosis is usually good even in the most severe form of the disease, with a slow but gradual recovery of lung function.

## Pulmonary arteriovenous malformations

The arteriovenous malformations consist of abnormal communications between the arterial and the venous circulation. PAVMs are rare vascular anomalies of the lung, in which abnormal dilated vessels provide a right-to-left shunt between the pulmonary artery and vein. A distinction can be made between macroscopic and microscopic PAVMs.

## Macroscopic PAVMs

### Overview and pathogenesis

In congenital cases, PAVMs are considered to result from a defect in the terminal capillary loops, which causes dilatation and the formation of thin-walled vascular sacs with a diameter ranging from 3 to 50 mm. Generally derived from an embryonic anomaly, they tend to be confined to the lung. PAVMs are more rarely caused by penetrating trauma, iatrogenic pulmonary artery penetration during right heart catheterization or as part of an inflammatory disease of the pulmonary vessels. Nevertheless, in 80% of cases, macroscopic PAVMs are observed as part of hereditary hemorrhagic telangiectasia (also known as Rendu–Osler–Weber disease), which is a genetic disease with autosomal dominant transmission [106]. Four types of mutations have been identified, including mutations in genes coding for endoglin (or *HHT1*, chromosome 9) [107], *ACVRL1* (or *HHT2*, chromosome 12) [108], and less frequently *HHT3* (chromosome 5) or genes coding for Smad4 protein (chromosome 18). These receptors, ligands or intracellular messengers are all part of the TGF-ß signaling pathways [109,110]. Thus, macroscopic PAVMs probably result from an aberrant signaling in the TGF-ß pathway during vascular development.

### Clinical presentation

The prevalence of the disease varies from 2 to 43 cases per 100,000 [111]. Only 15%–30% of patients with hereditary hemorrhagic telangiectasia will develop PAVMs (Table 7.5). Mucocutaneous anomalies are the

Table 7.5 Clinical manifestations of hereditary hemorrhagic telangiectasia

| Site | Frequency (%) | Age (years) | Clinical consequences |
| --- | --- | --- | --- |
| Nose | 90–95 | 3–20 | Epistaxis |
| PAVMs[a] | 15–30 | 3–20 | Hypoxemia, hemoptysis, and paradoxical embolism |
| Mucous telangiectasia | 50–80 | 15–30 | Aesthetic, bleeding |
| Facial telangiectasia | 30–50 | 30–50 | Aesthetic |
| Digestive telangiectasia | 20–40 | 40–60 | Anemia, digestive hemorrhage |
| Cerebral AVMs[a] | 10–20 | Variable | Epilepsy, hemorrhage |
| Hepatic AVMs[a] | 10–30 | Variable | Usually asymptomatic, high-output heart failure |

*Source:* Letteboer, T.G.W. et al., *J Med Genet.*, 43, 371–377, 2006.
AVM, arteriovenous malformation; PAVM, pulmonary arteriovenous malformation.
[a] Cerebral and pulmonary AVMs are more frequent in patients with the HHT1 mutation, while hepatic AMVS are more frequent in patients with HHT2 mutation.

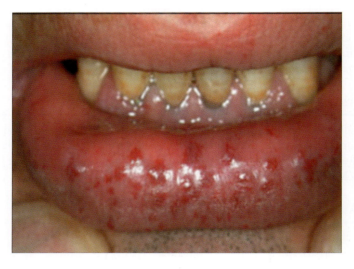

Figure 7.13 Oral mucous telangiectasia.

most common manifestation of Rendu–Osler–Weber disease (Figure 7.13). Clinical manifestations are variable in time and among members of the same family [112].

Most of PAVMs are symptomatic because of the right-to-left shunt physiology as well as the loss of capillary bed that acts as a filter for blood bound particles [113]. Thus, approximately 50% of patients will experience dyspnea, sometimes associated with cyanosis and hypoxemia. Rupture of abnormal blood vessels can seldom lead to hemoptysis and hemothorax. However, the most feared complications remain cerebral ischemia and abscesses. These complications occur when debris circulating in the venous circulation is allowed into the arterial circulation by the abnormal arteriovenous communication caused by PAVMs. Up to 20% of patients with PAVMs will experience an acute ischemic stroke, whereas 10% will experience a cerebral abcess [114]. To prevent such complications, most authors have recommended routine screening for PAVMs of all patients with hereditary hemorrhagic telangiectasia [115]. Importantly, clinical screening is clearly insufficient for detecting PAVMs since cyanosis, clubbing, and a pulmonary bruit are observed in <10% of patients with PAVMs. Contrast echocardiography remains the screening test of choice, with a sensitivity of >90% for the detection of PAVMs [116,117]. In healthy subjects, bubbles are captured by the pulmonary capillary bed, but with PAVMs they travel to the left atrium and to the systemic circulation. PAVMs can sometimes be apparent on the standard chest radiography. Computed tomography pulmonary angiogram is the current accepted diagnostic gold standard and is used to confirm and measure the size of PAVMs in patients with positive contrast echocardiography (Figure 7.14a) [115,118]. Standard pulmonary angiography, which has a lower resolution than current multidetector computed tomography angiogram, is now used for the definitive treatment of most PAVM using embolization of synthetic material (Figure 7.14b and c).

## Microscopic arteriovenous malformations

### Overview and pathogenesis

Microscopic PAVMs represent pulmonary capillary dilatation reaching diameters ranging from 80 to 100 μm. Thus, these are not true PAVMs. However, clinical consequences are somewhat similar and consist mainly of hypoxemia and more rarely paradoxal embolization of debris originating from the venous to the arterial circulation. The PAVMs are more commonly found as part of the hepatopulmonary syndrome, a syndrome which regroups hepatic disease, hypoxemia, and PAVMs (Table 7.6) [119–121]. Several mechanisms have been implied in the pathogenesis of hepatopulmonary syndrome. It is believed that some mediators produced or metabolized by the liver may influence the pulmonary circulation. This hypothesis is supported by the occurrence of a syndrome similar to hepatopulmonary syndrome in patients with congenital anomalies resulting in the direct passage of blood from the systemic to the pulmonary circulation, bypassing the hepatic circulation [122,123], or following a Fontan procedure (a palliative surgical procedure used in children with univentricular hearts that involves diverting the venous blood from the inferior and superior vena cava to the pulmonary arteries). There is also an overproduction of pulmonary nitric oxide (NO) due to an increase in inducible endothelial NO synthase found in the endovascular macrophages [124–126]. In hepatopulmonary syndrome experimental models, hypoxemia is corrected by the administration of NO synthase inhibitors [127]. The increase in NO production could result from and increased production of endothelin-1 by the liver in association with an overexpression of ET-B receptors on the pulmonary endothelial cells [128,129]. When stimulated, these receptors induce NO production. On the other hand, endovascular macrophages located in the pulmonary microcirculation are major producers of NO. During bacteremia due to intestinal translocation, portal hypertension, and portosystemic shunt reroute bacteria to the pulmonary

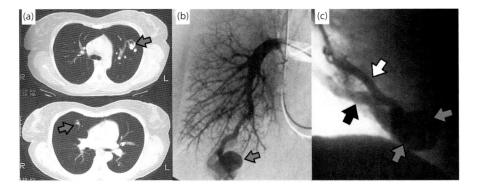

Figure 7.14 Pulmonary arteriovenous malformations (PAVMs). **(a)** PAVMs can generally be seen on chest tomography (gray arrows). **(b)** Conventional pulmonary angiography remains an essential exam to define the anatomy of PAVMs as well as to embolize them. **(c)** The feeding artery (white arrow), the vascular sack (gray arrows), and the draining vein (black arrow) are identified before definitive embolization.

Table 7.6 Diagnostic criteria and severity of hepatopulmonary syndrome

| Diagnostic criteria | Grade | Severity | |
|---|---|---|---|
| | | $P(A-a)\ O_2^{a,b}$ (mmHg) | $PaO_2^c$ (mmHg) |
| 1. **Hepatic disease** | Mild | ≥15 | ≥80 |
| 2. **P(A–a) O2 ≥15 mmHg** | Moderate | ≥15 | ≥60 and <80 |
| 3. **Positive contrast cardiac echography** | Severe | ≥15 | ≥50 and <60 |
| | Very severe | ≥15 | <50 |

Source: Rodríguez-Roisin, R. et al., *Eur Respir J.*, 24, 861–880, 2004.
P(A–a) O2, alveolo-arterial oxygen pressure gradient; $PaO_2$, oxygen partial arterial pressure.
[a] Simplified formula: $P(A-a)\ O_2 = FiO_2\ (P_{atm} - P_{H2O}) - PaCO_2 / QR - PaO_2$; where $FiO_2$ is the fraction of inspired oxygen, $P_{atm}$ is the atmospheric pressure, $P_{H2O}$ is the water vapor pressure, $PaCO_2$ is the carbon dioxide partial arterial pressure, and QR is the respiratory quotient.
[b] Normal value between 4 and 8 mmHg. For patients over 64 years old, a $P(A-a)\ O_2 \geq 20$ mmHg can be suggested as a diagnostic criteria.
[c] Normal value ≥80 mmHg.

circulation instead of being captured by the liver sinusoids, drawing the macrophages at this level [130,131]. More rarely, microscopic PAVMs are observed in association with schistosomiasis, mitral stenosis, actinomycosis, Fanconi syndrome, and metastatic thyroid carcinoma.

### Pathophysiology

The hepatopulmonary syndrome results from a decrease in vasomotor tone with the loss of hypoxic Vasoconstriction* [132,133]. These anomalies generally predominate in the lung bases. Three mechanisms cause hypoxemia in these patients: ventilation–perfusion mismatch, shunting, and diffusing capacity alterations. The first two mechanisms are due to excessive perfusion compared to ventilation in certain pulmonary areas. Alterations in diffusion are due to increased distance between alveoli and red blood cells travelling through the dilated capillaries. Because cardiac output is increased, as it is frequently seen in hepatic diseases, the transit time of the red blood cells through the capillary is diminished. These factors explain the incomplete equilibration of alveolar and blood gases [134]. Hypoxemia can be aggravated in supine or sitting position (orthodeoxia) since gravity privileges blood flow to the lung bases, where the PAVMs are most abundant.

### Clinical presentation

There is limited correlation between the severity of liver disease and the severity of hepatopulmonary syndrome [135,136]. Among cirrhotic patients, the reported prevalence is about 15%. In addition to events related to the liver disease, patients present with dyspnea and hypoxemia (Table 7.6) [119–121]. Since PAVMs are microscopic, they are generally invisible on the chest computed tomography or pulmonary angiography and it is unusual for debris (blood clot or bacteria) to travel from the venous to the systemic circulation. PAVMs are thus documented by contrast echography or by perfusion scintigraphy confirming the presence of an intrapulmonary right-to-left shunt.

The prognosis of patients with cirrhosis is impaired by the coexistence of a hepatopulmonary syndrome, with a median survival of 1 year [137]. Numerous pharmacological treatments with different mechanisms were evaluated but showed no significant or sustained improvement in oxygenation [130,138–143]. Oxygen therapy is indicated for patients with severe hypoxemia. Finally, liver transplantation leads to resolution of hepatopulmonary syndrome in 80% of patients in the months following the intervention. Therefore, many transplant centers consider severe hepatopulmonary syndrome as an indication for transplant [144]. However, perioperative morbidity is significantly increased [145].

## Conclusion

The pulmonary circulation is at the origin of multiple pathologies. Some are rare (arteriovenous malformations and PH), while others are very frequent (pulmonary embolism and pulmonary edema). Because of its important physiologic role, conditions affecting the pulmonary circulation are most commonly serious and associated with considerable morbidity and mortality. Over the past few decades, significant scientific breakthroughs have been made and greatly improved the diagnosis and management of pulmonary vascular diseases.

## References

1. Junod AF. Metabolism, production, and release of hormones and mediators in the lung. *Am Rev Respir Dis* 1975; **112**: 93–108.
2. Kovacs G, Berghold A, Scheidl S, Olschewski H. Pulmonary arterial pressure during rest and exercise in healthy subjects: A systematic review. *Eur Respir J* 2009; **34**: 888–94.
3. Vonk-Noordegraaf A, Haddad F, Chin KM, et al. Right heart adaptation to pulmonary arterial hypertension: Physiology and pathobiology. *J Am Coll Cardiol* 2013; **62**: D22–33.
4. Chemla D, Castelain V, Hervé P, Lecarpentier Y, Brimioulle S. Haemodynamic evaluation of pulmonary hypertension. *Eur Respir J* 2002; **20**: 1314–31.
5. Chemla D, Castelain V, Simonneau G, Lecarpentier Y, Hervé P. Pulse wave reflection in pulmonary hypertension. *J Am Coll Cardiol* 2002; **39**: 743–4.
6. Barer GR, Howard P, Shaw JW. Stimulus-response curves for the pulmonary vascular bed to hypoxia and hypercapnia. *J Physiol* 1970; **211**: 139–55.
7. Malik AB, Kidd BS. Independent effects of changes in H+ and CO 2 concentrations on hypoxic pulmonary vasoconstriction. *J Appl Physiol* 1973; **34**: 318–23.
8. Loeppky JA, Scotto P, Riedel CE, Roach RC, Chick TW. Effects of acid-base status on acute hypoxic pulmonary vasoconstriction and gas exchange. *J Appl Physiol* 1992; **72**: 1787–97.
9. Murray JF, Karp RB, Nadel JA. Viscosity effects on pressure-flow relations and vascular resistance in dogs' lungs. *J Appl Physiol* 1969; **27**: 336–41.
10. Barnes PJ, Liu SF. Regulation of pulmonary vascular tone. *Pharmacol Rev* 1995; **47**: 87–131.
11. Hoeper MM, Bogaard HJ, Condliffe R, et al. Definitions and diagnosis of pulmonary hypertension. *J Am Coll Cardiol* 2013; **62**: D42–50.
12. Azarian R, Wartski M, Collignon MA, et al. Lung perfusion scans and hemodynamics in acute and chronic pulmonary embolism. *J Nucl Med* 1997; **38**: 980–3.
13. Piazza G, Goldhaber SZ. Acute pulmonary embolism: part I: Epidemiology and diagnosis. *Circulation* 2006; **114**: e28–32.
14. Herve P, Lau EM, Sitbon O, et al. Criteria for diagnosis of exercise pulmonary hypertension. *Eur Respir J* 2015; **46**: 728–37.
15. Godinas L, Lau EM, Chemla D, et al. Diagnostic concordance of different criteria for exercise pulmonary hypertension in subjects with normal resting pulmonary artery pressure. *Eur Respir J* 2016; **48**: 254–7; published online March 30. doi:10.1183/13993003.01678-2015.
16. Goldhaber SZ, Haire WD, Feldstein ML, et al. Alteplase versus heparin in acute pulmonary embolism: Andomised trial assessing right-ventricular function and pulmonary perfusion. *Lancet* 1993; **341**: 507–11.
17. Naeije R. Assessment of right ventricular function in pulmonary hypertension. *Curr Hypertens Rep* 2015; **17**: 35.
18. Provencher S, Chemla D, Hervé P, Sitbon O, Humbert M, Simonneau G. Heart rate responses during the 6-minute walk test in pulmonary arterial hypertension. *Eur Respir J* 2006; **27**: 114–20.

19. Provencher S, Herve P, Jais X, et al. Deleterious effects of beta-blockers on exercise capacity and hemodynamics in patients with portopulmonary hypertension. *Gastroenterology* 2006; **130**: 120–6.
20. Vlahakes GJ, Turley K, Hoffman JI. The pathophysiology of failure in acute right ventricular hypertension: Hemodynamic and biochemical correlations. *Circulation* 1981; **63**: 87–95.
21. Vieillard-Baron A, Michard F, Chemla D. Définitions et rappels physiologiques concernant les déterminants du statut volémique. *Reanimation* 2004; **13**: 264–7.
22. D'Alonzo GE, Barst RJ, Ayres SM, et al. Survival in patients with primary pulmonary hypertension. Results from a national prospective registry. *Ann Intern Med* 1991; **115**: 343–9.
23. Potus F, Ruffenach G, Dahou A, et al. Downregulation of microRNA-126 contributes to the failing right ventricle in pulmonary arterial hypertension. *Circulation* 2015; **132**: 932–43.
24. Ryan JJ, Archer SL. The right ventricle in pulmonary arterial hypertension: Disorders of metabolism, angiogenesis and adrenergic signaling in right ventricular failure. *Circ Res* 2014; **115**: 176–88.
25. Chen X, Talati M, Fessel JP, et al. Estrogen metabolite 16α-hydroxyestrone exacerbates bone morphogenetic protein receptor type II-associated pulmonary arterial hypertension through microRNA-29-mediated modulation of cellular metabolism. *Circulation* 2016; **133**: 82–97.
26. Frump AL, Goss KN, Vayl A, et al. Estradiol improves right ventricular function in rats with severe angioproliferative pulmonary hypertension: Effects of endogenous and exogenous sex hormones. *Am J Physiol Lung Cell Mol Physiol* 2015; **308**: L873–90.
27. Ventetuolo CE, Mitra N, Wan F, et al. Oestradiol metabolism and androgen receptor genotypes are associated with right ventricular function. *Eur Respir J* 2016; **47**: 553–63.
28. Paulin R, Sutendra G, Gurtu V, et al. A miR-208-Mef2 axis drives the decompensation of right ventricular function in pulmonary hypertension. *Circ Res* 2015; **116**: 56–69.
29. Simonneau G, Gatzoulis MA, Adatia I, et al. Updated clinical classification of pulmonary hypertension. *J Am Coll Cardiol* 2013; **62**: D34–41.
30. Tuder RM, Archer SL, Dorfmüller P, et al. Relevant issues in the pathology and pathobiology of pulmonary hypertension. *J Am Coll Cardiol* 2013; **62**: D4–12.
31. Deng Z, Morse JH, Slager SL, et al. Familial primary pulmonary hypertension (gene PPH1) is caused by mutations in the bone morphogenetic protein receptor-II gene. *Am J Hum Genet* 2000; **67**: 737–44.
32. Lane KB, Machado RD, Pauciulo MW, et al. Heterozygous germline mutations in BMPR2, encoding a TGF-beta receptor, cause familial primary pulmonary hypertension. *Nat Genet* 2000; **26**: 81–4.
33. Thomson JR, Machado RD, Pauciulo MW, et al. Sporadic primary pulmonary hypertension is associated with germline mutations of the gene encoding BMPR-II, a receptor member of the TGF-beta family. *J Med Genet* 2000; **37**: 741–5.
34. Soubrier F, Chung WK, Machado R, et al. Genetics and genomics of pulmonary arterial hypertension. *J Am Coll Cardiol* 2013; **62**: D13–21.
35. Rudarakanchana N, Flanagan JA, Chen H, et al. Functional analysis of bone morphogenetic protein type II receptor mutations underlying primary pulmonary hypertension. *Hum Mol Genet* 2002; **11**: 1517–25.
36. Ma L, Roman-Campos D, Austin ED, et al. A novel channelopathy in pulmonary arterial hypertension. *N Engl J Med* 2013; **369**: 351–61.
37. Naeije R, Vachiery J-L, Yerly P, Vanderpool R. The transpulmonary pressure gradient for the diagnosis of pulmonary vascular disease. *Eur Respir J* 2013; **41**: 217–23.
38. Harvey RM, Enson Y, Ferrer MI. A reconsideration of the origins of pulmonary hypertension. *Chest* 1971; **59**: 82–94.
39. Vachiéry J-L, Adir Y, Barberà JA, et al. Pulmonary hypertension due to left heart diseases. *J Am Coll Cardiol* 2013; **62**: D100–8.
40. Zieliński T, Pogorzelska H, Rajecka A, Biedermavn A, Sliwiński M, Korewicki J. Pulmonary hemodynamics at rest and effort, 6 and 12 months after mitral valve replacement: A slow regression of effort pulmonary hypertension. *Int J Cardiol* 1993; **42**: 57–62.

41. Chaouat A, Kraemer J-P, Canuet M, et al. Hypertension pulmonaire des affections respiratoires chroniques. *Presse Med* 2005; **34**: 1465–74.
42. Seeger W, Adir Y, Barberà JA, et al. Pulmonary hypertension in chronic lung diseases. *J Am Coll Cardiol* 2013; **62**: D109–16.
43. Eddahibi S, Chaouat A, Morrell N, et al. Polymorphism of the serotonin transporter gene and pulmonary hypertension in chronic obstructive pulmonary disease. *Circulation* 2003; **108**: 1839–44.
44. Matsuoka S, Washko GR, Yamashiro T, et al. Pulmonary hypertension and computed tomography measurement of small pulmonary vessels in severe emphysema. *Am J Respir Crit Care Med* 2010; **181**: 218–25.
45. Kim NH, Delcroix M, Jenkins DP, et al. Chronic thromboembolic pulmonary hypertension. *J Am Coll Cardiol* 2013; **62**: D92–9.
46. Mehta S, Helmersen D, Provencher S, et al. Diagnostic evaluation and management of chronic thromboembolic pulmonary hypertension: A clinical practice guideline. *Can Respir J* 2010; **17**: 301–34.
47. Moser KM, Bloor CM. Pulmonary vascular lesions occurring in patients with chronic major vessel thromboembolic pulmonary hypertension. *Chest* 1993; **103**: 685–92.
48. Becattini C, Agnelli G, Pesavento R, et al. Incidence of chronic thromboembolic pulmonary hypertension after a first episode of pulmonary embolism. *Chest* 2006; **130**: 172–5.
49. Pengo V, Lensing AWA, Prins MH, et al. Incidence of chronic thromboembolic pulmonary hypertension after pulmonary embolism. *N Engl J Med* 2004; **350**: 2257–64.
50. Spiekerkoetter E, Fabel H, Hoeper MM. Effects of inhaled salbutamol in primary pulmonary hypertension. *Eur Respir J* 2002; **20**: 524–8.
51. Sitbon O, Humbert M, Jaïs X, et al. Long-term response to calcium channel blockers in idiopathic pulmonary arterial hypertension. *Circulation* 2005; **111**: 3105–11.
52. Humbert M, Ghofrani H-A. The molecular targets of approved treatments for pulmonary arterial hypertension. *Thorax* 2016; **71**: 73–83.
53. Galiè N, Manes A, Negro L, Palazzini M, Bacchi-Reggiani ML, Branzi A. A meta-analysis of randomized controlled trials in pulmonary arterial hypertension. *Eur Heart J* 2009; **30**: 394–403.
54. Lajoie AC, Lauzière G, Lega J-C, et al. Combination therapy versus monotherapy for pulmonary arterial hypertension: A meta-analysis. *Lancet Respir Med* 2016; **4**: 291–305.
55. Packer M, McMurray J, Massie BM, et al. Clinical effects of endothelin receptor antagonism with bosentan in patients with severe chronic heart failure: Results of a pilot study. *J Card Fail* 2005; **11**: 12–20.
56. Califf RM, Adams KF, McKenna WJ, et al. A randomized controlled trial of epoprostenol therapy for severe congestive heart failure: The Flolan International Randomized Survival Trial (FIRST). *Am Heart J* 1997; **134**: 44–54.
57. Hoendermis ES, Liu LCY, Hummel YM, et al. Effects of sildenafil on invasive haemodynamics and exercise capacity in heart failure patients with preserved ejection fraction and pulmonary hypertension: A randomized controlled trial. *Eur Heart J* 2015; **36**: 2565–73.
58. Bonderman D, Ghio S, Felix SB, et al. Riociguat for patients with pulmonary hypertension caused by systolic left ventricular dysfunction: A phase IIb double-blind, randomized, placebo-controlled, dose-ranging hemodynamic study. *Circulation* 2013; **128**: 502–11.
59. Raghu G, Behr J, Brown KK, et al. Treatment of idiopathic pulmonary fibrosis with ambrisentan: A parallel, randomized trial. *Ann Intern Med* 2013; **158**: 641–9.
60. Redfield MM, Chen HH, Borlaug BA, et al. Effect of phosphodiesterase-5 inhibition on exercise capacity and clinical status in heart failure with preserved ejection fraction: A randomized clinical trial. *JAMA* 2013; **309**: 1268–77.
61. Ghofrani H-A, D'Armini AM, Grimminger F, et al. Riociguat for the treatment of chronic thromboembolic pulmonary hypertension. *N Engl J Med* 2013; **369**: 319–29.

62. Ishiguro H, Kataoka M, Inami T, et al. Percutaneous transluminal pulmonary angioplasty for central-type chronic thromboembolic pulmonary hypertension. *JACC Cardiovasc Interv* 2013; **6**: 1212–3. doi:10.1016/j.jcin.2013.03.025.
63. Inami T, Kataoka M, Ando M, Fukuda K, Yoshino H, Satoh T. A new era of therapeutic strategies for chronic thromboembolic pulmonary hypertension by two different interventional therapies; pulmonary endarterectomy and percutaneous transluminal pulmonary angioplasty. *PLoS One* 2014; **9**: e94587.
64. Vincens JJ, Temizer D, Post JR, Edmunds LH, Herrmann HC. Long-term outcome of cardiac surgery in patients with mitral stenosis and severe pulmonary hypertension. *Circulation* 1995; **92**: II137–42.
65. Meyer P, Filippatos GS, Ahmed MI, et al. Effects of right ventricular ejection fraction on outcomes in chronic systolic heart failure. *Circulation* 2010; **121**: 252–8.
66. Kjaergaard J, Akkan D, Iversen KK, Køber L, Torp-Pedersen C, Hassager C. Right ventricular dysfunction as an independent predictor of short- and long-term mortality in patients with heart failure. *Eur J Heart Fail* 2007; **9**: 610–6.
67. Kjaergaard J, Akkan D, Iversen KK, et al. Prognostic importance of pulmonary hypertension in patients with heart failure. *Am J Cardiol* 2007; **99**: 1146–50.
68. Lam CSP, Roger VL, Rodeheffer RJ, Borlaug BA, Enders FT, Redfield MM. Pulmonary hypertension in heart failure with preserved ejection fraction: A community-based study. *J Am Coll Cardiol* 2009; **53**: 1119–26.
69. Damy T, Goode KM, Kallvikbacka-Bennett A, et al. Determinants and prognostic value of pulmonary arterial pressure in patients with chronic heart failure. *Eur Heart J* 2010; **31**: 2280–90.
70. Cappola TP, Felker GM, Kao WHL, Hare JM, Baughman KL, Kasper EK. Pulmonary hypertension and risk of death in cardiomyopathy: Patients with myocarditis are at higher risk. *Circulation* 2002; **105**: 1663–8.
71. Weitzenblum E, Hirth C, Ducolone A, Mirhom R, Rasaholinjanahary J, Pelletier A. The prognostic significance of pulmonary arterial hypertension in chronic obstructive airway disease. *Poumon Coeur* 1981; **37**: 177–84.
72. Leuchte HH, Baumgartner RA, Nounou M El, et al. Brain natriuretic peptide is a prognostic parameter in chronic lung disease. *Am J Respir Crit Care Med* 2006; **173**: 744–50.
73. Nadrous HF, Pellikka PA, Krowka MJ, et al. Pulmonary hypertension in patients with idiopathic pulmonary fibrosis. *Chest* 2005; **128**: 2393–9.
74. Nathan SD, Shlobin OA, Ahmad S, Urbanek S, Barnett SD. Pulmonary hypertension and pulmonary function testing in idiopathic pulmonary fibrosis. *Chest* 2007; **131**: 657–63.
75. Lettieri CJ, Nathan SD, Barnett SD, Ahmad S, Shorr AF. Prevalence and outcomes of pulmonary arterial hypertension in advanced idiopathic pulmonary fibrosis. *Chest* 2006; **129**: 746–52.
76. Riedel M, Stanek V, Widimsky J, Prerovsky I. Longterm follow-up of patients with pulmonary thromboembolism: Late prognosis and evolution of hemodynamic and respiratory data. *Chest* 1982; **81**: 151–8.
77. Pepke-Zaba J, Delcroix M, Lang I, et al. Chronic thromboembolic pulmonary hypertension (CTEPH): Results from an international prospective registry. *Circulation* 2011; **124**: 1973–81.
78. Humbert M, Sitbon O, Yaïci A, et al. Survival in incident and prevalent cohorts of patients with pulmonary arterial hypertension. *Eur Respir J* 2010; **36**: 549–55.
79. Humbert M, Sitbon O, Chaouat A, et al. Survival in patients with idiopathic, familial, and anorexigen-associated pulmonary arterial hypertension in the modern management era. *Circulation* 2010; **122**: 156–63.
80. Margaglione M, Brancaccio V, Giuliani N, et al. Increased risk for venous thrombosis in carriers of the prothrombin G--&gt;A20210 gene variant. *Ann Intern Med* 1998; **129**: 89–93.

81. Koster T, Blann AD, Briët E, Vandenbroucke JP, Rosendaal FR. Role of clotting factor VIII in effect of von Willebrand factor on occurrence of deep-vein thrombosis. *Lancet* 1995; **345**: 152–5.
82. Mélot C, Delcroix M, Closset J, et al. Starling resistor vs. distensible vessel models for embolic pulmonary hypertension. *Am J Physiol* 1995; **268**: H817–27.
83. Sharma G V, McIntyre KM, Sharma S, Sasahara AA. Clinical and hemodynamic correlates in pulmonary embolism. *Clin Chest Med* 1984; **5**: 421–37.
84. Lualdi JC, Goldhaber SZ. Right ventricular dysfunction after acute pulmonary embolism: Pathophysiologic factors, detection, and therapeutic implications. *Am Heart J* 1995; **130**: 1276–82.
85. Dantzker DR, Bower JS. Alterations in gas exchange following pulmonary thromboembolism. *Chest* 1982; **81**: 495–501.
86. D'Alonzo GE, Dantzker DR. Gas exchange alterations following pulmonary thromboembolism. *Clin Chest Med* 1984; **5**: 411–9.
87. Delcroix M, Mélot C, Vermeulen F, Naeije R. Hypoxic pulmonary vasoconstriction and gas exchange in acute canine pulmonary embolism. *J Appl Physiol* 1996; **80**: 1240–8.
88. Manier G, Castaing Y. Influence of cardiac output on oxygen exchange in acute pulmonary embolism. *Am Rev Respir Dis* 1992; **145**: 130–6.
89. Heit JA. The epidemiology of venous thromboembolism in the community: Implications for prevention and management. *J Thromb Thrombolysis* 2006; **21**: 23–9.
90. Elliott CG, Goldhaber SZ, Jensen RL. Delays in diagnosis of deep vein thrombosis and pulmonary embolism. *Chest* 2005; **128**: 3372–6.
91. Goldhaber SZ, Visani L, De Rosa M. Acute pulmonary embolism: clinical outcomes in the International Cooperative Pulmonary Embolism Registry (ICOPER). *Lancet* 1999; **353**: 1386–9.
92. Pollack C V., Schreiber D, Goldhaber SZ, et al. Clinical characteristics, management, and outcomes of patients diagnosed with acute pulmonary embolism in the emergency department: Initial report of EMPEROR (Multicenter Emergency Medicine Pulmonary Embolism in the Real World Registry). *J Am Coll Cardiol* 2011; **57**: 700–6.
93. Jiménez D, Aujesky D, Moores L, et al. Simplification of the pulmonary embolism severity index for prognostication in patients with acute symptomatic pulmonary embolism. *Arch Intern Med* 2010; **170**: 1383–9.
94. Lega J-C, Lacasse Y, Lakhal L, Provencher S. Natriuretic peptides and troponins in pulmonary embolism: A meta-analysis. *Thorax* 2009; **64**: 869–75.
95. Kearon C, Akl EA, Ornelas J, et al. Antithrombotic Therapy for VTE Disease: CHEST Guideline and Expert Panel Report. *Chest* 2016; **149**: 315–52.
96. Kahn SR, Houweling AH, Granton J, Rudski L, Dennie C, Hirsch A. Long-term outcomes after pulmonary embolism: Current knowledge and future research. *Blood Coagul Fibrinolysis* 2014; **25**: 407–15.
97. Nijkeuter M, Hovens MMC, Davidson BL, Huisman M V. Resolution of thromboemboli in patients with acute pulmonary embolism: A systematic review. *Chest* 2006; **129**: 192–7.
98. Suzuki S, Tanita T, Koike K, Fujimura S. Evidence of acute inflammatory response in reexpansion pulmonary edema. *Chest* 1992; **101**: 275–6.
99. Coalson JJ, Jaques WE, Campbell GS, Thompson WM. Ultrastructure of the alveolar-capillary membrane in congenital and acquired heart disease. *Arch Pathol* 1967; **83**: 377–91.
100. Staub NC. Pulmonary edema. *Physiol Rev* 1974; **54**: 678–811.
101. Lloyd TC. Reflex effects of left heart and pulmonary vascular distension on airways of dogs. *J Appl Physiol* 1980; **49**: 620–6.
102. Noble WH, Kay JC, Obdrzalek J. Lung mechanics in hypervolemic pulmonary edema. *J Appl Physiol* 1975; **38**: 681–7.
103. Snapper JR. Lung mechanics in pulmonary edema. *Clin Chest Med* 1985; **6**: 393–412.

104. Pelosi P, Cereda M, Foti G, Giacomini M, Pesenti A. Alterations of lung and chest wall mechanics in patients with acute lung injury: Effects of positive end-expiratory pressure. *Am J Respir Crit Care Med* 1995; **152**: 531–7.
105. Lamy M, Fallat RJ, Koeniger E, et al. Pathologic features and mechanisms of hypoxemia in adult respiratory distress syndrome. *Am Rev Respir Dis* 1976; **114**: 267–84.
106. Guttmacher AE, Marchuk DA, White RI. Hereditary hemorrhagic telangiectasia. *N Engl J Med* 1995; **333**: 918–24.
107. McAllister KA, Grogg KM, Johnson DW, et al. Endoglin, a TGF-beta binding protein of endothelial cells, is the gene for hereditary haemorrhagic telangiectasia type 1. *Nat Genet* 1994; **8**: 345–51.
108. Berg JN, Gallione CJ, Stenzel TT, et al. The activin receptor-like kinase 1 gene: Genomic structure and mutations in hereditary hemorrhagic telangiectasia type 2. *Am J Hum Genet* 1997; **61**: 60–7.
109. Abdalla SA, Letarte M. Hereditary haemorrhagic telangiectasia: Current views on genetics and mechanisms of disease. *J Med Genet* 2006; **43**: 97–110.
110. Cole SG, Begbie ME, Wallace GMF, Shovlin CL. A new locus for hereditary haemorrhagic telangiectasia (HHT3) maps to chromosome 5. *J Med Genet* 2005; **42**: 577–82.
111. Porteous ME, Burn J, Proctor SJ. Hereditary haemorrhagic telangiectasia: A clinical analysis. *J Med Genet* 1992; **29**: 527–30.
112. Letteboer TGW, Mager JJ, Snijder RJ, et al. Genotype-phenotype relationship in hereditary haemorrhagic telangiectasia. *J Med Genet* 2006; **43**: 371–7.
113. Gossage JR, Kanj G. Pulmonary arteriovenous malformations. A state of the art review. *Am J Respir Crit Care Med* 1998; **158**: 643–61.
114. White RI, Lynch-Nyhan A, Terry P, et al. Pulmonary arteriovenous malformations: Techniques and long-term outcome of embolotherapy. *Radiology* 1988; **169**: 663–9.
115. Faughnan ME, Granton JT, Young LH. The pulmonary vascular complications of hereditary haemorrhagic telangiectasia. *Eur Respir J* 2009; **33**: 1186–94.
116. Nanthakumar K, Graham AT, Robinson TI, et al. Contrast echocardiography for detection of pulmonary arteriovenous malformations. *Am Heart J* 2001; **141**: 243–6.
117. Cottin V, Plauchu H, Bayle J-Y, Barthelet M, Revel D, Cordier J-F. Pulmonary arteriovenous malformations in patients with hereditary hemorrhagic telangiectasia. *Am J Respir Crit Care Med* 2004; **169**: 994–1000.
118. Curie A, Lesca G, Cottin V, et al. Long-term follow-up in 12 children with pulmonary arteriovenous malformations: Confirmation of hereditary hemorrhagic telangiectasia in all cases. *J Pediatr* 2007; **151**: 299–306.
119. Rodríguez-Roisin R, Krowka MJ, Hervé P, Fallon MB, ERS Task Force Pulmonary-Hepatic Vascular Disorders (PHD) Scientific Committee. Pulmonary-Hepatic vascular Disorders (PHD). *Eur Respir J* 2004; **24**: 861–80.
120. Rodríguez-Roisin R, Agustí AG, Roca J. The hepatopulmonary syndrome: New name, old complexities. *Thorax* 1992; **47**: 897–902.
121. Fallon MB, Abrams GA. Pulmonary dysfunction in chronic liver disease. *Hepatology* 2000; **32**: 859–65.
122. Lee J, Menkis AH, Rosenberg HC, et al. Reversal of pulmonary arteriovenous malformation after diversion of anomalous hepatic drainage. *Ann Thorac Surg* 1998; **65**: 848–9.
123. Alvarez AE, Ribeiro AF, Hessel G, Baracat J, Ribeiro JD. Abernethy malformation: One of the etiologies of hepatopulmonary syndrome. *Pediatr Pulmonol* 2002; **34**: 391–4.
124. Rolla G, Brussino L, Colagrande P, et al. Exhaled nitric oxide and impaired oxygenation in cirrhotic patients before and after liver transplantation. *Ann Intern Med* 1998; **129**: 375–8.
125. Fallon M, Abrams G, Luo B, Hou Z, Dai J, Ku D. The role of endothelial nitric oxide synthase in the pathogenesis of a rat model of hepatopulmonary syndrome. *Gastroenterology* 1997; **113**: 606–14.
126. Nunes H, Lebrec D, Mazmanian M, et al. Role of nitric oxide in hepatopulmonary syndrome in cirrhotic rats. *Am J Respir Crit Care Med* 2001; **164**: 879–85.

127. Zhang X-J, Katsuta Y, Akimoto T, et al. Intrapulmonary vascular dilatation and nitric oxide in hypoxemic rats with chronic bile duct ligation. *J Hepatol* 2003; **39**: 724–30.
128. Luo B, Abrams GA, Fallon MB, et al. Endothelin-1 in the rat bile duct ligation model of hepatopulmonary syndrome: Correlation with pulmonary dysfunction. *J Hepatol* 1998; **29**: 571–8.
129. Ling Y, Zhang J, Luo B, et al. The role of endothelin-1 and the endothelin B receptor in the pathogenesis of hepatopulmonary syndrome in the rat. *Hepatology* 2004; **39**: 1593–602.
130. Rabiller A, Nunes H, Lebrec D, et al. Prevention of gram-negative translocation reduces the severity of hepatopulmonary syndrome. *Am J Respir Crit Care Med* 2002; **166**: 514–7.
131. Schraufnagel DE, Malik R, Goel V, Ohara N, Chang SW. Lung capillary changes in hepatic cirrhosis in rats. *Am J Physiol* 1997; **272**: L139–47.
132. Rodriguez-Roisin R, Roca J, Agusti AG, Mastai R, Wagner PD, Bosch J. Gas exchange and pulmonary vascular reactivity in patients with liver cirrhosis. *Am Rev Respir Dis* 1987; **135**: 1085–92.
133. Mélot C, Naeije R, Dechamps P, Hallemans R, Lejeune P. Pulmonary and extrapulmonary contributors to hypoxemia in liver cirrhosis. *Am Rev Respir Dis* 1989; **139**: 632–40.
134. Genovesi MG, Tierney DF, Taplin G V, Eisenberg H. An intravenous radionuclide method to evaluate hypoxemia caused by abnormal alveolar vessels. Limitation of conventional techniques. *Am Rev Respir Dis* 1976; **114**: 59–65.
135. Babbs C, Warnes TW, Haboubi NY. Non-cirrhotic portal hypertension with hypoxaemia. *Gut* 1988; **29**: 129–31.
136. Teuber G, Teupe C, Dietrich CF, Caspary WF, Buhl R, Zeuzem S. Pulmonary dysfunction in non-cirrhotic patients with chronic viral hepatitis. *Eur J Intern Med* 2002; **13**: 311–8.
137. Schenk P, Schöniger-Hekele M, Fuhrmann V, Madl C, Silberhumer G, Müller C. Prognostic significance of the hepatopulmonary syndrome in patients with cirrhosis. *Gastroenterology* 2003; **125**: 1042–52.
138. Agusti AG, Roca J, Bosch J, Garcia-Pagan JC, Wagner PD, Rodriguez-Roisin R. Effects of propranolol on arterial oxygenation and oxygen transport to tissues in patients with cirrhosis. *Am Rev Respir Dis* 1990; **142**: 306–10.
139. Cadranel JL, Milleron BJ, Cadranel JF, et al. Severe hypoxemia-associated intrapulmonary shunt in a patient with chronic liver disease: Improvement after medical treatment. *Am Rev Respir Dis* 1992; **146**: 526–7.
140. Krowka MJ, Cortese DA. Severe hypoxemia associated with liver disease: Mayo Clinic experience and the experimental use of almitrine bismesylate. *Mayo Clin Proc* 1987; **62**: 164–73.
141. Krowka MJ, Dickson ER, Cortese DA. Hepatopulmonary syndrome. Clinical observations and lack of therapeutic response to somatostatin analogue. *Chest* 1993; **104**: 515–21.
142. Rolla G, Bucca C, Brussino L. Methylene blue in the hepatopulmonary syndrome. *N Engl J Med* 1994; **331**: 1098.
143. Song JY, Choi JY, Ko JT, et al. Long-term aspirin therapy for hepatopulmonary syndrome. *Pediatrics* 1996; **97**: 917–20.
144. Collisson EA, Nourmand H, Fraiman MH, et al. Retrospective analysis of the results of liver transplantation for adults with severe hepatopulmonary syndrome. *Liver Transpl* 2002; **8**: 925–31.
145. Arguedas MR, Abrams GA, Krowka MJ, Fallon MB. Prospective evaluation of outcomes and predictors of mortality in patients with hepatopulmonary syndrome undergoing liver transplantation. *Hepatology* 2003; **37**: 192–7.

# 8

# Respiratory infections

NOËL LAMPRON

| | |
|---|---|
| Introduction | 149 |
| Normal host defense mechanisms | 150 |
| Anatomical and mechanical barriers of the upper respiratory tract | 150 |
| Humoral and cellular immunity | 150 |
| Phagocytosis and inflammatory reaction | 153 |
| Infections of the upper respiratory tract | 153 |
| Infections of the lower respiratory tract | 153 |
| Acute exacerbations of chronic obstructive pulmonary disease | 154 |
| Pneumonia | 156 |
| Community-acquired pneumonia | 157 |
| Viral pneumonia | 158 |
| Tuberculosis and other atypical mycobacteria | 158 |
| Tuberculosis | 159 |
| Atypical mycobacteria | 160 |
| Parasitic, fungal, and other infections in the immunocompromised host | 160 |
| Conclusion | 160 |
| References | 161 |

## Introduction

Respiratory tract infections, including pneumonia, are among the commonest causes of death worldwide. With a vast epithelial surface area of 70–100 m$^2$, the respiratory tract and lungs are constantly exposed to an environment made of various gases, foreign particles, and a myriad of microorganisms, some of them being pathogens and able to initiate respiratory infections. Approximately 15,000 L of air, and sometimes more in cases of sustained effort, are inhaled every day and come into contact with the respiratory tract and lungs. Moreover, contaminated oropharyngeal secretions are often aspirated into the lower respiratory tract. When people are awake, the glottis normally prevents aspiration but, during sleep, approximately 50% of normal individuals will have episodes of microaspiration. In a normal adult, 1 mL of oropharyngeal secretions has a content of $10^7$–$10^9$ bacteria, an amount which can increase by 100–1000 when the individual has periodontitis. Despite the fact that microscopic aspiration of oropharyngeal secretions is common, the lower respiratory tract is usually able to remain sterile not only because of performant host defense mechanisms but also because of the low virulence of the oropharyngeal bacterial flora [1,2].

## Normal host defense mechanisms

Although aspiration of oropharyngeal secretions is common, the host defense mechanisms are usually able to clear potential pathogens and thus prevent parenchymal infections. These defense mechanisms include the anatomical and mechanical barriers of the upper respiratory tract, the humoral and cellular immune systems, the phagocytosis by neutrophils and macrophages, and the inflammatory reaction. Thus, inhaled or aspirated pathogens meet several lines of defenses before reaching the distal lung. That the lung is routinely exposed to potential pathogens and yet generally able to maintain its sterility is a testimony to the effectiveness of the defenses of the respiratory system.

## Anatomical and mechanical barriers of the upper respiratory tract

A significant part of normal host defenses against pulmonary infection relates to the anatomical and mechanical barriers provided by the upper respiratory tract. The cough reflex and dynamic action of the epiglottis, for instance, prevent most large particles from reaching the distal airway while the airway aerodynamic filtration system and mucociliary clearance processes are effective against smaller particles. Of note, the majority of microorganisms in the atmosphere are in the form of aerosolized particles.

The nasopharynx, oropharynx, and larynx are the first structures to be exposed to the inhaled microorganisms. Particles with diameters greater than 100 μm are first filtrated by nasal hair and then, due to the configuration of the nasal turbinate and oropharynx, they quickly precipitate by impacting on the mucosal surface. Particles with a diameter of 10–100 μm are enmeshed in the mucus layer coating the nasal epithelium while those with a diameter of 5–10 μm are humidified in the trachea and enmeshed at tracheal level or in major bronchi. The branching and acute angulation of airways are efficient in trapping, either by impaction or adhesion, particles measuring between 2 and 10 μ. Once trapped, the particles are mixed with mucus and mechanically transported by mucociliary movement toward the oropharynx where they can either be swallowed or expectorated (Figure 8.1). The airway mucus is composed of pericilliary liquid that allows the cilia to beat and a gel phase on the surface. The mucus gel acts as a barrier for bacteria [3]. Only particles measuring between 1 and 5 μ will reach the alveolar space and, depending on their diameter, those particles carry an inoculum of 1–100 microorganisms. While the average bacterial diameter varies between 0.5 and 2.0 μ, the diameter of the *Mycoplasma*, *Chlamydia*, and *Coxiella* spp. is 5–100 times smaller than the average-sized bacteria. The better air flow to the lower lobes in the upright position favors the deposit of inhaled microorganisms in those lobes.

Normally, the phagocytic cells of the innate immune system (alveolar macrophages) will quickly eliminate those microorganisms but, in patients with impaired immune systems, the pathogens can reach the terminal airways and alveoli, where infection will be initiated [2,4].

## Humoral and cellular immunity

From the nasopharynx to the distal terminal bronchiole, the inner surface of the respiratory tract is lined with a pseudostratified ciliated epithelium interspersed with secreting cells (goblet cells) and other cells such as the dendritic cells. The alveolar area of the lung is made of two types of epithelial cells. The first type, called "type I pneumocytes," are important in gas exchange while the second type, "type II pneumocytes," which are type I precursors, are involved in the regulation of the immune system.

The secreting cells of the epithelial surface are mucus-producing cells. The main constituents of mucus are glycoproteic complexes called "mucins," which are responsible for mucus bacterial adherence making those microorganisms unable to adhere to the epithelial cells. Mucociliary clearance is then achieved through coordinated epithelial cells, cilia motion which propels mucus-trapped particles and microorganisms toward the oropharynx where they are either expectorated or swallowed up.

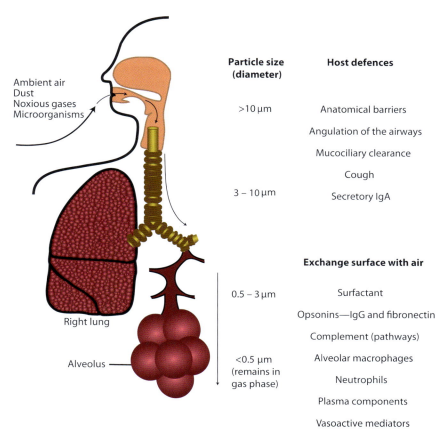

Figure 8.1 Mechanisms involved in the protection of the respiratory system. The naso and oropharynx filter inspired air thus preventing larger particles and most bacteria from gaining access to the lower respiratory tract. This is done through mucosal impaction and glottis reflex action. The particles thus trapped are either swallowed up or expectorated (cough or sneezing). Smaller particles or bacteria that have been able to filter through those first-line defenses and reach the respiratory tract are then submitted to the upper airway aerodynamic filtration process and most are trapped (impaction and sedimentation) at that level and then expelled by mucociliary clearance, cough or sneezing. The few particles that are able to reach the alveoli are dealt with by more sophisticated defense mechanisms such as phagocytosis by macrophages and polynuclear cells, and production of surfactant and complement. (Adapted from Reynolds, H.Y., *Chest.*, 95, 223s–230s, 1989).

When inhaled bacteria manage to adhere to the epithelial cell surface of the respiratory tract, two innate immune mechanisms are activated in order to eliminate them. The first of those mechanisms is mechanical and involves the process of mucociliary clearance while the second is chemical and involves epithelial cell-secreted organic antibiotics such as defensins, lysozymes, and transferrin that have a bacteriostatic or bactericidal effect on the microorganisms. In addition, the respiratory tract mucosa secretes a small inorganic molecule (OSCN) that enhances the bactericidal effect of organic antibiotics through an oxidative mechanism efficient against both Gram-negative and Gram-positive bacteria without significant host toxicity [2,3,5–8].

In the oropharynx, saliva secretion, epithelial cell desquamation, *in situ* bacterial flora interference, and local production of complement and immunoglobulins are all important parts of host defense mechanisms.

The mucosal immunoglobulin A (IgA), which has antibacterial and antiviral properties, is mostly produced at the level of the upper respiratory tract and accounts for approximately 10% of all nasal secretions proteins. Immunoglobulins G (IgG) and M (IgM) reach the respiratory tract through a transudation process from the systemic circulation. These immunoglobulins have a role in bacterial opsonization (coating), complement activation, and they also promote agglutination. Epithelial cells finally contribute to regulating the inflammatory response by producing cytokines such as tumor necrosis factor (TNF)-alpha, IL-6, IL-8, and other mediators that are helpful in activating the process of recruiting immunocompetent cells such as polynuclear cells and macrophages [2].

The naso- and oropharynx are normally colonized by a mixture of aerobic and anaerobic bacteria including *Streptococcus* spp., *Streptococcus pneumoniae*, *Neisseria* spp., *Fusobacterium* spp., Anaerobic streptococcus, and some *Bacteroides* spp. All of these bacteria are trapped in mucosal adhesion sites and thus play a role in protecting the respiratory tract from colonization by more virulent pathogens.

Modifications in bacterial adherence to the surface epithelium of the upper respiratory tract as a consequence of alterations in the secretion of fibronectin and lactoferrin is a crucial step in the colonization and subsequent modifications in the nature of the oropharyngeal bacterial flora which can potentially lead to respiratory infections. Alterations in fibronectin secretion and in the quality of adherence of the respiratory epithelium for various lectins usually occur as a response to an underlying disease process (respiratory or not) or following a viral infection [2]. On the surface of some bacteria, there are slender thread-like structures named "pili or flagella" which improve bacterial epithelial cell adherence. These structures can also secrete proteolytic enzymes that can degrade IgA and exotoxins thus allowing bacteria to bypass host defenses and initiate colonization. The risk of pathogen colonization of the upper respiratory tract in a given individual is directly proportional to the severity and duration of the underlying disease process and of prior antibiotic therapy.

Risk factors for upper airway colonization also include tobacco smoking, malnutrition, alcoholism, diabetes mellitus, impaired consciousness, low perfusion syndromes, surgery, endotracheal intubation and mechanical ventilation, tracheostomy, neutropenia, compromised immune system, and viral infection.

Bacterial species *Haemophilus influenzae* and *Haemophilus parainfluenzae* are often found in a smoker's upper respiratory tract where they can act as colonization agents. Patients suffering from chronic bronchitis also often have upper airway colonization with *H. influenzae*, *H. parainfluenza*e, *Moraxella catarrhalis*, *S. pneumoniae*, and sometimes Gram-negative bacteria.

Aspiration of oropharyngeal secretions is the most common route for colonization of the lower respiratory tract and, as a consequence, bacteria colonizing the upper respiratory tract are often also involved in the colonization of the lower respiratory tract.

Respiratory tract epithelial cells and secreting cells produce both mucus in the tracheobronchial tree and an alveolar-lining fluid—a thin aqueous film rich in proteins and peptides mixed with transudates from plasma. These proteins and peptides provide a powerful antimicrobial screen, in addition to inhibiting biofilm formation and preventing viral replication. They even have, in some cases, antifungal properties. The alveolar lining fluid contains lysozymes (cell wall degrading enzymes), lactoferrin, and proteinases which can inhibit the function of secreting lymphocytes. These substances have an antimicrobial action and also play a key role in the process of modulating inflammatory responses. The alveolar-lining fluid finally contains surfactant, fibronectin, IgG, and complement, all helpful in the process of opsonization and phagocytosis by macrophages. In addition, some of these molecules play a role in the expression of adherence substances and act as powerful antioxydative and antiproteinase agents. Recent and promising research on the therapeutic potential of these molecules as anti-inflammatory or anti-infectious agents has been carried out by several investigators [2,9,10].

The respiratory epithelial cells are also the source of powerful antimicrobial peptides such as the cathelicidins and human B defensins that can act as chemokines at the level of the T lymphocytes and dendritic cells. As such, they can be helpful in linking innate immunity (nonspecific and nonantibody mediated) and adaptive immunity (specific and antibody mediated) systems. Cellular immunity plays an important role in the defense against pathogens like viruses, intracellular parasites, and other bacteria such as mycobacteria and *Legionella pneumophila* that have the potential to survive inside macrophages. The respiratory system has bronchial-associated lymphoid tissue (BALT), which is similar to the intestinal Peyer plaques. This lymphoid tissue, which is present in both the bronchi and lung parenchyma, is considered to be a reflection of the adaptive immune system response to colonization.

Inhaled antigens can transgress the surface epithelium and stimulate B and T lymphocytes which, in the lung, will produce antibodies and inflammatory mediators in addition to themselves having a cytotoxic activity [9].

The most recent advances with regards to the understanding of host defenses are implicating the "pattern recognition receptors (PRRs)," such as "Toll-like receptors (TLRs)" and the more recently identified cytosolic "NOD-like receptors (NLRs)" [11]. These molecules, which are expressed in alveolar macrophages, epithelial cells, and dendritic cells (Figure 8.2), are able to initiate first-line defenses against pathogens and can also contribute to the activation of other inflammatory mechanisms.

## Phagocytosis and inflammatory reaction

Alveolar macrophages, which are monocytes derivatives, represent first-line defenses against pathogens that have reached the alveoli. In addition to their phagocytic action, the alveolar macrophages are also actively involved in the host inflammatory reaction. When the bacterial load is too important or the pathogens too virulent to be controlled, the macrophages can induce the recruiting of circulating blood neutrophils and monocytes by secreting cytokines, such as the TNF-alpha, IL-26, and the IL-8. In turn, the recruited neutrophils can modulate and mediate the inflammatory reaction by secreting a variety of cytokines [7,9,12]. The recruitment of neutrophils, at least in an acute setting, may be the major component of the host response to bacterial infection [9,13].

The monocyte-derived dendritic cells located in the respiratory epithelium, terminal bronchioles, alveolar septa, pulmonary blood vessels, and visceral pleura can also secrete a number of cytokines which will help to stimulate B- and T-lymphocytes [14].

Other cells such as fibroblasts, smooth muscle cells, and endothelial cells can finally be the source of pro- and anti-inflammatory substances (Figure 8.2).

## Infections of the upper respiratory tract

Infections of the upper respiratory tract are generally limited to mucosal infections and their origin is either bacterial or viral. Classically, these infections are mild and the associated mortality is low (Table 8.1). Even if they are limited to the mucosa, such infections can, however, activate the inflammatory cascade with cytokine and chemokine secretion and a systemic response with hyperthermia. Epiglottitis is, on the other hand, a potentially fatal illness. It is generally related to a Type B *H. influenzae* infection causing edema of the epiglottis with secondary upper airway obstruction and hypoxic respiratory failure. Since the introduction of anti-haemophilus vaccination, however, this type of infection is seldom encountered.

## Infections of the lower respiratory tract

The commonest lower respiratory tract infection is, usually secondary to a viral infection, acute bronchitis. It is essentially a mucosal infection with little or no systemic repercussions. The infection activates a complex signaling circuit to the host innate defense mechanisms which will stimulate cytokine and chemokine secretion and activation of local inflammatory response. This inflammatory response combined to the demise of infected epithelial cells disturbs the mucociliary clearance process and encourages bacterial colonization of the lower respiratory tract by facilitating epithelial cell bacterial adherence. The inflammatory reaction is responsible for the cough, a classical symptom of acute bronchitis, and can also induce a usually transitory bronchial hyperreactivity.

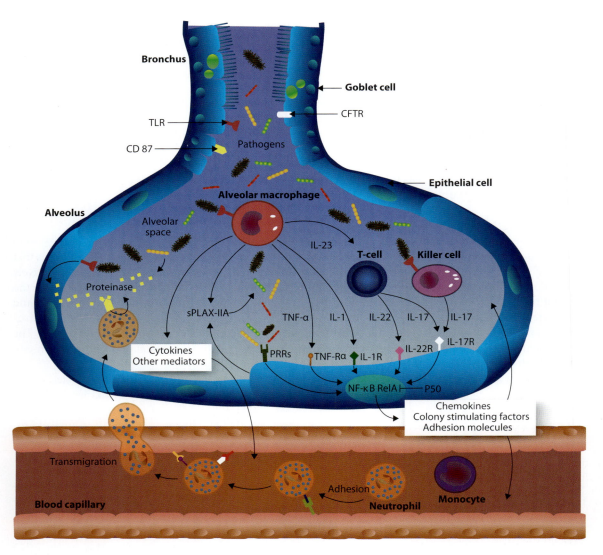

Figure 8.2 Immune and inflammatory defense mechanisms in the distal respiratory tract and alveoli. Cells of the respiratory tract and alveolar space are continuously exposed to large amounts of atmospheric particles and microorganisms. The TLRs and PRRs whose expression is in epithelial cells, alveolar macrophages, dendritic cells, and other cells are able to recognize pathogens and activate various anti-inflammatory and antimicrobial mechanisms through the secretion of multiple cytokines and peptides. Some of these cytokines are then able to initiate the recruiting of neutrophils from systemic capillaries and these neutrophils will enhance intra-alveolar defenses. (Adapted from Opitz, B. et al., *Am J Respir Crit Care Med.*, 181, 1294–1309, 2010).

## Acute exacerbations of chronic obstructive pulmonary disease

In individuals suffering from chronic obstructive pulmonary disease (COPD), the respiratory tract can be colonized without the actual presence of an active infection. The implantation of new bacterial strains or the proliferation of strains already present in the airway greatly facilitates the risk of infections which can

Table 8.1 Infections of the upper respiratory tract

| Infection | Pathogen |
| --- | --- |
| • Pharyngitis, tonsillitis, and laryngitis | Group A streptococcus<br>Adenovirus<br>Enterovirus<br>Epstein–Barr virus<br>Herpes hominis virus<br>Influenza virus<br>*Chlamydophila pneumoniae*<br>Respiratory viruses[a] |
| • Sinusitis | *Streptococcus pneumoniae*<br>*Chlamydophila pneumoniae*<br>*Haemophilus influenzae*<br>Anaerobic bacteria<br>Rhinovirus<br>*Pseudomonas aeruginosa* (rare) |
| • Epiglottitis | *Haemophilus influenzae*<br>*Haemophilus parainfluenzae*<br>*Staphylococcus aureus*<br>Group A streptococcus |
| • Croup | Parainfluenza virus<br>Syncytial respiratory virus<br>Adenovirus<br>*Mycoplasma pneumoniae* |

[a] Influenza A and B viruses, syncytial respiratory adenovirus, metapneumovirus, and parainfluenza virus.

initiate acute exacerbations of COPD, also called acute exacerbations of chronic bronchitis or emphysema. It has been clearly established that exposure to microorganisms, such as viruses or bacteria, is related to the occurrence of exacerbation in COPD patients, [15,16]. In fact, it has been demonstrated that a change in the lung microbiome is associated with COPD exacerbation and is potentially implicated in mediating host inflammatory responses at least in some subjects [17,18]. Moreover, recent studies in COPD patients revealed that the microbiome composition of the lung fluctuates with the severity of COPD [19]. In about 50% of cases, the pathogens are bacteria (Table 8.2). The type of bacteria involved depends on the severity of the underlying obstructive pulmonary disease, the frequency of exacerbations, the presence of associated comorbidities, and if the individual has recently received antibiotic treatment.

Patients presenting with infrequent and uncomplicated exacerbations and who have a baseline forced expiratory volume in 1 second ($FEV_1$) greater than 50% of predicted value are generally infected with *S. pneumoniae* or *H. influenzae*. In contrast, patients who have frequent (more than four episodes per year) and complicated exacerbations, who have a baseline $FEV_1$ smaller than 50% of predicted value, and who, in addition, have associated comorbidities (ischemic heart disease, diabetes, oxygen dependency, corticosteroid therapy, and recent antibiotic treatment) are more likely to be colonized with Gram-negative bacteria (Table 8.3). In these individuals, the superimposed infection will initiate or accentuate the already present inflammatory reaction, which will predispose to interstitial edema and accumulation of endobronchial secretions. These will, in turn, result in increased amount of respiratory work, pulmonary hyperinflation, ventilation/perfusion mismatches, and eventually hypoxic or hypercapnic respiratory failure [20].

Table 8.2 Infections of the lower respiratory tract

| Infection | Pathogen |
| --- | --- |
| Bronchitis and acute exacerbations of COPD | S. pneumoniae, H. influenzae, Moraxella catarrhalis, M. pneumoniae, C. pneumoniae, and respiratory viruses[a] |
| Community-acquired pneumonia | See Table 8.4 |
| Nosocomial pneumonia | S. pneumoniae, H. influenzae, S. aureus, Escherichia coli, Klebsiella spp., Proteus spp., Serratia marcescens, Acinetobacter spp., and P. aeruginosa |

[a] Influenza A and B viruses, syncytial respiratory adenovirus, metapneumovirus, and parainfluenzae virus.

Table 8.3 Acute exacerbations of chronic obstructive pulmonary disease

| Type | Risk factors | Pathogens |
| --- | --- | --- |
| Uncomplicated | None | H. influenzae<br>S. pneumoniae<br>M. catarrhalis |
| Complicated | $FEV_1$ <50% predicted<br>≥4 exacerbations per year<br>Coronary artery disease<br>Oxygen dependency<br>Use of systemic steroids<br>Antibiotic treatment over past 3 months | H. influenzae<br>S. pneumoniae<br>M. catarrhalis<br>Aerobic Gram-negative bacilli<br>Klebsiella spp.<br>P. aeruginosa |

# Pneumonia

Despite the advent of potent antibiotics and effective vaccines, pneumonia remains a potentially fatal illness, especially when it occurs in the very young or very old individuals. The aging of the population with its associated and often numerous comorbidities as well as the inappropriate usage of antibiotics are significant risk factors not only for the occurrence of pneumonia but also for the emergence of resistant to treatment bacterial strains.

Pneumonia is defined as an infection of the lower respiratory tract that involves the secondary lobules of the lung, the respiratory bronchioles, the alveolar ducts, and mostly the alveoli. It results from an infectious process which induces the occurrence of an intra-alveolar exudate second era to lower respiratory tract pathogen proliferation and invasion. The impairment of the host inflammatory and immune (local and systemic) responses may contribute to this phenomenon.

Clinically, patients present with a constellation of symptoms and signs that include fever, chills, cough with purulent sputum production, dyspnea, chest discomfort, tachycardia, and tachypnea with or without alterations in overall general condition depending on the severity of illness. Abnormal findings on physical examination include crepitation on auscultation (crackles) and signs of pulmonary consolidation such as dullness on percussion and bronchial breathing. Biologically, the majority of patients have leukocytosis as well as other nonspecific findings indicative of an inflammatory reaction such as an elevated C-reactive protein and sedimentation rate. The presence of a pulmonary alveolar-type infiltrate with an air bronchogram on a chest radiograph represents the gold standard for the diagnosis of pneumonia. Other possible radiographic patterns include segmental, lobar or multilobar distribution, and, on occasion, presence of an interstitial process. In approximately 20%–40% of cases, a pleural effusion called a parapneumonic effusion will be associated to the pneumonia [1,2,21].

## Community-acquired pneumonia

Community-acquired pneumonia (CAP) occurs in patients who have not recently (within 14 days) been hospitalized in an acute or chronic care facility (including nursing homes). By contrast, hospital-acquired pneumonia (HAP), also called nosocomial pneumonia, is defined as pneumonia occurring after 48–72 hours after hospital admission in a patient neither infected nor incubating an infection upon admission and less than 14 days following hospital discharge. Nosocomial pneumonia is sometimes called ventilation-associated pneumonia (VAP) because it often occurs in intubated patients under mechanical ventilation. In such cases, the pneumonia often results from aspiration which may have occurred during the intubation process or aspiration around the endotracheal tube.

CAP usually results from microaspiration of infected oropharyngeal secretions (bacteria) or inhalation of pathogens, such as viruses, atypical agents, mycobacteria, and fungal agents, in the lower respiratory tract. Less commonly, the pneumonia will result from direct extension of infectious foci located in contiguous areas such as the mediastinum or the subphrenic spaces, from hematogenous spread from a distant infected foci, or from traumatic implant such as can occur following biopsy or penetrating chest injuries. Pneumonia in immunocompromised hosts can occur when microorganisms, such as *Mycobacterium tuberculosis* or *Pneumocystis jiroveci*, who were in a latent phase become reactivated.

CAP causative agents are most commonly microorganisms that have already colonized the oropharynx (Table 8.4).

The presence of pathogens in the lower respiratory tract, their proliferation, and the beginning of the infectious process will trigger the release of previously described mediators of host defense mechanisms as well as that of an acute inflammatory reaction. Indeed, close contact between pathogen and epithelial

Table 8.4 Predominant pathogens in community-acquired and nosocomial pneumonia

| Pneumonia setting | Pathogens |
| --- | --- |
| Ambulatory patient | *S. pneumoniae* |
|  | *M. pneumoniae* |
|  | *H. influenzae* |
|  | *C. pneumoniae* |
|  | Respiratory viruses[a] |
| In-hospital patient (nonintensive care unit) | *S. pneumoniae* |
|  | *M. pneumoniae* |
|  | *C. pneumoniae* |
|  | *H. influenzae* |
|  | *Legionella* spp. |
|  | Anaerobic bacteria (aspiration) |
|  | Respiratory viruses[a] |
| In-hospital patient (intensive care unit) | *S. pneumoniae* |
|  | *S. aureus* |
|  | *Legionella* spp. |
|  | Virulent Gram-negative bacteria |
|  | *H. influenzae* |

[a] Influenzae viruses A and B, syncytial respiratory adenovirus, metapneumovirus, and parainfluenzae virus

surface (respiratory tract or alveolus) activates multiple circuits of complex signaling which, in turn, initiate chemokine expression by recruiting phagocytic cells and neutrophils to the infected area [4,7,9].

Locally, the inflammatory response can lead to decreased pulmonary compliance that can result, regionally, in ventilation/perfusion ($\dot{V}/\dot{Q}$) imbalances with subsequent right to left shunt. In patients with severe pneumonia, the hypoxemia resulting from impaired $\dot{V}/\dot{Q}$ ratios can initiate reflex pulmonary vasoconstriction which may reduce the significance of the shunt effect. The pneumonia-induced inflammatory reaction will generally stimulate cytokines and other mediators' production responsible for the systemic pneumonia-associated fever as well as other biological signs of acute inflammation.

If the pneumonia is not controlled, it can initiate a bacteremia with eventual multi-organ failure. Locally, pneumonia can be complicated by an acute lung injury (ALI) syndrome or adult respiratory distress syndrome (ARDS).

## Viral pneumonia

Viral pneumonia generally occurs in children and the most commonly involved pathogens are the syncytial respiratory viruses, the metapneumoviruses, the adenoviruses, the rhinoviruses, the enteroviruses, and the influenza virus. In the adult population, the common causative viruses include the influenza viruses A and B, the adenoviruses, and the syncytial respiratory viruses. These viruses can either be the only organisms involved in the infection or they can act, in synergy, with other pathogens such as *M. pneumoniae* or *Chlamydophila pneumoniae* [1,21]. Indeed, viral/bacteria mixed infections occur in approximately 20% of CAP and mixed infections involving rhinoviruses and *S. pneumoniae* bacteria are currently not uncommon. Patients so infected will often have more severe pneumonia and it has been shown that an infection with a rhinovirus may encourage Streptococcus adherence to the respiratory surface epithelium [22,23].

Viral respiratory infections often have a seasonal pattern and, clinically, their mode of presentation is similar to that of nonviral pneumonia with fever (sometimes low grade), cough (often nonproductive), and myalgia. Radiologically, the image may be that of a reticular interstitial pattern. Pathophysiologically, viruses invade epithelial cells, replicate, and the infection then spreads locally from one cell to the next. Viral pneumonia is usually caused by microdroplet inhalation and, in many cases, hands are involved in the transmission of infection. As in bacterial infections, T- and B-lymphocytes are part of the specific host defense mechanisms against viruses.

T "helper" lymphocytes and alveolar macrophages are involved in the production of a myriad of cytokines as well as interferon in attempting to prevent viral replication and draw in more phagocytic cells. Secreted antibodies slow down the propagation of infection and encourage the lysis of viruses through opsonization (coating), neutralization, complement activation, and activation of cytotoxic lymphocytes. At the alveolar level, the influx of inflammatory mediators increases capillary permeability and forming of an inflammatory exudate thus increasing the severity of V/Q ratio imbalances. Ultimately, these responses can lead to ARDS or to a systemic inflammatory syndrome. All viral respiratory infections can have complications, the commonest being bacterial supra-infections (secondary infections) generally caused by *Staphylococcus aureus* and *S. pneumoniae* [22].

## Tuberculosis and other atypical mycobacteria

Pulmonary mycobacterial diseases are pathologic processes in which the lung is infected with mycobacterial organisms. Tuberculosis is caused by *M. tuberculosis*, but species of mycobacteria other than tuberculosis (MOTT) can produce similar pathologic changes. The infections mainly involve the lungs where cell-mediated immunity results in the formation of granulomas.

# Tuberculosis

*M. tuberculosis* ( Tuberculosis or Koch bacillus) (MTB) infections are, after HIV, the second commonest cause of adult pulmonary infections worldwide, with nearly 8 million new cases being diagnosed every year, mostly in underdeveloped countries, and 1.7 million annual deaths directly related to the disease (statistics from the World Health Organization [24]). It is also known that approximately 5%–10% of contaminated individuals will go on to develop an active disease, usually within 2–3 years of the initial contact. For the remaining contaminated individuals, the bacillus can remain in a latent phase only to become reactivated several years later, a phenomenon known as "secondary tuberculosis" (Figure 8.3).

The transmission of tuberculosis usually occurs by way of an airborne or aerosol route. Droplets are expelled from infected people during cough and, if droplet diameter is large enough (5–10 μ) bronchial airflow will favor their deposition deep in the lung [25], usually in the basal segments of the lower lobes and apical and posterior segments of the upper lobes, areas known as the primary infection segments. In the first stage, nonactivated macrophages ingest the tubercle bacilli and, depending on the virulence of the bacilli and the macrophages microbicidal activity, bacilli multiplication is inhibited or the bacilli are destroyed. Infected macrophages release cytokines and chemokines that attract additional macrophages as well as neutrophils resulting in the formation of granulomas, called tubercles, a characteristic pathologic finding in tuberculosis. Tuberculous granulomas are characterized by the accumulation of

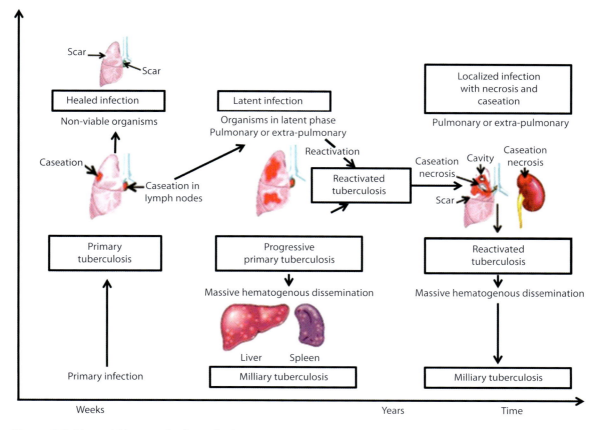

Figure 8.3 Natural history of tuberculosis.

blood-derived macrophages, epithelioid cells which are degenerating macrophages, and multinucleated giant cells (Langhans' cells), which are fused macrophages with nuclei around the periphery. If, at this stage, the infection is not quelled, tubercles will increase in size and the bacilli may contaminate adjacent lymph nodes, another typical feature of primary pulmonary tuberculosis. The pulmonary lesion and associated nodal involvement (usually calcified nodes) is called a Ghon complex which is often the only remaining evidence of the primary tuberculous infection.

When the number of bacilli reaches $10^3$–$10^4$, which occurs 2–6 weeks after the initial infection, cell-mediated immunity and delayed hypersensitivity with associated tissue repair will occur in order to prevent parenchymal destruction.

Macrophage death causes central caseation which is typical although not specific to MTB infections. Caseum, the Latin word for cheese, consists of cellular debris having the consistency of soft cheese. Various cytokines and enzymes secreted by cytotoxic cells also contribute to the occurrence of central caseation. The cell-mediated immunity reaction also involves CD4+ lymphocytes who will produce gamma interferon (INF-y)—a substance which will increase the ability of macrophages to ingest and destroy the tuberculous bacilli [26].

Extrapulmonary tuberculosis is secondary to hematogenous or lymphatic spread of pulmonary lesions and virtually any organ can become infected. Extrapulmonary sites of interest include the gastrointestinal tract (swallowed secretions), the pericardium where tuberculosis can cause a constrictive pericarditis, the pleural space (pleural tuberculosis), and the bones including the spine (Pott's disease).

In approximately 5%–10% of individuals infected primarily with tuberculosis, reactivation will occur some years later, a phenomenon called reactivated tuberculosis. Typically, but not exclusively, reactivated tuberculosis begins in the apical or posterior segments of the upper lobes where it is believed that the sites were seeded during the bacteremia of primary infection. Risk factors for reactivated tuberculosis include human immunodeficiency virus (HIV) infection, renal failure, diabetes, lymphomas, and corticosteroid or other immunosuppression or immunomodulatory drugs usage.

## Atypical mycobacteria

Several MOTT (mycobacteria other than tuberculosis) are present in the environment but most are human saprophytes. Some of these bacteria can, however, produce clinical infections and the ones most commonly associated with lung disease are *Mycobacterium avium-intracellulare* and *Mycobacterium Kansasii*. These infections can occur in individuals without systemic risk factors but who have bronchiectasis or cystic fibrosis [27,28].

Other than the lungs, the most common organs that can be affected by MOTT are the cervical lymph nodes, the soft tissues, the bones, and the joints.

## Parasitic, fungal, and other infections in the immunocompromised host

The reader is refered to reviews of this topic for more information [29].

## Conclusion

Respiratory infections are common and, represent one of the leading causes of death, worldwide. Through their virulence and pathogenicity, the infectious agents that are responsible for those respiratory infections have an unbelievable ability to quickly adjust to environmental conditions to maximize pathogenicity.

Faced with this constant threat, the respiratory system has powerful antimicrobial defenses as well as important anti-inflammatory properties, both being efficient in their fight against microbial aggression.

When evaluating patients with suspected respiratory infections, it is finally important to make judicious use of the various modalities, such as clinical examination, radiological and microbiological testing, available to clinicians to accurately diagnose and properly plan treatment of such individuals. Underlying disorders such as the presence of immunosuppression must also be carefully assessed because they represent significant risk factors for infection-related morbidity and mortality.

# References

1. Mason CM, Summer WR. Respiratory infection. *Pulmonary Pathophysiology*. New York, NY: McGraw Hill 2005, 2nd edition. Chapter 10; 169–192.
2. Donowitz GR. Acute pneumonia. *Mandell, Douglas, and Bennett's. Principles and Practice of Infectious Diseases*. Churchill Livingstone 2010, 7th edition. Chapter 64; 891–916.
3. Puchelle E, Girod-de-Bentzmann S, Jacquot J. Airway defence mechanisms in relation to biochemical and physical properties of mucus. *Eur Respir Rev* 1992; 2: 259–263.
4. Reynolds HY. Pulmonary host defenses. *Chest* 1989; 95: 223s–230s.
5. Sibille Y, Reynolds HY. Macrophage and polymorphonuclear neutrophils in lung defense and injury. *Am Rev Respir Dis* 1990; 141: 471–501.
6. Rogan MP, Gerarghty P, Greene CM et al. Antimicrobial proteins and polypeptides in pulmonary innate defense. *Respir Res* 2006; 7: 29–40.
7. Prince A, Mizgerd JP, Wiener-Kronish J, Bhattacharya J. Cell signaling underlying the pathophysiology of pneumonia. *Am J Physiol Lung Cell Mol Physiol* 2006; 291: L297–L300.
8. Akira S, Uematsu S, Takeuchi O. Pathogen recognition and innate immunity. *Cell* 2006; 124: 783–801.
9. Mizgerd JP. Mechanisms of disease: Acute lower respiratory tract infection. *N Engl J Med* 2008; 358: 716–727.
10. Diamond G, Legarda D, Ryan LK. The innate immune response of the respiratory epithelium. *Immunol Rev* 2000; 173: 27–38.
11. Opitz B, Van Laak V, Eitel J, Suttor N. Innate immune recognition in infectious and non-infectious disease of the lung. *Am J Respir Crit Care Med* 2010; 181: 1294–1309.
12. Che KE, Tengvall S, Levänen B et al. Interleukin-26 in antibacterial host defence of human lungs. Effects on neutrophil mobilization. *Am J Respir Crit Care Med* 2014; 190 (9): 1022–1031.
13. Mizgerd JP. Molecular mechanisms of neutrophil recruitment elicited by bacteria in the lung. *Sem Immunol* 2002; 14: 123–132.
14. Nicod L.P. Lung defences: An overview. *Eur Respir Rev* 2005; 14: 95, 45–50.
15. Papi A, Bellato CM, Braccioni F et al. Infection and airway inflammation in chronic obstructive pulmonary disease severe exacerbations. *Am J Respir Crit Care Med* 2006; 173: 1114–1121.
16. De Serre G, Lampron N, Laforge J et al. Importance of viral infection in chronic obstructive pulmonary disease exacerbation. *J Clinn Virol* 2009; 46: 129–133.
17. Wang Z, Bafadhel M, Haldar K et al. Lung microbiome dynamics in COPD exacerbations. *Eur Respir J* 2016; 47: 1082–1092.
18. Sze MA, Dimitriu PA, Hayashi S et al. The lung tissue microbiome in chronic obstructive pulmonary disease. *Am J Respir Crit Care Med* 2012; 185: 1073–1080.
19. Mammmen MJ, Sethi S. COPD and the microbiome. *Respirology* 2016; 21: 590–599.
20. O'Donnell DE, Hernandez P, Kaplan A et al. Canadian Thoracic Society recommendations for management of chronic obstructive pulmonary disease-2008 Updated. *Can Resp J* 2008; 15 (Suppl A): 1A–8A.
21. Lynch JP, Zhanel GG. Streptococcus pneumonia: Epidemiology, risk factors, and strategies for prevention. *Sem Respir Crit Care Med* 2009; 30: 189–209.
22. Olivier BGG, Lim S, Wark P et al. Rhinovirus exposure impairs immune response to bacterial products in human alveolar macrophage. *Thorax* 2008; 63: 519–525.
23. Jenning LC, Anderson TP, Beynon KA et al. Incidence and characteristics of viral community-acquired pneumonia in adults. *Thorax* 2008; 63: 42–48.
24. WHO Publications on Tuberculosis. http://www.who.int/tb/publications/en/.
25. Adler JJ, Rose DN. Transmission and pathogenesis of tuberculosis. In: Rom WN, Garey S, eds. *Tuberculosis*. Toronto, Canada: Little, Brown and Company 1996; 129–140.

26. Piessens WF, Nardell EA. Pathogenesis of tuberculosis. In: Reichman LB, Hershfield ES, eds. *Tuberculosis: A Comprehensive International Approach*. 2nd edition. New York, NY: Marcel Decker, Inc. 2000; 241–260.
27. Griffith DE, Aksamit T, Brown-Elliott BA et al. An official ATS/IDSA statement: Diagnosis, treatment, and prevention of nontuberculous mycobacterial diseases. *Am J Respir Crit Care Med* 2007; 175: 367–416.
28. Griffith DE, Aksamit TR. Bronchiectasis and nontuberculous mycobacterial disease. *Clin Chest Med* 2012; 33: 283–285.
29. Corti M, Palmero D, Eiguchi K. Respiratory infections in immunocompromised patients. *Curr Opin Pulm Med* 2009; 15: 209–217.

# 9
# Sleep-related breathing disorders

FRÉDÉRIC SÉRIÈS and WENYANG LI

| | |
|---|---|
| Introduction | 163 |
| Terminology and consequences of sleep-related breathing disorders | 164 |
| Pathophysiology of nocturnal hypoventilation | 164 |
| OSA/hypopnea syndrome | 165 |
| Efficiency of UA dilating muscle contraction | 166 |
|     Upper airway size and shape | 167 |
|     Factors interfering with UA muscle physiological properties | 167 |
|     Mechanical coupling between UA muscles and perimuscular soft tissues | 168 |
|     Consequences of sleep on respiratory and UA activity | 168 |
|     Fluctuations in the level of activity of respiratory and UA dilating muscles | 168 |
|     Role of tissue inflammation and surface tension forces | 169 |
|     Clinical applications | 169 |
| Central sleep apnea | 169 |
| Conclusions | 170 |
| References | 170 |

## Introduction

Sleep-related breathing disorders occur due to the effects of sleep on the central nervous respiratory control system and/or on upper airway (UA) patency. Sleep can thus initiate periods of hypoventilation in individuals already afflicted by disturbances of their ventilatory mechanics such as those suffering from chronic obstructive pulmonary disease, restrictive lung disease, neuromuscular disorders, and morbid obesity. Sleep can also be associated with respiratory instability which, in turn, can translate into the occurrence of respiratory disorders of central origin such as seen in patients with Cheyne–Stokes respiration. Finally, the occurrence of partial or complete UA obstruction during sleep characterizes the obstructive sleep apnea (OSA)/hypopnea syndrome. Interestingly, these various sleep-related breathing disorders can occur jointly, depending on the nature of the underlying disease process (obesity, restrictive thoracic disease, myopathy, and left-sided heart failure) that may be present. Proper understanding of all these patterns of sleep-breathing disorders is essential if one wants to initiate and implement the proper and personalized management.

## Terminology and consequences of sleep-related breathing disorders

Breathing (respiration), which is mainly under a behavioral or voluntary control system during awakening, is essentially under a metabolic or automated control system during sleep (stage I, II, and III). During rapid eye movement (REM) sleep, however, breathing loses this metabolic control and respiratory efficiency decreases by about 10% (reduction in ventilatory response to metabolic stimuli, increase in UA resistance, decreased ventilatory response to resistance loading), accounting for an increase in the partial pressure of carbon dioxide ($PaCO_2$) and a modest lowering of the partial pressure of oxygen ($PaO_2$) [1]. During the periods of light sleep (sleep stages I and II), respiration is irregular due to variations in tidal volume but it becomes remarkably regular during periods of slow wave sleep (delta sleep). The most irregular ventilatory pattern (amplitude and frequency) is seen during REM sleep.

The contribution of the thoracic cage to the overall respiration remains the same during wakefulness and nonrapid eye movement (NREM) sleep (+/−40%). However, it decreases significantly during REM sleep (+/−20%). The decrease in sleep-related tonic (inactive) and phasic (active) striated muscle activity is mostly seen in UA [2] and accessory respiratory muscles (intercostal) while diaphragmatic muscle activity is preserved. During sleep, lower intrathoracic airway resistance remains unchanged in contrast to that of the velo- and oropharyngeal airway which largely increase [3]. This decrease in muscle tone is more important during REM sleep than it is in NREM sleep and it is associated with reductions in lung volume.

Breathing disorders occurring during sleep include disturbances in gas exchange (hypoventilation with secondary hypoxemia/hypercapnia) and/or complete or partial transient reduction in $\dot{V}$ (apnea/hypopnea). Apnea and hypopnea are further classified as being of central origin (central sleep apnea) if they are secondary to a disturbance in the respiratory central control system or obstructive (OSA) or if they are related to UA closure with maintenance of respiratory efforts. In cases of partial UA obstruction, there is a plateauing in inspiratory air flow despite increases in intrathoracic pressures (flow limitation). Recovery of ventilation after episodes of OSA generally occurs in conjunction with awakening or arousal.

Each sleep-related breathing disorder can have short- and long-term consequences. Overnight nocturnal hypoventilation with secondary hypoxemia and hypercapnia, for instance, are associated with increases in pulmonary artery pressures that can, in turn, potentially lead to pulmonary hypertension and right-sided heart failure (chronic cor pulmonale). In patients already suffering from pulmonary diseases, nocturnal hypoventilation is also associated with increased morbidity and mortality [4,5]. Nocturnal episodes of apnea or hypopnea are associated with repetitive periods of arterial oxygen ($SaO_2$) desaturation and with short periods of electroencephalographic (EEG) awakening leading to fragmented sleep. The magnitude of arterial desaturation is variable but, in general, it is more significant in individuals with lower baseline $SaO_2$, in those with prolonged episodes of apnea/hypopnea, and in those with lower baseline lung volumes. Obstructive apnea/hypopnea is also associated with more significant episodes of desaturation than sleep-related breathing disorders of central origin. The effect of sleep apnea/hypopnea on the autonomic nervous system (increase in sympathetic activity and decrease in parasympathetic activity) also contributes to fluctuations in systemic arterial blood pressure. In addition to the cardiovascular risks associated with the hemodynamic consequences of OSA/hypopnea, periodic episodes of arterial desaturation/resaturation (intermittent hypoxia) and perturbations in neurovegetative activity could promote the occurrence of arteriosclerotic vascular disease as well as of metabolic complications, such as insulin resistance, possibly in relation with a systemic inflammatory response [6,7].

## Pathophysiology of nocturnal hypoventilation

Considering the importance of the metabolic regulation in the control of respiration during sleep, one can easily speculate that any change in the ventilatory response to hypoxic or hypercapnic stimuli (primary central hypoventilation or hypoventilation secondary to the use of respiratory depressive medication) will increase the magnitude of nocturnal hypoventilation episodes. On the other hand, nocturnal hypoventilation can improve during REM sleep when it is not related to mechanical disturbances of the respiratory system because respiration is not under metabolic control.

Other possible causes of nocturnal hypoventilation mostly relate to respiratory muscle weakness like that seen in neuromuscular disorders such as myotonic dystrophy, muscular dystrophy of Duchenne, congenital myopathies, Steinert's disease, and diaphragmatic paralysis. Nocturnal hypoventilation can also relate to unfavorable mechanical conditions that may prevail during the contraction of respiratory muscles such as is seen in patients with chronic obstructive pulmonary disease, restrictive lung disease, and morbid obesity. In such individuals, the efficiency of ventilation is maintained during wakefulness through the recruitment of accessory respiratory muscles. Even if diaphragmatic activity is relatively preserved during sleep, the reduction in accessory respiratory muscle activity occurring during sleep makes these individuals even more dependent on the efficiency of diaphragmatic contraction.

During REM sleep, the degree of hypoventilation increases in these patients in relation with the drop of skeletal muscle tone, reduction in lung volumes, and increase in UA resistance. These conditions explain why severe episodes of desaturation can be observed in patients with diaphragmatic paralysis during REM sleep. This also accounts for the differences in the magnitude of nocturnal desaturation episodes between subjects with emphysema-related respiratory failure (slim individuals with pulmonary hyperinflation) who mostly have desaturation episodes during REM sleep and those with chronic bronchitis (overweight individuals with little or no hyperinflation and low resting $SaO_2$) who have stable oxygen desaturation during non-REM sleep which is further increased during REM sleep [8].

Disturbances in gas exchange can become even more significant when added to ventilation/perfusion mismatches often seen in patients with decreased lung volumes (restrictive thoracic disorders, morbid obesity, and REM sleep). The occurrence of additional nocturnal apnea episodes increases the severity of desaturation as well as that of their hemodynamic consequences [9]. Any iatrogenic central respiratory depression (narcotics, hypnotics) will also increase the deleterious effects of sleep on nocturnal ventilation. The occurrence of nocturnal hypoventilation is often a turning point in the progression of any underlying disease which will necessitate the use of specific therapeutic strategies.

## OSA/hypopnea syndrome

UA are usually patent throughout the respiratory cycle and they behave in a manner similar to that of a Starling resistance model where a collapsible segment (pharynx) is located between two noncollapsible segments (osseous and cartilaginous nasal and laryngeal airway) (Figure 9.1). The negative inspiratory intraluminal pressure in the

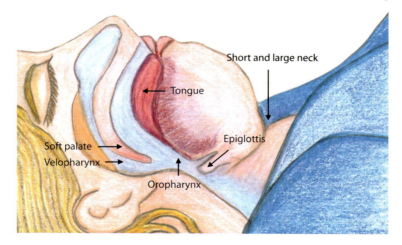

Figure 1. Schematic illustration of the different upper airway levels

UA and the weight of the soft tissues surrounding them tend to passively collapse the UA. This effect is, however, counterbalanced by the activation and contraction of oropharyngeal stabilizing muscles which precedes that of respiratory muscles [10], and whose activation is serotoninergic and adrenergic controlled [11]. Outside of sleep, other important factors that control dilating oropharyngeal muscle activity are metabolic (hypoxia, hypercapnia) [12] and mechanical (reflex activation of stabilizing oropharyngeal muscles in response to UA negative pressure) [13,14]. Of note, this reflex activation response has been shown to decrease during sleep [15].

These factors will influence UA cross-sectional area depending on the compliance of the UA and of its shape and cross-sectional area. Simultaneous recording of UA cross-sectional area and intraluminal pressure taken during nasopharyngoscopy allow for the measurement of the static compliance of various segments of the UA (naso-, velo-, oro-, and hypo-pharyngeal levels) [16]. The critical closing pressure (Pcrit) is the level of trans-pharyngeal pressure at which there is complete UA obstruction. This pressure is subatmospheric in normal individuals, less negative in snorers, and atmospheric or positive in apneic individuals [17].

The UA shape and cross-sectional area play an important role in the pathophysiology of sleep-induced UA closure because these parameters determine the efficiency of UA stabilizing forces. The UA cross-sectional area varies during the respiratory cycle (smaller at end-expiration, slowly getting larger at the beginning of inspiration, and stabilizing during the reminder of inspiration) [18]. Such changes are due to the influence of changes in lung volumes [19,20], on the positioning of the arch of the hyoid bone [21], and longitudinal traction of UA wall with tracheal traction [22]. Thus end-expiratory volume is an important factor involved in UA occlusion [23,24], as suggested by the gradual increase in UA resistance during the respiratory cycles preceding episodes of obstructive apnea [25]. The consequences of lung deflation on UA size are more significant in apneic patients than they are in normal individuals [26]. It has finally been shown that the variations in circulating blood volume and vascular tone can also influence UA cross-sectional area and collapsibility [27].

The forces involved in the stabilization or collapse of the UA have an impact on their propensity to close during sleep as documented by their influence on Pcrit. In an animal model, for instance, mass loading simulating excess fat tissue weight at the level of the cricothyroid membrane increases Pcrit in proportion to increases in weight [28]. In contrast, lowering the transmural pressure gradient by applying negative pressure in the tissues surrounding the neck will significantly lower UA resistance [29]. In anesthetized and paralyzed apneic subjects, positive or negative values of Pcrit correlate with respectively greater or lower proportions of UA adipose and muscular tissues [30]. Subatmospheric Pcrit levels documented in apneic patients in which airway collapsibility is measured in the absence of activation of muscle tone/activity highlight the importance of UA stabilizing forces [31,32]. Improvements in Pcrit observed after uvulopalatopharyngoplasty also demonstrate the influence of tissue weight on Pcrit [33]. With regards to stabilizing muscles effect on Pcrit, its value becomes less negative following the administration of diazepam [34], and more negative after hypercapnic stimulation [35] which respectively decrease and increase the tonic and phasic activity of UA muscles. The interaction between the numerous mechanisms involved in UA closing and reopening is detailed in figure 9.2.

The presence or absence of obstructive respiratory disorders during sleep depends on the dynamic interaction of the various factors determining Pcrit values. The previously described forces have an influence on UA patency not only through the amplitude of stabilizing forces but also depending on their mechanical effectiveness. The influence of the force generated by the contraction of stabilizing muscles cannot be separated from the mechanical characteristic of perimuscular soft tissues and UA size and shape.

## Efficiency of UA dilating muscle contraction

The stabilizing effect resulting from the contraction of pharyngeal dilating muscles depends on the intensity of their neuromuscular activity [36,37] and of the mechanical conditions prevailing when they contract.

Efficiency of UA dilating muscle contraction 167

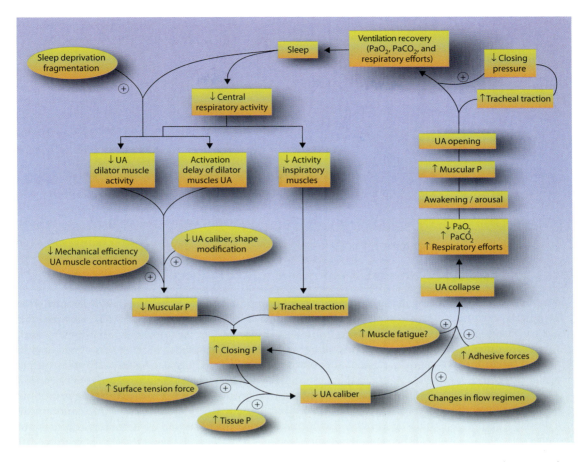

Figure 9.2 Interaction between the numerous mechanisms involved in upper airway (UA) closing and reopening.

## Upper airway size and shape

An increase in the thickness of the lateral pharyngeal walls [38] and the presence of fat deposits along those walls [39] can explain the differences in UA shape observed between normal individuals and apneic patients (elliptical configuration with coronal axis in normal individuals and sagittal axis in apneic patients) [40]. UA are more compliant in their lateral than posterior–anterior axis [41], and abovementioned differences in UA shape can alter muscle contraction efficiency by putting them in an unfavorable mechanical condition [42]. Other than what can be observed with soft tissue mechanical properties *per se*, dynamic factors can also alter UA size and shape. Indeed, some authors have recently reported that transferring blood volume from the lower limbs when recumbent (fluid shift) may reduce UA cross-sectional area and increase their collapsibility [43,44]. In apneic individuals, for instance, the severity of sleep-related breathing disorders is positively correlated with the amount of overnight fluid shift [45].

## Factors interfering with UA muscle physiological properties

Electromyography (EMG) measurements of UA muscle activity are useful to quantify the level of neuromuscular activation but much less useful in providing information on strength being developed. *In vitro* studies have shown that the musculus uvulae muscle is able to generate more tension in apneic patients than in snorers, without any difference in levels of fatigue between the two groups under hypoxic conditions [46]. The larger muscular cross-sectional area observed in apneic subjects can account for these results [3,16].

The histochemical features of UA muscles are consistent from one muscle to the other, the proportion of type II muscle fibers (middle pharyngeal constrictor muscle) being higher than that of type I fibers in snorers than in nonsnorers [47]. Similarly, this proportion is higher in apneic patients than in snorers as measured in the musculus uvulae muscle [16] and genioglossus [48]. The metabolic characteristics of the musculus uvulae muscle are, however, different between apneic subjects and simple snorers. Both pharyngeal and laryngeal muscles seem to have some degree of physiological adaptation in response to repeated, supramaximal, and prolonged stimuli in snorers and apneic subjects [49].

The characteristics of the contractility of UA muscles can be altered in vivo by changing the setting in which they contract such as during sustained severe hypoxia [50]. On the other hand, the suction (aspiration) effect secondary to the negative pressure developing in the UA during inspiratory loading can stretch them and generate passive inspiratory muscular lengthening (eccentric contraction) with secondary lowering of contractility efficiency [51].

## Mechanical coupling between UA muscles and perimuscular soft tissues

In the animal model, signs of myopathy, such as fibrosis, edema, fiber grouping, and fascicular atrophy, which are all indicative of muscular suffering, have been documented in some UA muscles [52,53]. Such muscular damage has also been documented in humans (musculus uvulae muscle, palatopharyngeal muscle) without any significant differences between nonapneic snorers and apneic individuals [54,55]. Signs of mucosal and submucosal inflammation and of interstitial and interfascicular fibrosis may also be present and are indicative of some degree of UA skeletal muscle trauma secondary to tissue vibration occurring during sleep [56–58]. These features may have an influence on the mechanical properties of UA muscles and be responsible for the increase in uvula stiffness as reported in vitro in apneic patients compared to nonapneic snorers [59]. Thus, despite a higher potential to generate tension, tissue displacement secondary to muscular contraction is less effective in apneic subjects because of the impediment in the transmission of these dilating forces as a consequence of the soft tissues stiffness.

## Consequences of sleep on respiratory and UA activity

Both tonic and phasic activities of UA muscles are lowered during sleep although the consequences of such reduction may vary from one muscle to the other [60–62]. UA closure occurs when the level of activity of each of these muscles is at its lowest [63]. During sleep [64,65] and mostly during wakefulness [66], genioglossal muscle activity is higher in apneic subjects than in normal controls. One cannot thus invoke a disproportionate sleep-related decrease in oropharyngeal dilating muscle neuromuscular activity in apneic patients as an explanation to the UA closure.

## Fluctuations in the level of activity of respiratory and UA dilating muscles

Obstructive sleep-related breathing disorders are mostly seen in conditions where respiration becomes unstable during sleep [67]. Several arguments can be put forward to support the hypothesis that, during sleep, respiratory instability facilitates secondary UA instability [68–70] through a reduction in oropharyngeal muscle activity and occurrence of an activation delay in UA dilating muscles when compared to that of the respiratory muscles [71]. Respiratory stability can be assessed by the ventilatory loop gain that quantified the responsiveness of the respiratory system to a breathing disturbance—the higher the loop gain the higher respiratory instability. The influence of this physiological marker is supported by the positive correlation observed between

AHI and loop gain in patients with minimal to moderate increase in UA collapsibility (Pcrit) [72] and by the drop in apnea–hypopnea index (AHI) with oxygen therapy in patients with high loop gain [73].

The influence of the activity level in UA stabilizing muscles on their collapsibility can be reproduced during wakefulness through phrenic nerve stimulation in the neck. When the stimulus is applied at end-expiration, the pattern of the resulting flow-pressure curve is indicative of the UA mechanical properties that are observed when there is no phasic activity of stabilizing UA muscles [74,75]. The implications of the phrenic nerve stimulation experiments have some physiological interest such as in the evaluation of the role of tonic activity of dilating muscles on UA stability [76], measurement of UA collapsibility [77], evaluation of the consequences of head and neck postural changes on UA dynamics [78], assessment of mechanical efficiency of the contraction of UA stabilizing muscles [79], and breathing route on UA collapsibility [80]. They can also have some clinical interest such as in the identification of apneic subjects [81], measurement of the level of efficient positive pressure through maneuvers done during awakening [82], and assessment of the success rate of treatment with an oral appliance depending on the level of obstruction (i.e., velo- or oropharyngnx) observed during phrenic nerve stimulation [83].

## Role of tissue inflammation and surface tension forces

The degree of UA muscle inflammation [84] observed in subjects with OSA/hypopnea syndrome is magnified by weight excess [85]. These inflammatory changes could also contribute to UA sensory impairment [86]. They influence UA collapsibility [87] and are reversible with OSA treatment [88]. Surface tension forces contribute to the maintenance of UA closure once they are occluded [89]. In awake normal human subjects, synthetic lung surfactant decreases UA patency and closing pressures [90], suggesting that UA surface tension forces contribute to the maintenance of UA patency. Reduction in UA resistance [91] and in the severity of snoring [92] observed after the administration of surfactant could thus be attributed to this phenomenon.

## Clinical applications

Reducing the amount of fluid going to the UA could be an interesting therapeutic approach. The clinical benefits that have been observed [93], however, appear to be somewhat less than what had been experimentally documented [45]. Nonetheless, it is noticeable that simple strategies such as wearing compression stocking may contribute to decrease the severity of OSA and then could be used in complement to other potentially effective treatment options. Once UA obstruction has occurred, normal breathing will be achieved if UA dilator muscles are sensitive to the increase in respiratory drive (through UA negative pressure), if this increase in neuromuscular activity translates into effective dilating forces and if breathing efforts do not provoke an arousal before UA opening has occurred. This pathophysiological model suggests that the balance between UA muscles neuromechanical responsiveness, arousal threshold, and ventilator loop gain contribute to determine UA patency independently of UA collapsibility. Thus, the identification of physiological characteristics that may, in given individuals, contribute to UA obstruction could potentially lead to personalized therapies [94] with the objectives of reducing the sensitivity of ventilatory loop gain (i.e., oxygen, acetazolamide), increasing UA cross-sectional area (i.e., surgery, mandibular advancement), lowering the awakening threshold (i.e., sedatives), and increasing the dilating force resulting from the contraction of UA stabilizing muscles (i.e., neuromediators, neuromuscular stimulation).

## Central sleep apnea

Nonobstructive respiratory disorders include those related to isolated central sleep apnea, or those associated with episodes of hyper/hypoventilation (Cheyne–Stokes breathing). Disorders that are central in origin generally occur during periods of sleep stages 1 and 2 and, by contrast to obstructive sleep disorders, they are uncommon during paradoxical sleep where ventilation is no longer under metabolic control.

Cheyne–Stokes respiration is mostly seen in individuals with left heart failure and, in such cases, this type of respiration is associated with worse prognosis [95]. Cheyne–Stokes respiration reflects the central respiratory instability which is associated to fluctuations in $PaCO_2$ secondary to ventilation changes. The pulmonary venous congestion observed in congestive heart failure also generates vagal-mediated hyperventilation [96].

The apnea threshold (level of $PaCO_2$ below which the central respiratory drive is no longer present) is higher during sleep than during wakefulness [97]. If the level of hypocapnia present when awaked is significant enough, it stimulates the occurrence of periods of central sleep apnea as soon as the subject falls sleep. The hypoxemia and hypercapnia that are secondary to these periods of central sleep apnea are responsible for ventilatory resumption once the $PaCO_2$ rises again above the apnea threshold. If, on the other hand, the ventilatory response overtakes the simple correction of those metabolic disorders (i.e., high loop gain), it will generate a bounce-back hypocapnia which will be followed by recurrence of central sleep apnea and persisting respiratory instability. This phenomenon of hyperventilation is even more severe when the degree of ventilatory response secondary to hypoxia and hypercapnia stimuli is more significant and when the level of hypoxemia/hypercapnia due to the apnea is more pronounced. The occurrence of periods of awakening or arousals during periods of hyperventilation will increase its magnitude by restoring an increased sensitivity to metabolic stimuli and increasing the phenomenon of bounce-back hyperventilation/hypocapnia [98]. The significance of hypocapnia in the genesis of central sleep apnea or of Cheyne–Stokes respiration is well documented by observing the correction of such events when the subjects are inhaling a $CO_2$-enriched gas mixture [99]. Moreover, circulation time is an important determining factor of postapneic hyperventilation because it influences the delay in transmission of $PaCO_2$ changes from pulmonary circulation to carotid body receptors. An increase in circulation time which is proportional to the alteration of left heart function increases the duration of hyperventilation and contributes to sustaining respiratory instability [100]. In patients with idiopathic central sleep apnea, the duration of hyperventilation is shorter than in patients with left heart failure because the ventilatory bounce-back phenomenon relates to an isolated increase in ventilatory response to metabolic stimuli without any increase in circulation time.

## Conclusions

The occurrence of sleep-related breathing disorders depends on various interrelated pathophysiological mechanisms, most of them involving the influence of sleep on respiratory control and level of activity of UA muscles. The occurrence of these breathing abnormalities during sleep contributes to maintaining a vicious cycle by worsening of the underlying pathogenic process (i.e., left heart failure) and thus increasing its propensity to worsen during sleep. The proper identification of sleep-related respiratory disorders in relation to chronic pulmonary diseases, neuromuscular diseases, obesity hypoventilation, or heart failure is thus an important step in the management of these patients. Adequate understanding of these pathogenic mechanisms will also bring about new therapeutic options for patients with OSA as well as the use of innovative positive pressure ventilatory modes in the treatment of those with central sleep apnea.

## References

1. Phillipson EA. Control of breathing during sleep. *Am Rev Resp Dis* 1978; 118: 909–939.
2. Lo YL, Jordan AS, Malhotra A, Wellman A, Heinzer RA, Eikerman M, Schory K, Dover L, White DP. The influence of wakefulness on pharyngeal airway muscle activity. *Thorax* 2007 Mar 27; 62(9): 799–805.
3. Hudgel DW, Martin RJ, Johnson B, Hill P. Mechanics of the respiratory system and breathing pattern during sleep in normal humans. *J Appl Physiol* 1984; 56: 133–137.
4. Agusti AG. Systemic effects of chronic obstructive pulmonary disease. *Proc Am Thorac Soc* 2005; 2: 367–370.

5. Sin DD, Man SFP. Why are patients with chronic obstructive pulmonary disease at increased risk of cardiovascular diseases? The potential role of systemic inflammation in chronic obstructive pulmonary disease. *Circulation* 2003; 107: 1514–1519.
6. Caples SM, Garcia-Touchard A, Somers VK. Sleep-disordered breathing and cardiovascular risk. *Sleep* 2007; 30: 291–303.
7. Marin JM, Carrizo SJ, Vincente E, Agusti AG. Long-term cardiovascular outcomes in men with obstructive sleep apnoea-hypopnea with or without treatment with continuous positive airway pressure: An observational study. *Lancet* 2005; 365: 1046–1053.
8. Weizenblum E, Chaouat A. Sleep and chronic obstructive pulmonary disease. *Sleep Med Rev* 2004; 8: 281–294.
9. Hawrylkiewicz I, Sliwinski P, Gorecka D, Plywaczewski R, Zielinski J. Pulmonary haemodynamics in patients with OSAS or an overlap syndrome. *Monaldi Arch Chest Dis* 2004; 6: 148–152.
10. Strohl KP, Hensley MJ, Hallett M, Saunders NA, Ingram RH. Activation of upper airway muscles before onset of inspiration in normal humans. *J Appl Physiol* 1980; 49: 638–642.
11. Kubin L, Tojima H, Davies RO, Pack AI. Serotonergic exicatory drive to hypoglossal motoneurons in the decerebrate cat. *Neuroscience Letter* 1992; 139: 243–248.
12. Parisi RA, Neubauer JA, Frank MM, Edelman NH, Santiago TV. Correlation between genioglossal and diaphragmatic responses to hypercapnia during sleep. *Am Rev Resp Dis* 1987; 135: 378–382.
13. Mathew OP, Abu-Osba YK, Thach BT. Influence of upper airway pressure changes in genioglossus muscle respiratory activity. *J Appl Physiol* 1982; 52: 438–444.
14. Van Der Touw T, O'Neil N, Brancatisano A, Amis T, Wheatley J, Engel LA. Respiratory-related activity of soft palate muscles: Augmentation by negative airway pressure. *J Appl Physiol* 1994; 76: 424–432.
15. Shea SA, Edwards JK, White DP. Effect of wake-sleep transitions and rapid eye movement sleep on pharyngeal muscle response to negative pressure in humans. *J Physiol* 1999; 520: 897–908.
16. Morrisson DL, Launois SH, Isono S, Feroah TR, Whitelaw WA, Remmers, JE. Pharyngeal narrowing and closing pressures in patients with obstructive sleep apnea. *Am Rev Resp Dis* 1993; 148: 606–611.
17. Schwartz AR, Smith PL, Kashima HK. Respiratory function of the upper airways. In: Murray JF, Nadel JA, Eds. *Textbook of Respiratory Medicine*. 2nd edition. Philadelphia, PA: WB Saunders, 1994: 1351–1470.
18. Schwab RJ, Gefer WB, Hoffman EA, Gupta KB, Pack AI. Dynamic upper airway imaging during awake respiration in normal subjects and patients with sleep disordered breathing. *Am Rev Resp Dis* 1993; 148: 1385–1400.
19. Burger CD, Stanson AW, Daniels BK, Shheedy PF, Shepard JW. Fast-CT evaluation of the effect of lung volume on upper airway size and function in normal men. *Am Rev Resp Dis* 1992; 146: 335–339.
20. Séries F, Cormier Y, Desmeules M, La Forge J. Influence of passive changes in lung volumes on upper airway aesistance in normal subjects. *J Appl Physiol*. 1990; 68: 2159–2164.
21. Van Der Graaff WB. Thoracic influence on upper airway patency. *J Appl Physiol* 1988; 65: 2084–2090.
22. Thut DC, Schwartz AR, Roach D, Wise RA, Permutt S, Smith PL. Tracheal and neck position influence upper airway airflow dynamics by altering airway length. *J Appl Physiol* 1993; 75: 2084–2090.
23. Mahadevia AK, Onal E, Lopata M. Effects of expiratory positive airway pressure on sleep-induced respiratory abnormalities in patients with hypersomnia-sleep apnea syndrome. *Am Rev Resp Dis* 1983; 128: 708–711.
24. Sanders MH, Kern N. Obstructive sleep apnea treated by independently adjusted inspiratory and expiratory airway pressures via nasal mask: Physiologic and clinical implications. *Chest* 1990; 98: 317–324.

25. Sanders MH, Moose SE. Inspiratory and expiratory partitioning of airway resistance during sleep in patients with sleep apnea. *Am Rev Resp Dis* 1983; 127: 554–558.
26. Bradley TD, Brown IG, Grossman RF, Zamel N, Martinez D, Phillipson E, Hoffstein V. Pharyngeal size in snorers, nonsnorers, and patients with obstructive sleep apnea. *N Engl J Med* 1986; 315: 1327–1331.
27. Wasicko MJ, Hutt DA, Parisi RA, Neubaeur JA, Mezrich R, Edelman NH. The role of vascular tone in the control of upper airway collapsibility. *Am Rev Resp Dis* 1990; 141: 1569–1577.
28. Koenig JS, Thach B. Effects of mass loading on the upper airway. *J Appl Physiol* 1988; 64: 2294–2299.
29. Wolin AD, Strohl KP, Acree BN, Fouke JM. Responses to negative pressure surrounding the neck in anesthetized animals. *J Appl Physiol* 1990; 68: 154–160.
30. Stauffer JL, Buick MK, Bixler EO, Sharkey FE, Abt AB, Manders EK, Kales A, Cadieux RJ, Barry JD, Zwillich CW. Morphology of the uvula in obstructive sleep apnea. *Am Rev Resp Dis* 1989; 140: 724–728.
31. Gleadhill IC, Schwartz CAR, Schubert N, Wise RA, Permutt S, Smith PL. Upper airway collapsibility in snorers and in patients with obstructive hypopnea and apnea. *Am Rev Resp Dis* 1991; 143: 1300–1303.
32. Smith PL, Wise RA, Gold AR, Schwartz AR, Permutt S. Upper airway pressure-flow relationships in obstructive sleep apnea. *J Appl Physiol* 1988; 64: 78–795.
33. Schwartz AR, Schubert N, Rothman W, Godley F, Marsh B, Eisele D, Nadeau J, Permutt L, Gleadhill I, Smith P. Effect of uvulopalatopharyngoplasty on upper airway collapsibility in obstructive sleep apnea. *Am Rev Resp Dis* 1982; 145: 527–532.
34. Philip-Joet F, Marc I, Sériès F. Effects of genioglossus response to continuous negative airway pressure on upper airway collapsibility. *J Appl Physiol* 1996; 80: 1466–1474.
35. Oliven A, Odeh M, Gavriely N. Effect of hypercapnia on upper airway resistance and collapsibility in anesthetized dogs. *Respir Physiol* 1989; 75: 29–38.
36. Remmers JE, De Groot WJ, Sauerland EK, Anch AM. Pathogenesis of upper airway occlusion during sleep. *J Appl Physiol* 1978; 44: 931–938.
37. Onal E, Leech J, Lopata M. Dynamics of respiratory drive and pressure during NREM sleep in patients with occlusive apneas. *J Appl Physiol* 1985; 58: 1971–1974.
38. Schwab RJ, Gupta KB, Gefter WB, Metzger LJ, Hoffman EA, Pack AI. Upper airway and soft tissue anatomy in normal subjects and patients with sleep-disordered breathing. Significance of the lateral pharyngeal walls. *Am J Crit Care Med* 1995; 152: 1673–1689.
39. Shelton KE, Woodson H, Gay S, Suratt PM. Pharyngeal fat in obstructive sleep apnea. *Am Rev Resp Dis* 1993; 148: 462–468.
40. Rodenstein DO, Dooms G, Thomas Y, Liistro G, Stanescu DC, Culee C, Aubert-Tulkens G. Pharyngeal shape and dimensions in healthy subjects, snorers, and patients with obstructive sleep apnoea. *Thorax* 45: 722–727.
41. Kuna ST, Bedi DG, Ryckman C. Effect of nasal airway positive pressure on upper airway size and configuration. *Am Rev Respir Dis* 1988; 138: 969–975.
42. Leiter JC. Analysis of pharyngeal resistance and genioglossal EMG activity using a model of orifice flow. *J Appl Physiol* 1992; 73: 576–583.
43. Shiota S, Ryan CM, Chiu KL, Ruttanaumpawan P, Haight J, Artz M, Floras JS, Chan C, Bradley TD. Alterations in upper airway cross-sectional area in response to lower body positive pressure in healthy subjects. *Thorax* 2997: 868–872.
44. Su MC, Chiu KL, Ruttanaumpawan P, Shiota S, Yumino D, Redolfi S, Haight JS, Bradley TD. Lower body positive pressure increases upper airway collapsibility in healthy subjects. *Resp Physiol Neurobiol* 2008; 161: 306–312.

45. Redolfi S, Yumino D, Ruttanaumpawan P, Yau B, Su MC, LamJ, Bradley TD. Relationship between overnight rostral fluid shift and obstructive sleep apnea in nonobese men. *Am J Respir Crit Care Med* 2009; 179: 241–246.
46. Séries F, Coté C, Simoneau JS, Gélinas Y, St-Pierre S, Leclerc J, Ferland R, Marc I. Physiologic and metabolic profile of musculus uvulae in sleep apnea syndrome and in snorers. *J Clin Invest* 1995; 95: 20–25.
47. Sminne S, Iannaccone S, Ferini-Strambi L, Comola M, Colombo E, Nemni R. Muscle fiber type and habitual snoring. *Lancet* 1991; 337: 597–599.
48. Séries F, Simoneau JA, St-Pierre S, Marc I. Genioglossus and musculous uvulae muscle characteristics in sleep apnea hypopnea syndrome and in snorers. *Cam J Respir Crit Care Med* 1996; 153: 1870–1874.
49. Simoneau JA, Allah CK, Giroux M, Boulay MR, Lagassé P, Thériault G, Bouchard C. Metabolic plasticity of skeletal muscle in black and white males subjected to high-intensity intermittent training. *Med Sci Sports Exerc* 1991; 23: S149.
50. Salomone RJ, Van Lunteren E. Effects of hypoxia and hypercapnia on genio-hyoid contractility and endurance. *J Appl Physiol* 1991; 71: 709–715.
51. Brennick MJ, Parisi RA, England SJ. Influence of preload and afterload on genioglossus muscle length in awake goats. *Am J Respir Crit Care Med* 1997; 155: 2010–2017.
52. Petrof BJ, Pack AI, Kelly AM, Eby J, Hendricks JC. Pharyngeal myopathy of loaded upper airway in dogs with sleep apnea. *J Appl Physiol* 1994; 76: 1746–1752.
53. Schotland HM, Insko EK, Panckeri KA, Leigh JS, Pack AI, Hendricks JC. Quantitative magnetic resonance imaging of upper airway musculature in an animal model of sleep apnea. *J Appl Physiol* 1996; 81: 1339–1346.
54. Woodson BT, Garancis JC, Toohill RJ. Histopathologic changes in snoring and obstructive sleep apnea syndrome. *Laryngoscope* 1991; 101: 1318–1322.
55. Friberg D, Ansved T, Borg K, Carlsson-Nordlander B, Larsson H, Svanborg E. Histological indications of a progressive snorers disease in an upper airway muscle. *Am J Respir Crit Care Med* 1998; 157: 586–593.
56. Myllyla RA, Salminen L, Peltonen TE, Tanaka S, Vihjo V. Collagen metabolism of the mouse skeletal muscle during the repair of exercise injuries. *Pfluegers Arch* 1986; 407: 64–70.
57. Holgate ST, DjukanovicR, Howarth PH, Montefort S, Roche W. The T cell and the airway's fibrotic response in asthma. *Chest* 1993; 193: 125S–128S.
58. Raghow R. The role of extracellular matrix in postinflammatory wound healing and fibrosis. *FASEB J* 1994; 8: 823–831.
59. Séries F, Côté C. Differences in uvular tissue mechanical properties during in vitro stimulation of musculus uvulae between SAHS and nonapneic snorers. *Am J Respir Crit Care Med* 1997; 155: 823–831.
60. Tangel DJ, Mezzanotte WS, White DP. Influence of sleep on tensor palatini EMG and upper airway resistance in normal men. *J Appl Physiol* 1991; 70: 2574–2581.
61. Tangel DJ, Mezzanotte WS, White DP. Influences of NREM sleep on activity of palatoglossus and levator palatini muscles in normal men. *J Appl Physiol* 1995; 78: 689–695.
62. Mezzanotte WS, Tangel DJ, White DP. Influence of sleep onset on upper airway muscle activity in apnea patients versus normal controls. *Am J Crit Care Med* 1996; 153: 1880–1887.
63. Carlson DM, Onal E, Carley DW, Lopata M, Basner RC. Palatal muscle electromyogram activity in obstructive sleep apnea. *Am J Respir Crit Care Med* 1995; 152: 1022–1027.
64. Hendricks JC, Petrof BJ, Panckeri K, Pack AI. Upper airway dilating muscle hyperactivity during non-rapid eye movement sleep in English bulldogs. *Am Rev Resp Dis* 1993; 148: 185–194.

65. Suratt PM, McTier RF, Wilhoit SC. Upper airway muscle activation is augmented in patients with obstructive sleep apnea compared with that in normal subjects. *Am Rev Resp Dis* 1988; 137: 889–894.
66. Mezzanotte WS, Tangel DJ, White DP. Waking genioglossal electromyogram in sleep apnea patients versus normal controls (a neuromuscular compensation mechanism). *J Clin Invest* 1992; 89: 1571–1579.
67. Cherniack NS. Respiratory dysrhythmia during sleep. *N Engl J Med* 1981; 305: 325–330.
68. Onal E, Burrows DL, Hart RH. Induction of periodic breathing causes upper airway obstruction in humans. *J Appl Physiol* 1986; 61: 1438–1443.
69. Onal E, Lopata M. Periodic breathing and the pathophysiology of occlusive sleep apneas. *Cam Rev Resp Dis* 1982; 126: 676–680.
70. Hudgel DW, Hendricks C, Dadley A. Alteration in obstructive apnea pattern induced by changes in oxygen and carbon dioxide inspired concentrations. *Am Rev Resp Dis* 1988; 138: 16–19.
71. Hudgel DW, Harasick T. Fluctuation in timing of upper airway and chest wall inspiratory muscle activity in obstructive sleep apnea. *J Appl Physiol* 1990; 69: 443–450.
72. Wellman A, Jordan AS, Malhotra A, Fogel RB, Katz ES, Schory K, Edwards JK, White DP. Ventilatory control and airway anatomy in obstructive sleep apnea. *Am J Respir Crit Care Med* 2004; 170: 1225–1232.
73. Wellman A, Malhotra A, Jordan AS, Stevenson KE, Gautam S, White DP. Effect of oxygen in obstructive sleep apnea: Role of loop gain. *Respir Physiol Neurobiol* 2008 Jul 31; 162(2): 144–151.
74. Sériès F, Demoule A, Marc I, Sanfaçon C, Derenne JP, Similowski T. Inspiratory flow dynamics during phrenic nerve simulation in awake normals. *Am J Respir Crit Care Med* 1999; 160: 614–620.
75. Sériès F, Straus C, Demoule A, Attali V, Arnulf I, Derenne JP, Similowski T. Assessment of upper airway dynamics in awaked sleep apnea patients with phrenic nerve stimulation. *Am J Respir Crit Care Med* 2000; 162: 795–800.
76. Sériès F, Marc I. Influence of genioglossus tonic activity on upper airway dynamics assessed by phrenic nerve stimulation. *J Appl Physiol* 2002; 92: 418–423.
77. Sanfaçon C, Marc I, Sériès F. Usefulness of phrenic nerve simulation to measure upper airway collapsibility in normal awake subjects. *Respir Physiol and Neurobiol* 2002; 130: 57–67.
78. Vérin E, Sériès F, Locher C, Straus C, Zelter M, Derenne J-Ph, Similowski T. Effects of neck flexion and mouth opening on inspiratory flow dynamics in awake man. *J Appl Physiol* 2002; 92: 84–92.
79. Sériès F, Ethier G. Assessment of upper airway stabilizing forces with the use of phrenic nerve stimulation in conscious humans. *J Appl Physiol* 2003; 94: 2289–2295.
80. Wang W, Verin E, Sériès F. Influences of the breathing route on upper airway dynamic properties in normal awake subjects with constant mouth opening. *Clin Sci (Lond)* 2006; 111: 349–355.
81. Vérin E, Similowski T, Teixeira A, Sériès F. Discriminative power of phrenic twitch-induced dynamic response for the diagnosis of sleep apnea during wakefulness. *J Appl Physiol* 2003; 94: 31–37.
82. Vérin E, Similowski T, Sériès F. CPAP-induced changes in upper airway dynamics assessed with magnetic phrenic nerve stimulation in awake obstructive sleep apnea syndrome. *J Physiol (Lond)* 2003; 546: 279–287.
83. Bosshard V, Masse JF, Sériès F. Prediction of oral appliance efficiency in patients with apnoea using phrenic nerve stimulation while awake. *Thorax* 2011 Mar; 66(3): 220–225. doi:10.1136/thx.2010.150334. Epub 2011 Jan 12.
84. Boyd JH, Petrof BJ, Hamid Q, Fraser R, Kimoff RJ. Upper airway muscle inflammation and denervation changes in obstructive sleep apnea. *Cam J Respir Crit Care Med* 2004; 170: 541–546.
85. Sériès F, Chakir J, Boivin D. Influence of weight and sleep apnea status on immunologic and structural features of the uvula. *Am J Respir Crit Care Med* 2004; 170: 1114–1119.
86. Nguyen AT, Jobin V, Payne R, Beauregard J, Naor N, Kimoff RJ. Laryngeal and velopharyngeal sensory impairment in obstructive sleep apnea. *Sleep* 2005; 28: 585–589.

87. Schwartz AR, Gold AR, Scubert N, Stryzak A, Wise RA, Permutt S, Smith P. Effect of weight loss on upper airway collapsibility in obstructive sleep apnea. *Am Rev Resp Dis* 1991; 144: 494–498.
88. Ryan CF, Lowe AA, Li D, Fleetham JA. Magnetic resonance imaging of the upper airway in obstructive sleep apnea before and after chronic nasal positive airway pressure therapy. *Am Rev Resp Dis* 1991; 144: 939–944.
89. Wilson S, Thach BT, Brouillette RT, Abu-Osba YK. Upper airway patency in the human infant: Influence of airway pressure and posture. *J Appl Physiol* 1980; 48(3): 500–504.
90. Van Der Touw T, Crawford ABH, Wheatley JR. Effects of a synthetic lung surfactant on pharyngeal patency in awake human subjects. *J Appl Physiol* 1997; 82: 78–85.
91. Miki H, Hida W, Kikuchi Y, Chonan T, Satoh M, Iwase N, Takishima T. Effects of pharyngeal lubrication on the opening of obstructed upper airway. *J Appl Physiol* 1992; 72: 2311–2316.
92. Hoffstein V, Mateiko S, Halko S, Taylor R. Reduction in snoring with phosphocholinamin, a long acting tissue-lubricating agent. *Am J Otolaryngol* 1987; 8: 236–240.
93. Redolfi S, Arnulf I, Pottier M, Bradley TD, Similowski T. Effects of venous compression of the legs on overnight rostral fluid shift and obstructive sleep apnea. *Respir Physiol Neurobiol* 2011; 175: 390–393.
94. Wellman A, Eckert DJ, Jordan AS, Edwards BA, Passaglia CL, Jackson AC, Gautam S, Owens RL, Malhotra A, White DP. A method for measuring and modeling the physiological traits causing obstructive sleep apnea. *J Appl Physiol* 2011; 110: 1627–1637.
95. Lanfranchi PA, Braghiroli A, Bosimini E, Mazzuero G, Colombo R, Donner CF, Giannuzzi P. Prognostic value of nocturnal Cheyne-Stokes respiration in chronic heart failure. *Circulation* 1999; 99: 1435–1440.
96. Roberts AM, Bhattachara J, Schultz HD, Coleridge HM, Coleridge JC. Stimulation of pulmonary vagal afferent C-fibers by lung edema in dogs. *Circ Res* 1986; 58: 512–522.
97. Datta AK, Shea SA, Horner RL, Guz A. The influence of induced hypocapnia and sleep on the endogenous respiratory rhythm in humans. *J Physiol* 1991; 440: 17–33.
98. Naughton MT, Bernard D, Tam CA. Role of hyperventilation in the pathogenesis of central sleep apnea in patients with congestive heart failure. *Am Rev Resp Dis* 1993; 148: 330–338.
99. Xie A, Rankin F, Rutherford R, Bradley TD. Effects of inhaled CO2 and added dead space on idiopathic central sleep apnea. *J Appl Physiol* 1997; 82: 918–926.
100. Hall MJ, Xie A, Rutherford R, Ando S, Floras JS, Bradley TD. Cycle length of periodic breathing in patients with or without heart failure. *Am J Resp Crit Care Med* 1996; 154: 376–381.

# 10

# Interstitial lung diseases

GENEVIÈVE DION, YVON CORMIER and LOUIS-PHILIPPE BOULET

| | |
|---|---|
| Introduction | 177 |
| ILDs of known cause | 180 |
|     a) Hypersensitivity pneumonitis | 180 |
|     b) Pneumoconiosis | 181 |
|     c) Lung diseases caused by toxic or physical exposures | 181 |
|     d) ILDs of infectious origin | 182 |
|     e) ILDs caused by drugs | 182 |
|     f) Connective tissue disease | 182 |
|     g) Vasculitis | 183 |
| Sarcoidosis | 184 |
| Idiopathic ILDs | 186 |
|     a) Idiopathic pulmonary fibrosis | 187 |
|     b) Nonspecific interstitial pneumonitis | 189 |
|     c) Cryptogenic organizing pneumonia | 190 |
|     d) Respiratory bronchiolitis-interstitial lung disease and desquamative interstitial pneumonia | 191 |
|     e) Acute interstitial pneumonia | 192 |
|     f) Pleuroparenchymal fibroelastosis | 192 |
| Rare specific interstitial pneumonitis | 192 |
|     a) Langerhans cells histiocytosis | 192 |
|     b) Lymphangioleiomyomatosis | 194 |
|     c) Eosinophilic lung disease | 194 |
|     d) Acute eosinophilic lung diseases | 194 |
|     e) Chronic eosinophilic lung diseases | 194 |
|     f) Pulmonary alveolar lipoproteinosis | 196 |
| Conclusion | 196 |
| References | 196 |

## Introduction

The term "interstitial lung diseases" (ILDs) includes a set of diseases characterized by a diffuse infiltration of the interstitium [1]. The various factors responsible for this abnormal infiltration are often unknown [2]. We estimate that there are approximately 60–80 cases of ILDs per 100,000 inhabitants [3]. After cancer and chronic obstructive pulmonary disease, they represent the third most frequent type of chronic pulmonary disease [4].

There are more than 200 causes of ILDs that are classified into four main categories: (a) interstitial pneumonitis of known cause, including those associated with a connective tissue disease, secondary to drug-related injury or from environmental exposure; (b) idiopathic ILDs; (c) granulomatous diseases—sarcoidosis; and (d) rare ILDs, including lymphangioleiomyomatosis (LAM), Langerhans cell histiocytosis (LCH), eosinophilic lung diseases, and pulmonary alveolar lipoproteinosis (PALP) (Table 10.1) [5,6].

The pulmonary interstitium is a collection of loose connective tissue surrounding the bronchovascular structures and extending into the inter/intralobular septas and the subpleural space (Figure 10.1). ILDs are characterized by an abnormal accumulation of cells (lymphocytes, neutrophils, alveolar macrophages, and/or eosinophils), fibroblasts, and extracellular matrix substances such as proteoglycans and collagen at the level of the lung interstitium. This accumulation results in a reduction in the elastic properties of the lung, a progressive reduction of lung volumes, and a thickening of the alveolar-capillary membrane.

On pulmonary function tests, there is classically a reduction in vital capacity, lung volumes, and *diffusing capacity of the lung for carbon monoxide* (DLCO). Forced expiratory flows are usually reduced proportionally, with a normal or increased forced expiratory volume in 1 second/forced vital capacity ($FEV_1$/FVC).

Table 10.1 Classification of interstitial lung diseases

1. **Interstitial lung diseases of known cause**
    1.1 Hypersensitivity pneumonitis
    1.2 Pneumoconiosis (e.g., asbestosis, silicosis, and berylliosis)
    1.3 Diseases due to toxic or physical exposures
    1.4 Lung diseases caused by toxic or physical exposures
    1.5 Interstitial lung diseases of infectious origin
    1.6 Drug-induced interstitial lung diseases
    1.7 Interstitial lung diseases in the context of a connective tissue disease or vasculitis
    1.8 Others (e.g., interstitial lung diseases associated with an inflammatory disease of the gastrointestinal tract, malignant proliferations [e.g., carcinomatous lymphangitis, lepidic predominant adenocarcinoma, lymphoma, and amyloidosis], exogenous lipidosis, genetic pneumopathies [Niemann–Pick disease, Gaucher's disease, neurofibromatosis, Hermansky–Pudlak syndrome, Birt–Hogg–Dubé syndrome, etc.], and chronic cardiogenic pulmonary edema)
2. **Idiopathic interstitial lung diseases**
    2.1 Idiopathic pulmonary fibrosis (IPF)
    2.2 Idiopathic nonspecific interstitial pneumonia (NSIP)
    2.3 Cryptogenic organizing pneumonia (COP)
    2.4 Desquamative interstitial pneumonia (DIP)
    2.5 Respiratory bronchiolitis-interstitial lung disease (RB-ILD)
    2.6 Acute interstitial pneumonia (AIP)
    2.7 Idiopathic lymphoid interstitial pneumonia (LIP)
    2.8 Idiopathic pleuroparenchymal fibroelastosis
    2.9 Unclassifiable idiopathic interstitial pneumonias
3. **Granulomatous diseases—sarcoidosis**
4. **Rare specific interstitial lung diseases**
    4.1 Langerhans cell histiocytosis
    4.2 Lymphangioleiomyomatosis
    4.3 Eosinophilic pneumonia
    4.4 Pulmonary alveolar lipoproteinosis

*Source:* Adapted from American Thoracic Society (ATS) and the European Respiratory Society (ERS) Joint Statement. *American Journal of Respiratory and Critical Care Medicine*, 165, 277–304, 2002. Expert consensus and revised Travis, W.D. et al., *American Journal of Respiratory and Critical Care Medicine*, 188, 733–748, 2013.

Introduction 179

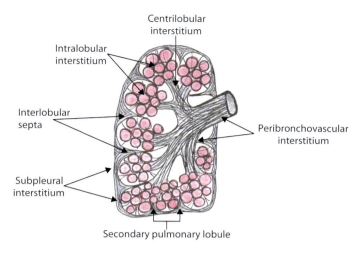

Figure 10.1 Pulmonary interstitium.

Airway hyperresponsiveness is generally not associated with interstitial lung diseases apart from few exceptions such as in some cases of sarcoidosis and hypersensitivity pneumonitis (HP).

Patients suffering from ILDs will usually present with a slowly progressive dyspnea and a dry cough. They will have a rapid shallow breathing pattern and a variable degree of hypoxemia on effort. In advanced stages, hypoxemia at rest with cyanosis, $CO_2$ retention, and right heart failure can be observed. As the initial symptoms are not specific, there is often a delay of approximately 2 years between the beginning of the symptoms and the diagnosis [7].

High-resolution chest tomodensitometry (HRCT) remains the test of choice for the investigation of ILDs. In comparison to the standard chest radiograph, the HRCT is much more sensitive and allows a better evaluation of the pulmonary secondary lobule.

The various findings on imaging include four main categories:

1. Nodular lesions
2. Widespread hyperdensities (alveolar condensation, ground glass opacities)
3. Linear or reticular opacities
4. Areas of hyperlucency (cysts, honeycombing, and emphysema) [8]

Occasionally, a bronchoalveolar lavage (BAL) will be done. A BAL is performed during a flexible bronchoscopy and consists in the instillation of about 150 mL of saline within a distal bronchus with partial recovery of the instilled liquid [9]. This test will allow the recovery of cells from the bronchioalveolar compartments and documentation of the immune, inflammatory, neoplastic, and/or infectious processes occurring at this level. In ILDs, BAL findings are often nonspecific, but they may occasionally be suggestive of a particular condition (e.g., HP, eosinophilic pneumonia) and sometimes can help to confirm a diagnosis (e.g., alveolar hemorrhage, malignancy, opportunistic infection, and PALP).

Biopsies can be performed during a flexible bronchoscopy. Transbronchial biopsies can be done to obtain lung tissue samples. This test is mostly useful for the diagnosis of sarcoidosis, some types of cancer (carcinomatous lymphangitis, lepidic predominant adenocarcinoma), and some opportunistic infections (*Pneumocystis jiroveci* pneumonia, miliary tuberculosis). As the samples obtained are small, transbronchial biopsies are not useful for the diagnosis of idiopathic ILDs. Biopsies or needle aspiration of lymph nodes can also be realized under ultrasonographic visualization (endobronchial ultrasound (EBUS) or endoscopic ultrasound (EUS)) or in the operating room during a mediastinoscopy. Biopsies/aspirations of lymph nodes are mainly useful in the diagnosis of sarcoidosis, lung cancer, and lymphoma.

Finally, a lung biopsy could occasionally be necessary to confirm a diagnosis. It is mainly useful when the diagnosis remains uncertain despite the standard investigation mentioned above.

Treatment of diffuse ILDs will vary according to their etiology. It could vary from simple observation, as in some cases of sarcoidosis, to the use of systemic corticosteroids, immunosuppressive agents, or antifibrotic treatments. The prognosis will also be variable from one pathology to another.

## ILDs of known cause

### Hypersensitivity pneumonitis

HP, also called extrinsic allergic alveolitis, is a disease caused by an immune response to an antigen usually made of proteins [10]. It is often characterized by nonspecific symptoms such as dyspnea, cough, weight loss, asthenia, and fever, sometimes in the form of episodes considered wrongly to be caused by a respiratory infection. These subjects can show precipitating antibodies against causal microorganisms (Table 10.2). The high resolution chest tomodensitometry (HRCT) scan could show some centrilobular nodules and ground glass infiltrations with zones of hyperlucency (air trapping) of the parenchyma.

All environments where there is a production of antigen aerosol of the types mentioned in Table 10.2 can cause a HP. According to the classification of Gell and Coombs, the immune response involved in HP is of type III or IV. The initial response will be close to a type III hypersensitivity reaction (antigen/antibody), but a late response will be associated with the production of granuloma and is therefore more suggestive of a type IV reaction (cellular). Among subjects exposed to an antigen that could cause an HP, only a minority will develop this disease. Some factors such as a genetic predisposition, or coexposure, for example, to endotoxins, could explain this observation.

Our understanding of the pathophysiology of HP has improved since BAL became more widely available [11]. In this disease, there is a marked increase in most cell types in BAL, mainly lymphocytes [12]. The proportion of lymphocytes is usually between 5% and 10% in normal individuals, although it can increase by more than 25% in HP. The number of alveolar macrophages is also increased but their % ratio is reduced. Neutrophils will increase during the acute phase, a few hours after exposure, and will disappear thereafter. Their role is unknown. They could contribute to the initial release of various cytokines and also possibly release some elastases, which could sometimes make the alveolitis evolve toward pulmonary emphysema. Lymphocytes are quite more numerous in HP than in sarcoidosis [13]. They are polyclonal and often have a cytotoxic/suppressor phenotype (CD8+) contrary to sarcoidosis, where we find an increase in CD4 cells. However, this characteristic is not universal and can vary according to the mode of presentation of the disease. In a more chronic form, there is an increase in CD4+ as in sarcoidosis. Also when the exposure to the antigen has stopped, we could see the progressive reduction in CD8+ and an increase in CD4+ cells.

Other types of lymphocytes, natural killer (NK) lymphocytes and memory cells (CD45R0) or T-regulator cells can increase in the lung and probably play a role in the pathophysiology of this disease. In HP, the

Table 10.2 Agents that could induce hypersensitivity pneumonitis

| Type of antigen | Example of sources |
| --- | --- |
| Fungi and yeasts | Moldy wood, humidifiers, and central heating |
| Bacteria | Dairy farm (farmer's lung) |
| Mycobacteria | Cutting fluid, sauna, and spa |
| Avian proteins | Breeders of pigeons, ducks, and canaries; down pillows |
| Chemical substances (linked to the subject proteins) | Isocyanates (automotive paints), zinc, and dyes |

absolute number of alveolar macrophages is increased and they are activated [14]. There is an overexpression of co-stimulatory molecules of the B7 family and the release of many inflammatory cytokines. Mast cells are slightly increased but their role in this context is still unknown.

In the BAL of patients with HP, there is an increase in immunoglobulins, various inflammatory factors, antiproteases, and growth factors. In HP, cytokines such as tumor necrosis factor (TNF), IL-1 (interleukin 1), IL-2, IL-5, and IL-8 are found in increased quantity in the BAL. Monocyte chemotactic protein (MCP-1) and the granulocyte-macrophage colony-stimulating factor (GM-CSF) are also increased. The role of each of these cytokines is still uncertain. Regarding immunoglobulins, an increase in IgA and IgG in the BAL can be found. Immunoglobulins G are also increased in the cells [15]. These immunoglobulins are specific to the causal antigen. They are markers of exposure and their specific role in the genesis of the disease is controversial.

The surfactant, a naturally immunosuppressive substance, seems to have lost its capacity in HP [16]. Contrary to a normal individual, the surfactant is no more able to control inflammation in suppressing macrophage activity. Various components of the cellular matrix, such as hyaluronic acid, fibronectin, vascular endothelial growth factor (VEGF), and collagen type 3, are also increased.

In conclusion, many mediators and cells are involved in the pathophysiology of HP. Their specific role in the development of this disease remains to be determined.

## Pneumoconiosis

These occupational diseases are caused by the chronic inhalation of mineral particles. They are discussed in Chapter 12.

## Lung diseases caused by toxic or physical exposures

Many chemical agents (e.g., chlorine, ammonia, acids) and physical aggressions (e.g., radiations) can affect the lungs and cause a pneumonitis [17,18]. In general, they will cause a lung inflammatory reaction by damaging the alveolar-capillary membrane. They can also induce a plasma transudation that can result in severe noncardiogenic pulmonary edema. There is a progressive recovery in most cases although some patients can remain with long-term sequelae, more often in the form of fibrosis.

Radiotherapy used for the treatment of some neoplasms, such as cancer of the lung, breast, esophagus, and for lymphoma, can cause an ILD. Lung histopathological changes induced by radiotherapy can be divided in three stages: (1) early stage, (2) intermediary stage, and (3) late stage [19,20]. Free radicals produced by ionizing radiations result in some structural and functional abnormalities at the level of DNA, as well as cell membrane lesions [21]. These modifications cause cell dysfunction and death (apoptosis). The cells with a marked mitotic activity such as type II pneumocytes and capillary endothelial cells are the most often affected. Damage observed in the early stages of exposure, such as during the first 2 months following radiotherapy, is mainly characterized by vascular endothelial lesions at the level of small vessels and capillaries, therefore resulting in an increase in vascular permeability and development of perivascular edema [22]. Hyaline membranes develop secondary to the damage caused to type II pneumocytes. In the intermediary stage, 2–9 months following radiotherapy, there is a blockade of the pulmonary capillaries by platelets, fibrin, and collagen [22]. Alveolar cells become hyperplastic and alveolar walls are infiltrated by fibroblasts. If secondary damage caused by radiation is mild, the inflammatory cells will gradually disappear and lung histology will revert to normal. However, if the damage is severe, a chronic phase (>9 months following radiotherapy) can develop, characterized by septal thickening, interstitial fibrosis, and progressive vascular sclerosis [23].

At the clinical level, there are three main types of presentations: (1) radiation pneumonitis, (2) radiation fibrosis, and (3) postradiation organized pneumonia. The radiation pneumonitis develops usually within 6 months following radiotherapy. Generally, the lung infiltration is well circumscribed, corresponding to the radiotherapy field and is visible on the chest radiograph [23]. Occasionally, the infiltration spreads out of the irradiated zone, suggesting a late hypersensitivity response [24]. The radiation fibrosis can develop

6–24 months following radiotherapy. HRCT will show typically a loss of volume in the affected zone, architectural distortion, and traction bronchiectasis [23]. Finally, in rare cases, an organizing pneumonia can develop in the year following radiotherapy [25]. Its radiologic features include alveolar opacities, sometimes migrating, that could spread to nonirradiated zones.

Factors predisposing to the development of radiation pneumonitis and fibrosis are mainly the volume of irradiated lung tissue, the total dose of radiation administered, the number of fractions (the risk is lower with fractionated treatment), a previous history of thoracic radiotherapy, concomitant administration of chemotherapy, and cessation of a previous treatment with high doses of corticosteroids [21].

## ILDs of infectious origin

Acute and subacute ILDs can also be caused by various infectious agents, including viruses, mycoplasma, mycosis, and parasites. These infections mostly affect immunocompromised patients but could also affect the general population (see Chapter 8).

## ILDs caused by drugs

A large number of drugs can cause a diffuse ILD (Table 10.3). This can take the form of an acute, subacute, or chronic pneumopathy. It rarely presents as alveolar hemorrhage or vasculitis [26]. This etiology is considered if there is a temporal relationship between the lung infiltrates and intake of the medication. It remains a diagnosis of exclusion [27]. The website of Pneumotox (www.pneumotox.com) lists the main causes of drug-induced lung diseases.

## Connective tissue disease

Connective tissue diseases are a heterogeneous group of diseases secondary to immune disorders. Table 10.4 shows the connective tissue diseases that can be associated with a pulmonary interstitial disease. Six main

Table 10.3 Main causes of interstitial pneumonitis caused by medication[a]

- Chemotherapy agents (bleomycine,[b] busulfan, chlorambucil, cyclophosphamide, fludarabine, paclitaxel, and mitocyclin C)
- Amiodarone[b]
- Beta-blockers
- Statins
- Inhibitors of the angiotensin-converting enzyme (IACE)
- Nonsteroidal anti-inflammatory drugs (NSAIDs)
- Methotrexate[b]
- Azathioprime
- Gold salts
- D-penicillamine
- Sulfasalazine
- Nitrufurantoin
- Ergot derivatives
- Antidepressives
- Carbamazepine
- Phenytoin

[a] This table is an incomplete list of the main causes of interstitial lung diseases caused by medication. For a more detailed list, consult the website of Pneumotox at www.pneumotox.com.
[b] More frequent causal drugs.

Table 10.4 Connective tissue diseases associated with interstitial lung diseases (CTD-ILD)

- Rheumatoid polyarthritis
- Scleroderma
- Polymyositis-dermatomyositis
- Systemic lupus erythematosus
- Gougerot–Sjögren syndrome
- Mixed connectivitis

histological forms can be found in this category: (1) usual interstitial pneumonia (UIP), (2) nonspecific interstitial pneumonia (NSIP) (the most common), (3) organizing pneumonia (COP), (4) acute interstitial pneumonia (AIP), (5) desquamative interstitial pneumonia (DIP), and (6) lymphocytic interstitial pneumonia [28]. The prevalence of interstitial damage varies according to the underlying connective tissue disease and the diagnostic criteria used (e.g., clinical, radiological, or histological [lung biopsy or autopsy] analysis). The rheumatologic symptoms usually precede the pulmonary affection, but, more rarely, the pulmonary interstitial damage is the first clinical demonstration of the connective tissue disease and precedes this one by several months to years.

We have few data on the pathophysiologic mechanisms underlying ILDs in the context of connective tissue disease, the majority of studies concerning scleroderma. Still, the exact mechanisms are not fully understood. A genetic predisposition, mainly the presence of some HLA haplotypes [29,30], environmental factors still unknown, and the presence of autoantibodies, could be involved in the development of the lung damage. Among others, the presence of anti-topoisomerase-I antibody in scleroderma [31], antisynthetase antibodies for polymyositis/dermatomyositis [32,33], anti-Ro/SSa in the Gougerot–Sjögren syndrome and lupus [34], and the presence of an increased titre of rheumatoid factor during rheumatoid arthritis [35] are particularly associated with the development of ILD.

Current knowledge about fibrosing alveolitis associated with scleroderma suggests that persistent and repeated damage to the epithelial and/or endothelial cells at the alveolar membrane is the initial mechanism initiating the fibrosis process [36]. Such damage to the alveolar membrane would lead to an alteration of the alveolar microenvironment, the release of multiple cytokines, particularly of Th2 type (e.g., IL-4, IL-5, IL-10, and IL-13), as well as many growth factors and soluble mediators, including tumor growth factor-beta (TGF-β), platelet-derived growth factor (PDGF), and endothelin-1 [36–40]. TGF-β could play a major role in the synthesis and accumulation of extracellular matrix and in the development of fibrosing alveolitis. TGF-β inhibits the synthesis of metalloproteinase to the matrix (enzymes involved in the degradation of components of the alveolar membrane and in remodeling the latter). TGF-β also favors the recruitment/activation of myofibroblasts, and reduces their apoptosis [4,41–43]. Myofibroblasts are key cells in the healing process, mainly via the deposition of extracellular matrix (e.g., collagen). In lung fibrosis, this deposition is more than necessary and results in the accumulation of extracellular matrix and scarring [44].

A recent study has shown loss of telocytes in the lung of systemic sclerosis (SSc) patients. Telocytes are a type of stromal cell, which may have a role in the regulation of tissue homeostasis, suggesting that this loss could be implicated in the pathogenesis of fibrosis [45].

Finally, circulating antiendothelial cell antibodies have been found in 30%–54% of patients with scleroderma, which is highly correlated with the presence of pulmonary fibrosis [46,47]. Their precise role is still unknown but they could be involved in the development of microvascular pulmonary damage. Other studies will be needed to establish precisely their role in the physiopathology of fibrosis.

## Vasculitis

Wegener's necrotizing granulomatous vasculitis (now called granulomatosis with polyangiitis [GPA]) and microscopic polyangiitis are two systemic vasculitis that can affect the lungs and are characterized by inflammation of the small vessels (Table 10.5). The vasculitic process can also involve many other organs

Table 10.5 Chapel Hill classification of vasculitis

**Vasculitis of large vessels**
Giant cell temporal arteritis
Takayasu arteritis

**Vasculitis of middle caliber vessels**
Polyarteritis nodosa
Kawasaki disease

**Vasculitis of small vessels**
Granulomatosis with polyangiitis (Wegener)
Eosinophilic granulomatosis with polyangiitis (Churg–Strauss Syndrome)
Microscopic polyangiitis
Schönlein–Henoch disease
Essential cryoglobulinemic vasculitis
Cutaneous leukocytoclastic angeiitis

Source: From Hunder, G.G. et al., *Arthritis and Rheumatism*, 33, 1065–1067, 1990; Kallenberg, C.G. et al., *Nature Clinical Practice Rheumatology*, 2, 661–670, 2006.

(sinus, kidneys, heart, skin, intestines, nerves, etc.) and can be life-threatening as in the case of alveolar hemorrhage, glomerulonephritis, and myocarditis. The most common pulmonary manifestations are lung nodules, lung cavities, pulmonary fibrosis, and alveolar hemorrhage [48,49].

These vasculitis are immune-mediated disorders. In most of cases, they are associated with the presence of antineutrophil cytoplasmic antibodies (ANCA). In GPA, ANCA show a cytoplasmic fluorescence and are more commonly targeted against proteinase 3 (PR3) while in the microscopic polyangiitis, the fluorescence is mostly perinuclear and they are specific for anti-myeloperoxidase (MPO). A new subtype of ANCA, anti-LAMP-2 antibodies, has been described. They are ANCA directed against lysosome-associated membrane protein-2. They often coexist with anti-PR3 and anti-MPO antibodies [50] and are present in >90% of patients with ANCA-positive pauci-immune necrotizing glomerulonephritis [51]. They also can be detected in patients with ANCA-negative pauci-immune focal necrotizing glomerulonephritis suggesting a role in the pathogenesis of ANCA-negative vasculitis [52].

The mechanisms by which ANCA develop, and the role of these autoantibodies in causing disease, are still unclear. Environmental exposure (silica dusts, mercury, lead exposure) [53,54], drugs (e.g., allopurinol, hydralazine, rifampicin, propylthiouracil), infectious agents, and/or genetic factors may be possible initiating events. Patients with alpha-1 antitrypsin (AAT) deficiency could also be at increased risk of GPA. In fact, AAT is the primary *in vivo* inhibitor of PR3, suggesting that deficient PR3 clearance from sites of inflammation may be implicated in the pathophysiology of the disease [55–57].

*In vitro*, ANCA can interact with neutrophils, monocytes, and epithelial cells to cause tissue damage. Studies on animals suggest a direct pathogenic effect of ANCA, especially anti-MPO, in leading to a necrotizing vasculitis and a glomerulonephritis as we can see in microscopic polyangiitis [58]. Their role is more uncertain for ANCA with specificity against PR3. GPA (Wegener) is not well explained. T cells may be involved but their specific role remains to be determined. The activation of neutrophils, endothelial cells, and B cells may also be involved.

## Sarcoidosis

Sarcoidosis or Besnier–Boeck–Schaumann disease is a multisystemic disease of unknown etiology characterized by the production of granuloma and infiltration of lung tissue by inflammatory cells, mainly lymphocytes [59,60] (Figure 10.2). Granuloma can be found in any organ, but the lung and lymph nodes are

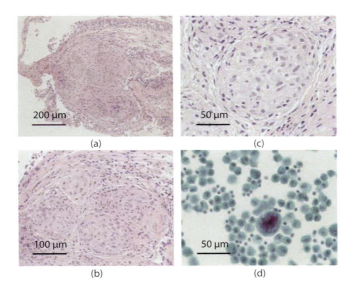

Figure 10.2 Histology of sarcoidosis. (a through c) Histology of an endobronchial biopsy at various magnifications. Non-necrotizing granuloma observed in the submucosa is voluminous, cohesive, and associated with or without the fibrosis. Hemotoxylin and eosin staining. (d). Cytology of bronchioloalveolar lavage. Multinucleated giant cell lymphocytosis. Papanicolaou staining. (Courtesy of Dr. Christian Couture.)

most frequently implicated. Sarcoidosis affects people from any age and any race. Its incidence is higher in women, in Nordic regions, in black people, as well as those in the 20th or 30th year of life [61].

Etiology of sarcoidosis is still unknown. A response of the immune system to various environmental substances, such as respiratory irritants, allergens, inorganic particles, insecticides, construction materials, and microorganisms, mainly bacteria, has been suggested [62]. A genetic predisposition to develop this disease is probable. Indeed, some studies have shown an increased prevalence of this disease in first- and second-degree relatives of index cases [63]. Various alleles could predispose to the development of the disease such as class I antigens (e.g., human leukocyte antigen – HLA-B8) and class II (e.g., HLA-DRB1 and DQB1) antigens [63,64], as well as some mutations at the level of coding gene for the co-stimulatory molecule BTNL2 [65].

In sarcoidosis, granulomas accumulate in the affected tissues. Those granulomas are noncaseating and made of various cells, such as macrophages, lymphocytes, epithelial, and multinucleated giant cells. In the lung, the majority of granulomas are localized close to or within bronchi at the subpleural level or in peribobular spaces (lymphatic distribution) [66]. Although the initiating event is still unknown, an antigen (infectious agent, organic or inorganic substance) has been suspected to be involved in the development of the disease (Figure 10.3). This antigen would be presented to T-lymphocytes, mainly CD4+ type, via antigen-presenting cells. This interaction would lead to the secretion of TNF-α; IL-12, IL-15, and IL-18; macrophage inflammatory protein-1 (MIP-1); as well as MCP-1 and GM-CSF [67]. Then, activated CD4+ T-lymphocytes would produce mainly Th-1 type cytokines (e.g., IL-2 and interferon-gamma [INF-γ]), activating and recruiting alveolar macrophages and other inflammatory cells to produce granuloma [68]. For an unknown reason, a shift of the phenotype toward a predominant Th-2 type can also happen, leading to the release of IL-4, IL-5, IL-6, and IL-10, proliferation of fibroblasts, and deposition of collagen, resulting in fibrotic lesions.

Clinically, the main respiratory symptoms are dyspnea and cough. There are four radiologic stages, without temporal relationship between them (i.e. one stage does not necessarily lead to the next) [59]:

- Stage 1: Bilateral hilar lymphadenopathy without pulmonary infiltrates
- Stage 2: Bilateral hilar lymphadenopathy with pulmonary infiltrates

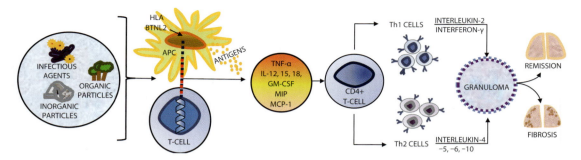

Figure 10.3 Physiopathology of sarcoidosis. APC, antigen-presenting cells; BTNL2, butyrophiline-like 2; GM-CSF, granulocyte-macrophage colony-stimulating factor; HLA, human leukocyte agents; MCP, monocyte chemotactic protein; MIP, macrophage inflammatory protein; TNF, tumor necrosis factor.

- Stage 3: Isolated lung parenchyma infiltrates
- Stage 4: Fibrosis of the lung with retractile lesions, predominant at the middle or upper parts of the lung

A CD4+-type lymphocytic alveolitis with an increased CD4+/CD8+ ratio is generally found on BAL [52]. On the contrary, we usually find a lymphopenia on blood tests with a reduction of CD4+ T cells and a reduction in the CD4+/CD8+ ratio resulting from a redistribution of lymphocytes from the peripheral blood toward the disease organs. A secondary hyperglobulinemia can be observed following an increase in the activation of B-lymphocytes [69].

At the level of lung function tests, patients with sarcoidosis usually have a restrictive syndrome, with a reduction of the total lung capacity. An obstructive pattern is found in 30%–50% of patients, with a reduction of $FEV_1/FVC$ ratio. The mechanisms of this airway obstruction are diverse and may include: (1) a reduction of bronchial caliber from bronchial granulomatosis, bronchial stenosis, distal bronchiolitis, or peribronchial fibrosis, (2) a bronchial distortion secondary to pulmonary fibrosis, and/or (3) a bronchial compression from hypertrophic thoracic adenopathy [70]. Airway hyperresponsiveness can also be observed. In addition to the thoracic features, many other organs may be involved with different frequencies (Table 10.6).

Organ damage by sarcoidosis can resolve spontaneously in 1 or 2 years or, in some cases, progress toward an evolving pulmonary fibrosis and irreversible damage to the affected organs. Many factors will influence the evolution of the disease, mainly the race (black race is associated with an increased prevalence of severe multisystemic disease), the initial radiologic stage (Table 10.7), and some genetic factors (e.g., alleles of types HLA-DQB1*0201 and HLA-DRB1*0301 are associated with a good prognosis) [71]. In the majority of cases, no treatment will be needed but in some specific situations, particularly when granulomas affect organ function, corticosteroid and/or immunosuppressive treatment can be indicated.

## Idiopathic ILDs

Idiopathic ILDs are a heterogeneous group of inflammatory and fibrosing pulmonary diseases of unknown cause. Table 10.8 shows the classification established according to the multidisciplinary international consensus conducted in 2002 and revised in 2013 by the American Thoracic Society and European Respiratory Society [5,6]. Histopathologic characteristics of these various diseases provide the basis of this classification.

Proper classification of idiopathic interstitial pneumonias requires a multidisciplinary discussion with input from pulmonologists, thoracic radiologists, and lung pathologists with an expertise in the diagnosis of ILDs. Despite this multidisciplinary review, approximately 10% of patients cannot be confidently classified with a specific ILD subtype. These patients are generally labeled as having an "unclassifiable ILD" [72].

Table 10.6 Types of organ damage in sarcoidosis

| Organs | Frequency (%) |
|---|---|
| Mediastinal lymphatic nodes | 95–98 |
| Lungs | 90–95 |
| Liver | 5–15[a] vs. 50–80[b] |
| Spleen | 5–15[a] vs. 40–80[b] |
| Eyes | 10–80 |
| Musculosqueletic system | 25–40 |
| Skin | 25–35 |
| Peripheral adenopathies | 30 |
| Central nervous system | 10[a] vs. 25[b] |
| Heart | 5[a] vs. 25[b] |
| Kidneys/hypercalcemia | 2–10 |
| Gastrointestinal system | <1 |

[a] Clinical
[b] Biopsy (liver) or autopsy (spleen, central nervous system, and heart)

Table 10.7 Probability of spontaneous remission of sarcoidosis at 24 months according to the radiologic stage

| Radiologic stage | Probability of spontaneous remission (%) |
|---|---|
| Stage I | 55–90 |
| Stage II | 40–70 |
| Stage III | 20 |
| Stage IV | 0 |

Table 10.8 Classification of idiopathic interstitial pneumopathies

| Clinicoradiologic diagnosis | Histologic diagnosis |
|---|---|
| Idiopathic pulmonary fibrosis (IPF) | Usual interstitial pneumonia (UIP) |
| Idiopathic nonspecific interstitial pneumonia (NSIP) | Nonspecific interstitial pneumonia (NSIP) |
| Cryptogenetic organized pneumonia (COP) | Organized pneumonia (OP) |
| Acute interstitial pneumonia (AIP) | Diffuse alveolar damage (DAD) |
| Respiratory bronchiolitis–interstitial lung disease (RB–ILD) | Respiratory bronchiolitis (RB) |
| Desquamative interstitial pneumonia (DIP) | Desquamative interstitial pneumonia (DIP) |
| Idiopathic lymphoid interstitial pneumonia (LIP) | Lymphoid interstitial pneumonia (LIP) |
| Idiopathic pleuroparenchymal fibroelastosis | Pleuroparenchymal fibroelastosis |

## Idiopathic pulmonary fibrosis

Idiopathic pulmonary fibrosis (IPF) is a chronic fibrosing disease limited to the lung and affecting mainly adults aged over 50 years. It represents, with sarcoidosis, one of the two most frequent ILDs [73]. On histology, we can observe UIP pattern characterized by an excessive and heterogeneous deposition of collagen, zones of abnormal parenchyma alternating with zones of normal appearance [5,74] (Figure 10.4). Classically, the lung lesions have also a temporal heterogeneity, being of different age [5,74]. Lesions are found in both lungs, preferentially at lung bases and at the periphery (subpleural zone) of the lungs. Honeycombing and fibroblastic foci are common.

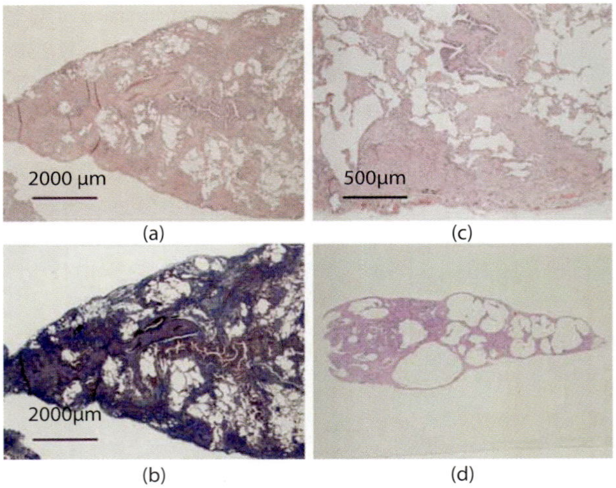

Figure 10.4 Histology of cuneiform lung biopsies illustrating the active phases of IPF and the terminal stage. (a–c) Active disease characterized by alternating areas of normal lung, interstitial fibrosis and honeycomb cysts mainly in the subpleural areas. The fibrotic areas are mainly made of fibroblastic foci dense collagen with positive staining on Masson's trichrome. (d) Terminal fibrosis with honeycombing and dense collagen scars without heterogeneity and active fibrosis. (Courtesy of Dr. Christian Couture.)

Many hypotheses have been proposed to explain its development, but no specific factor has been found until now to explain the inflammatory and fibrotic responses observed in UIP. Some risk factors have been identified, such as smoking, infections, exposure to environmental pollutants, gastroesophageal reflux, and genetic factors [75]. Research is needed to better understand its pathogenesis.

For many years, the main hypothesis has been that an inflammatory response was preceding the lung fibrosis. This hypothesis was first based on animal models suggesting that inflammation could be observed before the fibrotic process and that the suppression of this alveolitis decreased the subsequent fibrosis. Furthermore, BALs of patients with IPF at an early stage showed a predominance of inflammatory cells, including alveolar macrophages, neutrophils, eosinophils, and lymphocytes [76]. Anti-inflammatory treatments and systemic corticosteroids were however unable to modify the natural history of the disease [76–83]. Furthermore, other studies showed that, in the majority of IPF cases, inflammation was not a predominant finding [84] and that fibrosis could be induced in laboratory animals in the absence of inflammation [85,86]. In this context, new hypotheses and a new classification of interstitial pneumopathies were proposed. So, the term "IPF" was restricted to the idiopathic histological pattern of UIP, while a new condition until then poorly characterized and showing a more predominant inflammatory pattern, the nonspecific interstitial pneumonitis (NSIP), was added as a separate entity (see on "Nonspecific interstitial pneumonitis" on page 189).

Emergent concepts now suggest that IPF is mainly the result of repeated insults to the alveolar epithelial cells, followed by an aberrant scarring process with defective repair of the epithelium [85,87,88]. This process would be initiated by an epithelial injury with epithelial shedding and alveolar basement membrane lesions. The damaged alveolar epithelial cells and alveolar macrophages would then trigger the production and release of many soluble mediators such as PDGF, TGF-β, TNF-α, endothelin-1, and so on, allowing the recruitment and accumulation of fibroblasts and myofibroblasts in the lung interstitium and resulting in the formation of fibroblastic foci [85,87–93]. These myofibroblasts would then be involved in the overproduction of extracellular matrix proteins (e.g., collagen type I) and the subsequent fibrosis.

Epithelial lesions also activate the coagulation cascade with the release of thrombin and fibrin deposition [94–97]. This fibrin acts as a temporary matrix and reservoir of fibroblast and inflammatory cells growth factors. Furthermore, thrombin would favor fibroblast proliferation and their transformation into myofibroblasts, leading to extracellular matrix deposition in the lung interstitium [97].

Many factors contributing to this increased collagen production have been identified. First, a disequilibrium could exist between interstitial collagenases and tissue inhibitors of metalloproteinases [85,98]. This phenomenon could result in a reduction of the proteolytic activity and then lead to the progressive deposition of extracellular matrix proteins. Furthermore, signals responsible for myofibroblast apoptosis seem delayed or absent in IPF. This increased survival of myofibroblasts could explain their persistence in the damaged epithelial zones [85]. Finally, fibroblasts could be resistant to the antiproliferative properties of prostaglandins E2 [99]. Such uninhibited proliferation would then contribute to the excessive deposition of collagen.

To complete this process, patients with IPF would have an abnormal alveolar membrane repair process. Indeed, in addition to the secretion of proteins of the extracellular matrix responsible for the fibrosis observed, myofibroblasts would produce free radicals (oxidants) promoting alveolar epithelial cell apoptosis [100]. TGF-β could also contribute to this oxidative stress in inhibiting glutathione synthesis, a potent antioxidant [101]. Furthermore, alveolar epithelial cells would have a procoagulant activity that could compromise normal migration of cells necessary to the extracellular matrix repair.

IPF is associated with a poor prognosis with a median survival time of 2–3 years. In the last two decades, the prognosis of this condition has not been significantly changed despite an increase in knowledge of its underlying mechanisms. With the recognition of the role of fibroblasts, strategies are now oriented toward various agents with antifibrotic properties, hoping to inhibit this process, once initiated.

## Nonspecific interstitial pneumonitis

Before the 2012 ATS/ERS consensus, a number of patients initially considered as having IPF showed in fact a better prognosis and distinct histological characteristics [102]. A new classification of idiopathic interstitial pneumopathies was then considered necessary and a new entity, the NSIP, was described [5,103]. In comparison to IPF, NSIP is classically characterized by an earlier age of onset (40–50 years for NSIP vs. >50 years for IPF) [76,104], a female and nonsmoker predominance, common serologic abnormalities [105], a better response to corticosteroids, as well as a more favorable prognosis [106]. Contrary to the UIP pattern, the histological substratum of IPF, histopathology of NSIP is characterized by a spatial and temporal homogeneity of lesions. There is typically an inflammatory cell infiltrate and fibrosis of variable intensity. Honeycombing is rare and usually associated with the fibrosing form [5,102]. Most cases of NSIP are idiopathic but some are related to connective tissue disease, to antigenic exposure (e.g., avian proteins), to drugs, or follow an episode of acute respiratory distress syndrome (ARDS) [102].

As in IPF, epithelial injury and dysregulated repair are likely to play a role in the pathogenesis of NSIP. While NSIP was previously considered a possible early stage of IPF, more recent studies suggest that immune mechanisms are probably involved in its pathogenesis. In fact, NSIP is the more common histological pattern in ILDs associated with connective tissue diseases [107–110] and a number of patients with NSIP have serum autoantibodies [104,111]. Furthermore, many cases of NSIP initially considered idiopathic have serological or clinical features of connective tissue diseases even if they do not show the classical criteria for such diseases [112] and some patients will develop a connective tissue disease in the future. On histology, involvement of the immune system is suggested by the presence of lymphocytes in the alveolar septa and in BAL. Dendritic cells, which play a role in the immune response through antigen presentation, have also been noted in greater numbers in biopsies of patients with NSIP compared to UIP [113].

Table 10.9 Causes of and diseases associated with organized pneumonia

- Idiopathic
- Infections (bacteria, viruses, mycosis, and parasites)
- Drugs
- Connective tissue diseases
- Inflammatory diseases of the intestine
- Organ transplant (bone marrow, lung, liver, and kidney)
- Malignant hemopathies (myelodysplasia, leukemia, and myeloproliferative syndromes)
- Radiotherapy
- Aspiration pneumonia
- Hypersensitivity pneumonitis
- Environmental exposures (paints, toxic fumes)
- Other rare associations (HIV, IgA nephropathies, Sweet syndrome, thyroiditis, hepatitis C, common variable immune-deficiency syndrome, polymyalgia rheumatica, Behçet disease, and mesangiocapillary glomerulonephritis)

As a probable immune response is considered at the origin of this disease and inflammation is more marked than in IPF on histology, the treatment of this disease usually consists of steroids and immunosuppressive drugs.

## Cryptogenic organizing pneumonia

Organizing pneumonia is an ILD characterized by the presence of granulation tissue buds, mainly made of fibroblasts, myofibroblasts, and connective tissue, in distal airspaces (alveoli, alveolar ducts, and sometimes distal bronchioles) [114]. To make this diagnosis, the organized pneumonia should be a predominant feature on biopsy and not only an accessory finding of another condition such as in NSIP or granulomatosis with polyangiitis, for example. Many etiologies can cause or be associated with an organized pneumonia (Table 10.9). It is considered cryptogenic when there is no obvious cause.

The initial event leading to the formation of organized pneumonia is an injury to alveolar epithelial cells, causing a desquamation of pneumocytes, followed by denudation of the basement membrane [115]. This process will cause the formation of gaps in the basement membrane from which inflammatory cells (lymphocytes, neutrophils, eosinophils, plasma cells, and mast cells), and then fibroblasts, will infiltrate the alveolar interstitium, forming clusters (buds) of fibroinflammatory cells [116]. Following activation of the coagulation cascade, intra-alveolar deposition of fibrin will be observed, promoting migration of cells such as fibroblasts and favoring the fibrinogenesis. Progressively, the inflammatory cells will decrease in number at the alveolar interstitium and most of the fibroblasts will transform to myofibroblasts, leading to the production of collagen (e.g., type III collagen) and leaving room for endoalveolar fibrotic buds made of concentric layers of myofibroblasts and connective tissue cells [117]. Finally, an alveolar cell proliferation will allow a progressive re-epithelialization of the basement membrane and a return to its initial integrity.

Despite the fact that IPF and COP share similar pathophysiological features, their radiological and histopathological appearance as well as their response to treatments are quite different (Table 10.10). The cause of these differences remains unknown but some hypotheses have been raised. One of these is that there is a marked expression of the VEGF with a marked capillarization of the endoalveolar buds in COP, contrary to the lesser vascularization of young fibroblastic foci in UIP. This marked capillarization could allow a better repair process [118,119]. Otherwise, other studies have suggested an increased apoptotic activity in COP in comparison to IPF [120], which may contribute to the disappearance of fibroblasts and myofibroblasts from epithelial damage sites, with a return to a normal architecture.

Table 10.10 Comparative characteristics of COP, idiopathic NSIP, and IPF

| | COP | Idiopathic NSIP | IPF |
|---|---|---|---|
| Histopathological pattern | OP | NSIP | UIP |
| Histopathological characteristics | • Preserved lung architecture<br>• Patchy lesions<br>• Endoalveolar buds of granulation tissue<br>• Mild interstitial inflammation<br>• No HC<br>• No YFF | • *Homogeneity* in time and distribution of lesions<br>• Mild to moderate interstitial inflammation<br>• No or rare HC<br>• No or rare YFF | • *Heterogeneity* in time and distribution of lesions<br>• Destruction of the lung architecture<br>• Interstitial fibrosis with HC<br>• Presence of YFF |
| Mean age (years) | 50–60 | 40–50 | 60–70 |
| Onset | Subacute | Chronic/subacute | Chronic |
| Smoking | NS + PS >> S | NS > S | S + PS >> NS |
| Clinical manifestations | • Mild dyspnea, cough, fever, anorexia, and weight loss<br>• Focal crackles<br>• No clubbing | • Moderate to severe dyspnea, cough<br>• Diffuse crackles<br>• Rare clubbing | • Severe dyspnea, cough<br>• Diffuse crackles<br>• Common clubbing |
| Chest TDM | • Alveolar consolidations<br>• Bilateral<br>• Sometimes migrating | • Ground glass opacities<br>• Reticulations<br>• Basal predominance | • Reticulations and honeycombing >> GG<br>• Traction bronchiectasis<br>• Peripheral and basal predominance of lesions |
| Prognosis | Excellent, without sequelae | Variable | Poor |
| Response to corticosteroids | Excellent | Variable | Poor |

Source: From Cordier, J.F. European Respiratory Journal: Official Journal of the European Society for Clinical Respiratory Physiology, 28, 422–446, 2006.
COP, cryptogenic organizing pneumonia; GD, ground glass opacities; HC, honeycombing; IPF, idiopathic pulmonary fibrosis; NS, nonsmokers; NSIP, nonspecific interstitial pneumonia; PS, past smokers; S, smokers; UIP, usual interstitial pneumonia; YFF, young fibroblastic foci.

# Respiratory bronchiolitis-interstitial lung disease and desquamative interstitial pneumonia

Respiratory bronchiolitis-interstitial lung disease (RB-ILD) and desquamative interstitial pneumonia (DIP) are two rare idiopathic interstitial pneumonias, associated in more than 90% of cases with smoking [120]. These two interstitial pathologies are characterized by an accumulation of pigmented macrophages. In RB-ILD, this accumulation is greater in the lumen of the respiratory bronchioles while it predominates in the alveolar spaces in DIP [5]. Centrilobular emphysema is often associated [121]. In regard to its strong association with smoking, the first treatment is smoking cessation.

## Acute interstitial pneumonia

AIP, sometimes named Hamman–Rich syndrome, is an idiopathic interstitial pneumonia of rapid evolution. Its exact pathogenic mechanisms are still unknown but many inflammatory mediators seem to be involved (e.g., cytokines, oxygen free radicals) [122]. Pulmonary histopathology is characterized by diffuse alveolar damage (DAD).

There are two main consecutive phases: (1) an exudative phase developing the first week following the initial insult and (2) an organization phase starting during the second week. The exudative phase is characterized by the presence of edema, hyaline membranes, hyperplasia of type II pneumocytes, intra-alveolar hemorrhage, and acute interstitial inflammation [123,124]. The organization phase is characterized by a fibroblastic proliferation within the alveolar septum and in the interstitium, a pneumocyte type II hyperplasia, and the presence of thrombi at the level of small caliber arterioles [5,123].

The clinical and histopathological presentation is similar to the acute respiratory distress syndrome (ARDS), but contrary to this latter, there is no underlying evident cause. The beginning of symptoms is acute (1–3 weeks) with a rapid evolution toward hypoxemic respiratory insufficiency and the need for mechanical ventilation in the vast majority of individuals [124]. Mortality is quite high (>70% in the first 6 months). Survivors can recover a normal pulmonary function but some will present some recurrence of the disease and/or an evolution toward chronic fibrosing pneumopathy.

## Pleuroparenchymal fibroelastosis

The 2002 ATS/ERS classification for idiopathic ILDs was revised in 2013 and a rare entity, pleuroparenchymal fibroelastosis (PPFE), was introduced [6]. PPFE is a rare disorder characterized by predominantly upper lobe pleural fibrosis with accompanying elastosis of the alveolar walls and dense fibrous thickening of the visceral pleura [125]. Occasionally, it coexists with different patterns of ILD (e.g., HP, UIP, and NSIP). Most cases are considered idiopathic, although few cases are familial or have nonspecific antibodies. Approximately half of patients have experienced recurrent infections. The physiopathology underlying this disease is still unknown.

## Rare specific interstitial pneumonitis

## Langerhans cells histiocytosis

LCH, commonly called histiocytosis X, is a nonneoplastic proliferative disease associated with an accumulation of Langerhans cells at the level of tissues [124]. There are three clinical pictures according to the type of defect (diffuse, multifocal, or localized) [126]. Disseminated acute LCH (Letterer–Siwe disease) involves mainly young children. The disease is multisystemic, involving the skin, bones, bone marrow, lungs, liver, spleen, lymph nodes, and pituitary gland. Its prognosis is generally poor. Multifocal LCH (Hans–Schüller–Christian syndrome) affects mainly older children and teenagers. The disease is also multisystemic, often associated with an exophthalmia and diabetes insipidus. Its prognosis is variable but generally better than the Letterer–Siwe disease. Finally, LCH can be localized, affecting the lungs (pulmonary Langerhans histiocytosis), bones (eosinophilic granuloma) or skin. Pulmonary Langerhans histiocytosis affects mainly smoking young adults and is characterized by proliferation and infiltration of Langerhans cells in the respiratory and terminal bronchioles [127] (Figure 10.5). Langerhans cells, macrophages, lymphocytes, eosinophils, plasma cells, and fibroblasts will produce granulomas and nodules. Over time, the nodules will cavitate and eventually form pulmonary cysts [128]. Two-thirds of patients have a dry cough,

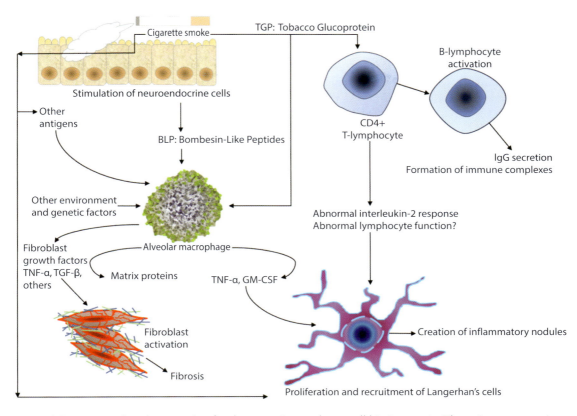

Figure 10.5 Proposed pathogenesis of pulmonary Langerhans cell histiocytosis. The primary event in the pathogenesis of pulmonary Langerhans cell histiocytosis probably involves cigarette smoke-induced recruitment and activation of Langerhans cells to the lung, a process that may result from a variety of potential mechanisms. Cigarette smoke may activate alveolar macrophages through bombesin-like peptides (BLP) released from airway neuroendocrine cells. Other antigens in cigarette smoke, including tobacco glycoprotein (TGP), may stimulate alveolar macrophages to produce cytokines (such as tumor necrosis factor-α [TNF-α] or granulocyte–macrophage colony-stimulating factor [GM-CSF]) or other factors that enhance recruitment and activation of Langerhans cells. Cigarette smoke may also directly activate Langerhans cells to secrete cytokines (such as TNF-α or GM-CSF) that mediate local accumulation of inflammatory cells, with resultant formation of nodules. Uptake of cigarette smoke antigens by alveolar macrophages or Langerhans cells may also promote local expansion of T-lymphocytes and further inflammation. Through the action of tobacco glycoprotein, reduced interleukin-2 secretion by lymphocytes may occur, thereby enhancing local survival and proliferation of Langerhans cells. T-lymphocytes may further stimulate B-lymphocyte activation, promoting secretion of antibodies and immune complex formation. Fibroblast activation and fibrosis may result from the local synthesis of transforming growth factor β (TGF-β) and TNF-α by alveolar macrophages. BLP, bombesin-like peptides; TGP, tobacco glycoprotein.

shortness of breath, chest pain, and systemic symptoms such as asthenia, fever, night sweats and weight loss [128]. Spontaneous pneumothorax has been described in 10%–20% of patients during the initial clinical presentation [126]. More rarely, a cystic bone defect, diabetes insipidus from involvement of posterior pituitary gland, and cutaneous lesions can be found. The main treatment is smoking cessation, which usually allows a resolution or stabilization of the disease in the majority of patients. For some severe cases not responding to smoking cessation, corticosteroids and sometimes even cytotoxic agents (e.g., vinblastine, methotrexate, cyclophosphamide, and etoposide) could be tried.

## Lymphangioleiomyomatosis

LAM is a rare ILD characterized by the proliferation of atypical smooth muscles at the level of the lungs and lymphatic vessels [129,130]. In the majority of case, LAM is sporadic and mainly found in childbearing-age women. More rarely, it is associated with Bourneville tuberous sclerosis. Its etiology is still unknown but a genetic predisposition is suspected. In LAM, the muscular cells are characterized by mutations of suppressor genes of tumor, the hamartine gene (TSC1) and the tuberine gene (TSC2). The hamartine-tuberine complex regulates normally the activity of mammalian target of rapamycin (mTOR), which regulates signaling pathways that control growth mobility and cell survival. In case of mutation, this regulation is abolished and there is a cell accumulation. These cells also express factors for lymphangiogenesis such as VEGF-C and D [131–136]. Otherwise, estrogens could have a role to play in this disease as they occur mostly in childbearing women.

The accumulation of atypical smooth muscle cells at the level of the distal airways creates a check valve phenomenon that leads to a distension of the distal airways, the formation of pulmonary cysts, and in two-thirds of cases, the occurrence of pneumothorax [135,136]. Otherwise, the progressive closure of lymphatic vessels by smooth muscle cells leads to the formation of cystic lymphatic masses (lymphangioleiomyoma), chylothorax (chylous pleural effusions), and chylous ascites [130]. Finally, renal angiomyolipoma (benign tumor containing soft tissue, blood vessels, and fatty tissue) can be found in about 50% of cases [135]. No cure currently exists. It is generally recommended to avoid oral contraceptives and hormonal replacement treatments at menopause, as they are associated with a worsening of the disease. In some patients with a rapid decline in lung function, a treatment with sirolimus (inhibitor of the mTOR) can be considered [136]. In this regard, McCormack et al. observed the stabilization of lung function and an improvement in symptoms and quality of life in patients with LAM treated with sirolimus [137].

## Eosinophilic lung disease

Many entities are included in the term "eosinophilic lung disease" or "pulmonary infiltrates with eosinophilia" (PIE) [138,139]. They can be categorized in acute or chronic pneumopathies. They have in common abnormal accumulation of eosinophils at the level of the pulmonary interstitium.

## Acute eosinophilic lung diseases

The *Löffler syndrome* is characterized by shortness of breath, nonproductive cough, peripheral blood eosinophilia, and transient migratory pulmonary infiltrates [139]. This syndrome can be due to a pulmonary hypersensitivity response to intestinal parasites such as Ascaris or to some drugs. Cessation of the causal drug or treatment of the underlying parasitic infection allows, in the majority of cases, a rapid resolution of the disease.

A most severe form is the *acute eosinophilic pneumonia* [140]. It is characterized by an acute onset of fever, shortness of breath, nonproductive cough, pleural-type thoracic pain, and hypoxemia. It is idiopathic in the majority of cases, but it can be secondary to the intake of drugs and some cases have also been reported following the inhalation of various substances (e.g., World Trade Center dust, fume from fire, indoor renovation work, compulsive smoking with massive inhalation, etc.). Blood eosinophilia is usually not observed at the initial presentation but may occur later. The chest radiograph shows diffuse interstitial infiltrates and pleural effusions in more than 50% of cases. Pulmonary function tests can show a restrictive syndrome with a reduction of the diffusing capacity of the lungs for carbon monoxide ($D_L CO$). BAL liquid shows an increased number of eosinophils (>25% of cells). A clinical improvement is shown quickly with the use of corticosteroids (within 24–48 hours) and recurrences are rare.

## Chronic eosinophilic lung diseases

*Chronic eosinophilic pneumonia (Carrington's disease)* [141] can be found at any age. It is more common in woman and atopic asthmatic people. In the majority of cases, no cause is found. It can rarely follow radiotherapy treatment for breast cancer. It is characterized by an insidious onset of fatigue, dyspnea on exercise, and nonproductive cough. It can affect all organs but its manifestations are mostly respiratory. The radiologic features suggest a reverse pattern of acute pulmonary edema, most of the infiltrates being at the periphery of the lung. There is also a peripheral blood eosinophilia in more than 90% of cases and a strong increase in eosinophils in the BAL fluid (>25% eosinophils). Response to corticosteroids is usually rapid, in less than 48 hours, but recurrences are frequent during weaning or cessation of this treatment.

*Parasitic pneumonia* [142], also named *tropical pulmonary eosinophilia*, is caused by parasites such as filariasis and characterized by an eosinophilic alveolitis of variable intensity.

*Allergic bronchopulmonary aspergillosis (ABPA)* is secondary to an allergic response to the fungus *Aspergillus*. It is often found in patients with asthma or cystic fibrosis and is characterized by an increased number of eosinophils in blood, an elevated total serum IgE level, IgE antibodies (precipitins) against *Aspergillus fumigatus* antigens, a positive cutaneous response to *Aspergillus*, and perihilar lung infiltrates with sometimes "finger-in-glove" images and central bronchiectasis at the lung tomodensitometry [143,144]. These features are due to the infiltration of bronchi by large quantity of eosinophils. In cystic fibrosis, the alteration of the mucociliary function can make difficult the elimination of fungal spores and promote its proliferation. Also, some proteolytic substances produced by *Aspergillus* can affect the bronchial epithelium. For asthma, we do not know if their coexistence represents common predisposing factors or the influence of a condition over the other (although most of the time, ABPA occurs in long-term asthma). About one-quarter of asthmatics are sensitized to *Aspergillus* but few patients will develop ABPA. The presence of this microorganism causes lymphocyte activation, particularly of the Th2 type with a production of cytokines and IgE, which will activate the mast cells present in the bronchial tree. This activation, associated with the production of IL-5, will induce the recruitment of eosinophils at the inflammatory site. Generally, in this condition, the airways show eosinophilic and lymphocytic infiltrations, goblet cell hyperplasia, bronchocentric granulomas with distal exudative bronchiolitis, mucoid impactions, and in some terminal cases, fibrotic changes [145].

ABPA is often associated with airway obstruction on lung function tests. Lung volumes and CO diffusion can be reduced in the presence of a secondary lung disease. This condition usually responds well to corticosteroids. Occasionally, if there is a resistance to the treatment, intolerance to corticosteroids, or frequent exacerbations of ABPA, itraconazole, an antifungal agent or omlizumab (anti-IgE therapy) can be useful [146].

*Churg and Strauss vasculitis*, now called *eosinophilic granulomatosis with polyangiitis (EGPA)*, is an autoimmune disease causing a chronic inflammation of small- and medium-caliber arteries (Table 10.5). Patients classically present severe asthma that can precede the vasculitic phase by many years. In addition to lungs, the disease can also affect many other organs such as the sinus, the skin, intestine, nerves, and heart [146]. Its etiology is still unknown. Antinuclear cytoplasmic antibodies (ANCA) are found in about half of patients [147]. Many abnormalities of the immune system are found, such as different allergic manifestations (asthma, allergic rhinitis, etc.) suggesting an increase in Th2 immune response, angiocentric pulmonary granulomatosis suggesting also an increase in Th1 immune reaction, as well as an increase in T-regulatory lymphocytes CD4+ CD25+ [148–151]. An hypergammaglobulinemia, particularly of the IgE type, and in some patients, a positive rheumatoid factor can be found. Eosinophil function is normal with, however, an increase in their recruitment and a reduced apoptosis of these cells [150]. Genetic factors could be involved in this disease. The assumption that there could be a link between some drugs and EGPA has been not confirmed [150].

The *hypereosinophilic syndromes (HESs)* are a group of disorders characterized by a sustained overproduction of eosinophils and, subsequently, an eosinophilic infiltration and damage to multiple organs [152,153]. Common target organs include the skin, lung, gastrointestinal tract, heart, and nervous system.

There are three main categories of HES: primary, secondary, and idiopathic. In *primary HES*, the eosinophilic expansion is clonal and secondary to an underlying neoplastic process. In *secondary HES*, the eosinophilic expansion is polyclonal and secondary to an overproduction of eosinophilopoietic cytokines such as IL-5. Defect in the regulation of survival and activation of eosinophils has been also suggested [153,154]. Typical examples are parasitic infection and certain solid tumors. In *idiopathic HES*, the underlying cause of HE remains unknown despite an extensive etiologic work-up.

Relevant subtypes include the myeloproliferative variants, the cell lymphocytic variants, and familial eosinophilia.

## Pulmonary alveolar lipoproteinosis

Pulmonary alveolar lipoproteinosis (PALP) is a rare disease characterized by the accumulation of periodic acid-Schiff (PAS)-positive lipoproteinaceous material in the alveoli and the peripheral bronchioles [155–157]. The lipoproteinaceous material is similar to surfactant and the underlying lung architecture is normally preserved with little or no lung inflammation.

Much evidence suggests that diminished GM-CSF protein or function plays a key role in PALP and is responsible for the observed impairments in surfactant processing. In fact, genetically engineered mice that lack the gene for GM-CSF have an abnormal accumulation of surfactant in the alveolar spaces and their treatment with aerosolized GM-CSF corrects the alveolar proteinosis [158]. Deficiency of GM-CSF could inhibit the normal activation and lead to dysfunction of alveolar macrophages. Thus, the dysfunctional alveolar macrophages are no longer able to eliminate the surfactant, which subsequently accumulates in the lung. They are also less efficient as a defense mechanism against infections, which means that patients are more susceptible to develop unusual infections such as nocardiosis, aspergillosis, or crytococcosis.

Three forms of PALP are recognized: congenital, secondary, and acquired. The *congenital form* is likely related to mutations in the genes for surfactant or in the GM-CSF receptor. The clinical presentation arrives early, in the neonatal period. The *acquired form* is the most common and is associated with a high prevalence of anti-GM-CSF antibodies. The *secondary form* is associated with a high level of dust exposure (e.g., silica, aluminum, titanium, and indium-tin oxide), hematologic malignancies, and after allogenic bone marrow transplantation. It is likely related to a relative deficiency of GM-CSF.

Most patients will present nonspecific symptoms, mostly in the form of dyspnea and cough. Physical examination is often normal but cyanosis and clubbing are found in about a third of cases [159]. The chest radiograph shows bilateral symmetric alveolar opacities without air bronchogram. These images can mimic an acute pulmonary edema but there is no pleural effusion or cardiomegaly. The chest tomodensitometry reveals ground-glass opacification with thickened intra- and interlobular septa in typical polygonal shapes, referred to as the "crazy paving" pattern. BAL will yield typically a milky appearance liquid, rich in proteins and lipids and alveolar macrophages that are engorged with PAS-positive material. Whole lung lavage is the most efficient treatment [160], although new experimental therapies with GM-CSF have been used in patients with PALP with some success [161–164].

## Conclusion

There are more than 200 causes of diffuse ILDs. For most of those, their physiopathology is not completely understood. The combination of a thorough questionnaire, HRCT imaging, blood tests, pulmonary function tests, and, occasionally, bronchoscopic techniques will allow, in most cases, a specific diagnosis. However, in some cases, lung biopsy will be necessary. Treatment and prognosis will vary according to the underlying disease. The new physiopathological concepts currently under study will allow development of new targeted therapies for these rare conditions.

## References

1. Ryu JH, Daniels CE, Hartman TE, Yi ES. Diagnosis of interstitial lung diseases. *Mayo Clinic Proceedings* 2007;82: 976–86.
2. Crystal RG. Research opportunities and advances in lung disease. *JAMA* 2001;285: 612–8.
3. Thomeer MJ, Costabe U, Rizzato G, Poletti V, Demedts M. Comparison of registries of interstitial lung diseases in three European countries. *European Respiratory Journal Supplement* 2001;32: 114s–8s.

4. Coultas DB, Zumwalt RE, Black WC, Sobonya RE. The epidemiology of interstitial lung diseases. *American Journal of Respiratory and Critical Care Medicine* 1994;150: 967–72.
5. American Thoracic Society, European Respiratory Society, American Thoracic Society/European Respiratory Society International Multidisciplinary Consensus Classification of the Idiopathic Interstitial Pneumonias. This joint statement of the American Thoracic Society (ATS), and the European Respiratory Society (ERS) was adopted by the ATS board of directors, June 2001 and by the ERS Executive Committee, June 2001. *American Journal of Respiratory and Critical Care Medicine* 2002;165: 277–304.
6. Travis WD, Costabel U, Hansell DM, King TE, Jr., Lynch DA, Nicholson AG, Ryerson CJ, Ryu JH, Selman M, Wells AU, Behr J, Bouros D, Brown KK, Colby TV, Collard HR, Cordeiro CR, Cottin V, Crestani B, Drent M, Dudden RF, Egan J, Flaherty K, Hogaboam C, Inoue Y, Johkoh T, Kim DS, Kitaichi M, Loyd J, Martinez FJ, Myers J, Protzko S, Raghu G, Richeldi L, Sverzellati N, Swigris J, Valeyre D, ATS/ERS Committee on Idiopathic Interstitial Pneumonias. An official American Thoracic Society/European Respiratory Society statement: Update of the international multidisciplinary classification of the idiopathic interstitial pneumonias. *American Journal of Respiratory and Critical Care Medicine* 2013;188: 733–48.
7. Lamas DJ, Kawut SM, Bagiella E, Philip N, Arcasoy SM, Lederer DJ. Delayed access and survival in idiopathic pulmonary fibrosis: A cohort study. *American Journal of Respiratory and Critical Care Medicine* 2011;184: 842–7.
8. Brauner M, Brillet P. Pathophysiological approach to infiltrative lung diseases on CT. *Journal de Radiologie* 2009;90: 1841–53.
9. King TE. The handling and analysis of bronchoalveolar lavage specimens. In: Baughman RP, ed. *Bronchoalveolar Lavage*. St. Louis, MO: Mosby, 1992: 3–25.
10. Cormier Y, Schuyler M. Hypersensitivity pneumonitis and organic dust toxic syndrome. In: Bernstein DI, Chann-Yeung M, Mala Jh, Bernsteing L, eds. Dekker 2005: 875.
11. Schuyler M, Gott K, Cherne A. Mediators of hypersensitivity pneumonitis. *Journal of Laboratory and Clinical Medicine* 2000;136: 29–38.
12. Cormier Y, Belanger J, LeBlanc P, Laviolette M. Bronchoalveolar lavage in farmers' lung disease: Diagnostic and physiological significance. *British Journal of Industrial Medicine* 1986;43: 401–5.
13. Drent M, Grutters JC, Mulder PG, van Velzen-Blad H, Wouters EF, van den Bosch JM. Is the different T helper cell activity in sarcoidosis and extrinsic allergic alveolitis also reflected by the cellular bronchoalveolar lavage fluid profile? *Sarcoidosis, Vasculitis, and Diffuse Lung Diseases : Official Journal of WASOG/World Association of Sarcoidosis and Other Granulomatous Disorders* 1997;14: 31–8.
14. Israel-Assayag E, Dakhama A, Lavigne S, Laviolette M, Cormier Y. Expression of costimulatory molecules on alveolar macrophages in hypersensitivity pneumonitis. *American Journal of Respiratory and Critical Care Medicine* 1999;159: 1830–4.
15. Patterson R, Wang JL, Fink JN, Calvanico NJ, Roberts M. IgA and IgG antibody activities of serum and bronchoalveolar fluid from symptomatic and asymptomatic pigeon breeders. *American Review of Respiratory Disease* 1979;120: 1113–8.
16. Israel-Assayag E, Cormier Y. Surfactant modifies the lymphoproliferative activity of macrophages in hypersensitivity pneumonitis. *American Journal of Physiology* 1997;273: L1258–64.
17. Andujar P, Nemery B. Acute and subacute chemical pneumonitis. *Revue des Maladies Respiratories* 2009;26: 867–85.
18. Boulet LP, Bowie, D. Acute occupational respiratory diseases. In: Mapp CE, ed. *Occupational Lung Disorders*. Sheffield, UK: European Respiratory Society 1999; 355.
19. Gross NJ. Pulmonary effects of radiation therapy. *Annals of Internal Medicine* 1977;86: 81–92.
20. Davis SD, Yankelevitz DF, Henschke CI. Radiation effects on the lung: Clinical features, pathology, and imaging findings. *AJR American Journal of Roentgenology* 1992;159: 1157–64.
21. Movsas B, Raffin TA, Epstein AH, Link CJ, Jr. Pulmonary radiation injury. *Chest* 1997;111: 1061–76.

22. Roswit B, White DC. Severe radiation injuries of the lung. *AJR American Journal of Roentgenology* 1977;129: 127–36.
23. Park KJ, Chung JY, Chun MS, Suh JH. Radiation-induced lung disease and the impact of radiation methods on imaging features. *Radiographics: A Review Publication of the Radiological Society of North America* 2000;20: 83–98.
24. Roberts CM, Foulcher E, Zaunders JJ, Bryant DH, Freund J, Cairns D, Penny R, Morgan GW, Breit SN. Radiation pneumonitis: A possible lymphocyte-mediated hypersensitivity reaction. *Annals of Internal Medicine* 1993;118: 696–700.
25. Crestani B, Valeyre D, Roden S, Wallaert B, Dalphin JC, Cordier JF. Bronchiolitis obliterans organizing pneumonia syndrome primed by radiation therapy to the breast. The Groupe d'Etudes et de Recherche sur les Maladies Orphelines Pulmonaires (GERM"O"P). *American Journal of Respiratory and Critical Care Medicine* 1998;158: 1929–35.
26. Camus PH, Foucher P, Bonniaud PH, Ask K. Drug-induced infiltrative lung disease. *European Respiratory Journal Supplement* 2001;32: 93s–100s.
27. Camus P, Fanton A, Bonniaud P, Camus C, Foucher P. Interstitial lung disease induced by drugs and radiation. *Respiration* 2004;71: 301–26.
28. Antoniou KM, Margaritopoulos G, Economidou F, Siafakas NM. Pivotal clinical dilemmas in collagen vascular diseases associated with interstitial lung involvement. *European Respiratory Journal: Official Journal of the European Society for Clinical Respiratory Physiology* 2009;33: 882–96.
29. Briggs DC, Vaughan RW, Welsh KI, Myers A, duBois RM, Black CM. Immunogenetic prediction of pulmonary fibrosis in systemic sclerosis. *Lancet* 1991;338: 661–2.
30. Gilchrist FC, Bunn C, Foley PJ, Lympany PA, Black CM, Welsh KI, du Bois RM. Class II HLA associations with autoantibodies in scleroderma: A highly significant role for HLA-DP. *Genes and Immunity* 2001;2: 76–81.
31. Diot E, Giraudeau B, Diot P, Degenne D, Ritz L, Guilmot JL, Lemarie E. Is anti-topoisomerase I a serum marker of pulmonary involvement in systemic sclerosis? *Chest* 1999;116: 715–20.
32. Hochberg MC, Feldman D, Stevens MB, Arnett FC, Reichlin M. Antibody to Jo-1 in polymyositis/dermatomyositis: Association with interstitial pulmonary disease. *Journal of Rheumatology* 1984;11: 663–5.
33. Yoshida S, Akizuki M, Mimori T, Yamagata H, Inada S, Homma M. The precipitating antibody to an acidic nuclear protein antigen, the Jo-1, in connective tissue diseases. A marker for a subset of polymyositis with interstitial pulmonary fibrosis. *Arthritis and rheumatism* 1983;26: 604–11.
34. Boulware DW, Hedgpeth MT. Lupus pneumonitis and anti-SSA(Ro) antibodies. *Journal of Rheumatology* 1989;16: 479–81.
35. Anaya JM, Diethelm L, Ortiz LA, Gutierrez M, Citera G, Welsh RA, Espinoza LR. Pulmonary involvement in rheumatoid arthritis. *Seminars in Arthritis and Rheumatism* 1995;24: 242–54.
36. du Bois RM. Mechanisms of scleroderma-induced lung disease. *Proceedings of the American Thoracic Society* 2007;4: 434–8.
37. Luzina IG, Atamas SP, Wise R, Wigley FM, Xiao HQ, White B. Gene expression in bronchoalveolar lavage cells from scleroderma patients. *American Journal of Respiratory Cell and Molecular Biology* 2002;26: 549–57.
38. Ludwicka A, Ohba T, Trojanowska M, Yamakage A, Strange C, Smith EA, Leroy EC, Sutherland S, Silver RM. Elevated levels of platelet derived growth factor and transforming growth factor-beta 1 in bronchoalveolar lavage fluid from patients with scleroderma. *Journal of Rheumatology* 1995;22: 1876–83.
39. Abraham DJ, Vancheeswaran R, Dashwood MR, Rajkumar VS, Pantelides P, Xu SW, du Bois RM, Black CM. Increased levels of endothelin-1 and differential endothelin type A and B receptor expression in scleroderma-associated fibrotic lung disease. *American Journal of Pathology* 1997;151: 831–41.
40. Atamas SP, Yurovsky VV, Wise R, Wigley FM, Goter Robinson CJ, Henry P, Alms WJ, White B. Production of type 2 cytokines by CD8+ lung cells is associated with greater decline in pulmonary function in patients with systemic sclerosis. *Arthritis and Rheumatism* 1999;42: 1168–78.

41. Kissin EY, Lemaire R, Korn JH, Lafyatis R. Transforming growth factor beta induces fibroblast fibrillin-1 matrix formation. *Arthritis and Rheumatism* 2002;46: 3000–9.
42. Varga J, Rosenbloom J, Jimenez SA. Transforming growth factor beta (TGF beta) causes a persistent increase in steady-state amounts of type I and type III collagen and fibronectin mRNAs in normal human dermal fibroblasts. *The Biochemical Journal* 1987;247: 597–604.
43. Zhang HY, Phan SH. Inhibition of myofibroblast apoptosis by transforming growth factor beta(1). *American Journal of Respiratory Cell and Molecular Biology* 1999;21: 658–65.
44. Bagnato G, Harari S. Cellular interactions in the pathogenesis of interstitial lung diseases. *European Respiratory Review : An Official Journal of the European Respiratory Society* 2015;24: 102–14.
45. Manetti M, Rosa I, Messerini L, Guiducci S, Matucci-Cerinic M, Ibba-Manneschi L. A loss of telocytes accompanies fibrosis of multiple organs in systemic sclerosis. *Journal of Cellular and Molecular Medicine* 2014;18: 253–62.
46. Rosenbaum J, Pottinger BE, Woo P, Black CM, Loizou S, Byron MA, Pearson JD. Measurement and characterisation of circulating anti-endothelial cell IgG in connective tissue diseases. *Clinical and Experimental Immunology* 1988;72: 450–6.
47. Ihn H, Sato S, Fujimoto M, Igarashi A, Yazawa N, Kubo M, Kikuchi K, Takehara K, Tamaki K. Characterization of autoantibodies to endothelial cells in systemic sclerosis (SSc): Association with pulmonary fibrosis. *Clinical and Experimental Immunology* 2000;119: 203–9.
48. Hunder GG, Arend WP, Bloch DA, Calabrese LH, Fauci AS, Fries JF, Leavitt RY, Lie JT, Lightfoot RW, Jr., Masi AT. The American College of Rheumatology 1990 criteria for the classification of vasculitis. Introduction. *Arthritis and Rheumatism* 1990;33: 1065–7.
49. Kallenberg CG, Heeringa P, Stegeman CA. Mechanisms of disease: Pathogenesis and treatment of ANCA-associated vasculitides. *Nature Clinical Practice Rheumatology* 2006;2: 661–70.
50. Salama AD, Pusey CD. Shining a LAMP on pauci-immune focal segmental glomerulonephritis. *Kidney International* 2009;76: 15–7.
51. Kain R, Exner M, Brandes R, Ziebermayr R, Cunningham D, Alderson CA, Davidovits A, Raab I, Jahn R, Ashour O, Spitzauer S, Sunder-Plassmann G, Fukuda M, Klemm P, Rees AJ, Kerjaschki D. Molecular mimicry in pauci-immune focal necrotizing glomerulonephritis. *Nature Medicine* 2008;14: 1088–96.
52. Peschel A, Basu N, Benharkou A, Brandes R, Brown M, Dieckmann R, Rees AJ, Kain R. Autoantibodies to hLAMP-2 in ANCA-negative pauci-immune focal necrotizing GN. *Journal of the American Society of Nephrology* 2014;25: 455–63.
53. Hogan SL, Satterly KK, Dooley MA, Nachman PH, Jennette JC, Falk RJ, Glomerular Disease Collaborative Network. Silica exposure in anti-neutrophil cytoplasmic autoantibody-associated glomerulonephritis and lupus nephritis. *Journal of the American Society of Nephrology* 2001;12: 134–42.
54. Albert D, Clarkin C, Komoroski J, Brensinger CM, Berlin JA. Wegener's granulomatosis: Possible role of environmental agents in its pathogenesis. *Arthritis and Rheumatism* 2004;51: 656–64.
55. Audrain MA, Sesboue R, Baranger TA, Elliott J, Testa A, Martin JP, Lockwood CM, Esnault VL. Analysis of anti-neutrophil cytoplasmic antibodies (ANCA): Frequency and specificity in a sample of 191 homozygous (PiZZ) alpha1-antitrypsin-deficient subjects. *Nephrology, Dialysis, Transplantation: Official Publication of the European Dialysis and Transplant Association—European Renal Association* 2001;16: 39–44.
56. Elzouki AN, Segelmark M, Wieslander J, Eriksson S. Strong link between the alpha 1-antitrypsin PiZ allele and Wegener's granulomatosis. *Journal of Internal Medicine* 1994;236: 543–8.
57. Mahr AD, Edberg JC, Stone JH, Hoffman GS, St Clair EW, Specks U, Dellaripa PF, Seo P, Spiera RF, Rouhani FN, Brantly ML, Merkel PA. Alpha(1)-antitrypsin deficiency-related alleles Z and S and the risk of Wegener's granulomatosis. *Arthritis and Rheumatism* 2010;62: 3760–7.
58. Chen M, Kallenberg CG. New advances in the pathogenesis of ANCA-associated vasculitides. *Clinical and Experimental Rheumatology* 2009;27: S108–14.

59. Iannuzzi MC, Rybicki BA, Teirstein AS. Sarcoidosis. *New England Journal of Medicine* 2007;357: 2153–65.
60. Newman LS, Rose CS, Maier LA. Sarcoidosis. *New England Journal of Medicine* 1997;336: 1224–34.
61. Rybicki BA, Major M, Popovich J, Jr., Maliarik MJ, Iannuzzi MC. Racial differences in sarcoidosis incidence: A 5-year study in a health maintenance organization. *American Journal of Epidemiology* 1997;145: 234–41.
62. Newman LS, Rose CS, Bresnitz EA, Rossman MD, Barnard J, Frederick M, Terrin ML, Weinberger SE, Moller DR, McLennan G, Hunninghake G, DePalo L, Baughman RP, Iannuzzi MC, Judson MA, Knatterud GL, Thompson BW, Teirstein AS, Yeager H, Jr., Johns CJ, Rabin DL, Rybicki BA, Cherniack R, ACCESS Research Group. A case control etiologic study of sarcoidosis: Environmental and occupational risk factors. *American Journal of Respiratory and Critical Care Medicine* 2004;170: 1324–30.
63. Rybicki BA, Iannuzzi MC, Frederick MM, Thompson BW, Rossman MD, Bresnitz EA, Terrin ML, Moller DR, Barnard J, Baughman RP, DePalo L, Hunninghake G, Johns C, Judson MA, Knatterud GL, McLennan G, Newman LS, Rabin DL, Rose C, Teirstein AS, Weinberger SE, Yeager H, Cherniack R, ACCESS Research Group. Familial aggregation of sarcoidosis. A case-control etiologic study of sarcoidosis (ACCESS). *American Journal of Respiratory and Critical Care Medicine* 2001;164: 2085–91.
64. Brewerton DA, Cockburn C, James DC, James DG, Neville E. HLA antigens in sarcoidosis. *Clinical and Experimental Immunology* 1977;27: 227–9.
65. Rybicki BA, Walewski JL, Maliarik MJ, Kian H, Iannuzzi MC, ACCESS Research Group. The BTNL2 gene and sarcoidosis susceptibility in African Americans and Whites. *American Journal of Human Genetics* 2005;77: 491–9.
66. The American Thoracic Society (ATS), the European Respiratory Society (ERS), the World Association of Sarcoidosis, and the ATS Board of Directors and by the ERS Executive Committee. Statement on sarcoidosis. *American Journal of Respiratory and Critical Care Medicine* 1999;160: 736–55.
67. Agostini C, Adami F, Semenzato G. New pathogenetic insights into the sarcoid granuloma. *Current Opinion in Rheumatology* 2000;12: 71–6.
68. Zissel G, Prasse A, Muller-Quernheim J. Sarcoidosis—Immunopathogenetic concepts. *Seminars in Respiratory and Critical Care Medicine* 2007;28: 3–14.
69. Miyara M, Amoura Z, Parizot C, Badoual C, Dorgham K, Trad S, Kambouchner M, Valeyre D, Chapelon-Abric C, Debre P, Piette JC, Gorochov G. The immune paradox of sarcoidosis and regulatory T cells. *Journal of Experimental Medicine* 2006;203: 359–70.
70. Naccache JM, Lavole A, Nunes H, Lamberto C, Letoumelin P, Brauner M, Valeyre D, Brillet PY. High-resolution computed tomographic imaging of airways in sarcoidosis patients with airflow obstruction. *Journal of Computer Assisted Tomography* 2008;32: 905–12.
71. Sato H, Grutters JC, Pantelidis P, Mizzon AN, Ahmad T, Van Houte AJ, Lammers JW, Van Den Bosch JM, Welsh KI, Du Bois RM. HLA-DQB1*0201: A marker for good prognosis in British and Dutch patients with sarcoidosis. *American Journal of Respiratory Cell and Molecular Biology* 2002;27: 406–12.
72. Ryerson CJ, Urbania TH, Richeldi L, Mooney JJ, Lee JS, Jones KD, Elicker BM, Koth LL, King TE, Jr., Wolters PJ, Collard HR. Prevalence and prognosis of unclassifiable interstitial lung disease. *European Respiratory Journal: Official Journal of the European Society for Clinical Respiratory Physiology* 2013;42: 750–7.
73. Valeyre D, Freynet O, Dion G, Bouvry D, Annesi-Maesano I, Nunes H. Epidemiology of interstitial lung diseases. *Presse Medicale* 2010;39: 53–9.
74. Gross TJ, Hunninghake GW. Idiopathic pulmonary fibrosis. *New England Journal of Medicine* 2001;345: 517–25.
75. Geist LJ, Hunninghake GW. Potential role of viruses in the pathogenesis of pulmonary fibrosis. *Chest* 1993;103: 119S–20S.

76. American Thoracic Society. Idiopathic pulmonary fibrosis: Diagnosis and treatment. International consensus statement. American Thoracic Society (ATS), and the European Respiratory Society (ERS). *American Journal of Respiratory and Critical Care Medicine* 2000;161: 646–64.
77. Collard HR, Ryu JH, Douglas WW, Schwarz MI, Curran-Everett D, King TE, Jr., Brown KK. Combined corticosteroid and cyclophosphamide therapy does not alter survival in idiopathic pulmonary fibrosis. *Chest* 2004;125: 2169–74.
78. Collard HR, King TE, Jr. Treatment of idiopathic pulmonary fibrosis: The rise and fall of corticosteroids. *American Journal of Medicine* 2001;110: 326–8.
79. Richeldi L, Davies HR, Ferrara G, Franco F. Corticosteroids for idiopathic pulmonary fibrosis. *Cochrane Database of Systematic Reviews* 2003;3: CD002880.
80. Mapel DW, Samet JM, Coultas DB. Corticosteroids and the treatment of idiopathic pulmonary fibrosis. Past, present, and future. *Chest* 1996;110: 1058–67.
81. Douglas WW, Ryu JH, Swensen SJ, Offord KP, Schroeder DR, Caron GM, DeRemee RA. Colchicine versus prednisone in the treatment of idiopathic pulmonary fibrosis. A randomized prospective study. Members of the Lung Study Group. *American Journal of Respiratory and Critical Care Medicine* 1998;158: 220–5.
82. Selman M, Carrillo G, Salas J, Padilla RP, Perez-Chavira R, Sansores R, Chapela R. Colchicine, D-penicillamine, and prednisone in the treatment of idiopathic pulmonary fibrosis: A controlled clinical trial. *Chest* 1998;114: 507–12.
83. Douglas WW, Ryu JH, Schroeder DR. Idiopathic pulmonary fibrosis: Impact of oxygen and colchicine, prednisone, or no therapy on survival. *American Journal of Respiratory and Critical Care Medicine* 2000;161: 1172–8.
84. Katzenstein AL, Myers JL. Idiopathic pulmonary fibrosis: Clinical relevance of pathologic classification. *American Journal of Respiratory and Critical Care Medicine* 1998;157: 1301–15.
85. Selman M, King TE, Pardo A, American Thoracic S, European Respiratory Society, American College of Chest Physicians. Idiopathic pulmonary fibrosis: Prevailing and evolving hypotheses about its pathogenesis and implications for therapy. *Annals of Internal Medicine* 2001;134: 136–51.
86. Adamson IY, Young L, Bowden DH. Relationship of alveolar epithelial injury and repair to the induction of pulmonary fibrosis. *American Journal of Pathology* 1988;130: 377–83.
87. Thannickal VJ, Toews GB, White ES, Lynch JP, 3rd, Martinez FJ. Mechanisms of pulmonary fibrosis. *Annual Review of Medicine* 2004;55: 395–417.
88. White ES, Lazar MH, Thannickal VJ. Pathogenetic mechanisms in usual interstitial pneumonia/idiopathic pulmonary fibrosis. *Journal of Pathology* 2003;201: 343–54.
89. Strieter RM, Mehrad B. New mechanisms of pulmonary fibrosis. *Chest* 2009;136: 1364–70.
90. Antoniades HN, Bravo MA, Avila RE, Galanopoulos T, Neville-Golden J, Maxwell M, Selman M. Platelet-derived growth factor in idiopathic pulmonary fibrosis. *Journal of Clinical Investigation* 1990;86: 1055–64.
91. Kapanci Y, Desmouliere A, Pache JC, Redard M, Gabbiani G. Cytoskeletal protein modulation in pulmonary alveolar myofibroblasts during idiopathic pulmonary fibrosis. Possible role of transforming growth factor beta and tumor necrosis factor alpha. *American Journal of Respiratory and Critical Care Medicine* 1995;152: 2163–9.
92. Nash JR, McLaughlin PJ, Butcher D, Corrin B. Expression of tumour necrosis factor-alpha in cryptogenic fibrosing alveolitis. *Histopathology* 1993;22: 343–7.
93. Khalil N, O'Connor RN, Unruh HW, Warren PW, Flanders KC, Kemp A, Bereznay OH, Greenberg AH. Increased production and immunohistochemical localization of transforming growth factor-beta in idiopathic pulmonary fibrosis. *American Journal of Respiratory Cell and Molecular Biology* 1991;5: 155–62.
94. Magro CM, Allen J, Pope-Harman A, Waldman WJ, Moh P, Rothrauff S, Ross P, Jr. The role of microvascular injury in the evolution of idiopathic pulmonary fibrosis. *American Journal of Clinical Pathology* 2003;119: 556–67.

95. Kotani I, Sato A, Hayakawa H, Urano T, Takada Y, Takada A. Increased procoagulant and antifibrinolytic activities in the lungs with idiopathic pulmonary fibrosis. *Thrombosis Research* 1995;77: 493–504.
96. Ward PA, Hunninghake GW. Lung inflammation and fibrosis. *American Journal of Respiratory and Critical Care Medicine* 1998;157: S123–9.
97. Chambers RC. Role of coagulation cascade proteases in lung repair and fibrosis. *European Respiratory Journal Supplement* 2003;44: 33s–35s.
98. Selman M, Montano M, Ramos C, Chapela R. Concentration, biosynthesis and degradation of collagen in idiopathic pulmonary fibrosis. *Thorax* 1986;41: 355–9.
99. Sheppard MN, Harrison NK. New perspectives on basic mechanisms in lung disease. 1. Lung injury, inflammatory mediators, and fibroblast activation in fibrosing alveolitis. *Thorax* 1992;47: 1064–74.
100. Cantin AM, North SL, Fells GA, Hubbard RC, Crystal RG. Oxidant-mediated epithelial cell injury in idiopathic pulmonary fibrosis. *Journal of Clinical Investigation* 1987;79: 1665–73.
101. Arsalane K, Dubois CM, Muanza T, Begin R, Boudreau F, Asselin C, Cantin AM. Transforming growth factor-beta1 is a potent inhibitor of glutathione synthesis in the lung epithelial cell line A549: Transcriptional effect on the GSH rate-limiting enzyme gamma-glutamylcysteine synthetase. *American Journal of Respiratory Cell and Molecular Biology* 1997;17: 599–607.
102. Katzenstein AL, Fiorelli RF. Nonspecific interstitial pneumonia/fibrosis. Histologic features and clinical significance. *American Journal of Surgical Pathology* 1994;18: 136–47.
103. Katzenstein AL. *Katzenstein and Askin's Surgical Pathology of Non-Neoplastic Lung Disease.* 3rd revised edition. Philadelphia, PA: WB Saunders, 1997.
104. Cottin V, Loire R, Chalabreysse L, Thivolet F, Cordier JF. Nonspecific interstitial pneumonitis: A new anatomoclinical entity among idiopathic diffuse interstitial pneumonias. *Revue des Maladied Respiratoires* 2001;18: 25–33.
105. Morice AH, Fontana GA, Sovijarvi ARA, Pistolesi M, Chung KF, Widdicombe J, O'Connell F, Geppetti P, Gronke L, De Jongste J, Belvisi M, Dicpinigaitis P, Fischer A, McGarvey L, Fokkens WJ, Kastelik J. The diagnosis and management of chronic cough. *European Respiratory Journal* 2004;24: 481–92.
106. Daniil ZD, Gilchrist FC, Nicholson AG, Hansell DM, Harris J, Colby TV, du Bois RM. A histologic pattern of nonspecific interstitial pneumonia is associated with a better prognosis than usual interstitial pneumonia in patients with cryptogenic fibrosing alveolitis. *American Journal of Respiratory and Critical Care Medicine* 1999;160: 899–905.
107. Bouros D, Wells AU, Nicholson AG, Colby TV, Polychronopoulos V, Pantelidis P, Haslam PL, Vassilakis DA, Black CM, du Bois RM. Histopathologic subsets of fibrosing alveolitis in patients with systemic sclerosis and their relationship to outcome. *American Journal of Respiratory and Critical Care Medicine* 2002;165: 1581–6.
108. Douglas WW, Tazelaar HD, Hartman TE, Hartman RP, Decker PA, Schroeder DR, Ryu JH. Polymyositis-dermatomyositis-associated interstitial lung disease. *American Journal of Respiratory and Critical Care Medicine* 2001;164: 1182–5.
109. Ito I, Nagai S, Kitaichi M, Nicholson AG, Johkoh T, Noma S, Kim DS, Handa T, Izumi T, Mishima M. Pulmonary manifestations of primary Sjogren's syndrome: A clinical, radiologic, and pathologic study. *American Journal of Respiratory and Critical Care Medicine* 2005;171: 632–8.
110. Kinder BW, Collard HR, Koth L, Daikh DI, Wolters PJ, Elicker B, Jones KD, King TE, Jr. Idiopathic nonspecific interstitial pneumonia: Lung manifestation of undifferentiated connective tissue disease? *American Journal of Respiratory and Critical Care Medicine* 2007;176: 691–7.
111. Fujita J, Ohtsuki Y, Yoshinouchi T, Yamadori I, Bandoh S, Tokuda M, Miyawaki H, Kishimoto N, Ishida T. Idiopathic non-specific interstitial pneumonia: As an "autoimmune interstitial pneumonia." *Respiratory Medicine* 2005;99: 234–40.
112. Colby TV. Pathologic aspects of bronchiolitis obliterans organizing pneumonia. *Chest* 1992;102: 38S–43S.

113. Shimizu S, Yoshinouchi T, Ohtsuki Y, Fujita J, Sugiura Y, Banno S, Yamadori I, Eimoto T, Ueda R. The appearance of S-100 protein-positive dendritic cells and the distribution of lymphocyte subsets in idiopathic nonspecific interstitial pneumonia. *Respiratory Medicine* 2002;96: 770–6.
114. Myers JL, Katzenstein AL. Ultrastructural evidence of alveolar epithelial injury in idiopathic bronchiolitis obliterans-organizing pneumonia. *American Journal of Pathology* 1988;132: 102–9.
115. Basset F, Ferrans VJ, Soler P, Takemura T, Fukuda Y, Crystal RG. Intraluminal fibrosis in interstitial lung disorders. *American Journal of Pathology* 1986;122: 443–61.
116. Cordier JF. Cryptogenic organising pneumonia. *European Respiratory Journal: Official Journal of the European Society for Clinical Respiratory Physiology* 2006;28: 422–46.
117. Lappi-Blanco E, Kaarteenaho-Wiik R, Soini Y, Risteli J, Paakko P. Intraluminal fibromyxoid lesions in bronchiolitis obliterans organizing pneumonia are highly capillarized. *Human Pathology* 1999;30: 1192–6.
118. Lappi-Blanco E, Soini Y, Kinnula V, Paakko P. VEGF and bFGF are highly expressed in intraluminal fibromyxoid lesions in bronchiolitis obliterans organizing pneumonia. *Journal of Pathology* 2002;196: 220–7.
119. Lappi-Blanco E, Soini Y, Paakko P. Apoptotic activity is increased in the newly formed fibromyxoid connective tissue in bronchiolitis obliterans organizing pneumonia. *Lung* 1999;177: 367–76.
120. Nagai S, Hoshino Y, Hayashi M, Ito I. Smoking-related interstitial lung diseases. *Current Opinion in Pulmonary Medicine* 2000;6: 415–9.
121. Downey GP, Granton JT. Mechanisms of acute lung injury. *Current Opinion in Pulmonary Medicine* 1997;3: 234–41.
122. Katzenstein AL, Myers JL, Mazur MT. Acute interstitial pneumonia. A clinicopathologic, ultrastructural, and cell kinetic study. *American Journal of Surgical Pathology* 1986;10: 256–67.
123. Bouros D, Nicholson AC, Polychronopoulos V, du Bois RM. Acute interstitial pneumonia. *European Respiratory Journal: Official Journal of the European Society for Clinical Respiratory Physiology* 2000;15: 412–8.
124. Vassallo R, Ryu JH, Colby TV, Hartman T, Limper AH. Pulmonary Langerhans'-cell histiocytosis. *New England Journal of Medicine* 2000;342: 1969–78.
125. Reddy TL, Tominaga M, Hansell DM, von der Thusen J, Rassl D, Parfrey H, Guy S, Twentyman O, Rice A, Maher TM, Renzoni EA, Wells AU, Nicholson AG. Pleuroparenchymal fibroelastosis: A spectrum of histopathological and imaging phenotypes. *European Respiratory Journal: Official Journal of the European Society for Clinical Respiratory Physiology* 2012;40: 377–85.
126. Vassallo R, Ryu JH. Pulmonary Langerhans' cell histiocytosis. *Clinics in Chest Medicine* 2004;25: 561–71, vii.
127. Colby TV, Lombard C. Histiocytosis X in the lung. *Human Pathology* 1983;14: 847–56.
128. Tazi A. Adult pulmonary Langerhans' cell histiocytosis. *European Respiratory Journal: Official Journal of the European Society for Clinical Respiratory Physiology* 2006;27: 1272–85.
129. Johnson SR. Lymphangioleiomyomatosis. *European Respiratory Journal: Official Journal of the European Society for Clinical Respiratory Physiology* 2006;27: 1056–65.
130. McCormack FX. Lymphangioleiomyomatosis: A clinical update. *Chest* 2008;133: 507–16.
131. Carsillo T, Astrinidis A, Henske EP. Mutations in the tuberous sclerosis complex gene TSC2 are a cause of sporadic pulmonary lymphangioleiomyomatosis. *Proceedings of the National Academy of Sciences of the United States of America* 2000;97: 6085–90.
132. Smolarek TA, Wessner LL, McCormack FX, Mylet JC, Menon AG, Henske EP. Evidence that lymphangiomyomatosis is caused by TSC2 mutations: Chromosome 16p13 loss of heterozygosity in angiomyolipomas and lymph nodes from women with lymphangiomyomatosis. *American Journal of Human Genetics* 1998;62: 810–5.
133. Astrinidis A, Khare L, Carsillo T, Smolarek T, Au KS, Northrup H, Henske EP. Mutational analysis of the tuberous sclerosis gene TSC2 in patients with pulmonary lymphangioleiomyomatosis. *Journal of Medical Genetics* 2000;37: 55–7.

134. Johnson SR, Tattersfield AE. Clinical experience of lymphangioleiomyomatosis in the UK. *Thorax* 2000;55: 1052–7.
135. Avila NA, Kelly JA, Chu SC, Dwyer AJ, Moss J. Lymphangioleiomyomatosis: Abdominopelvic CT and US findings. *Radiology* 2000;216: 147–53.
136. Johnson SR, Cordier JF, Lazor R, Cottin V, Costabel U, Harari S, Reynaud-Gaubert M, Boehler A, Brauner M, Popper H, Bonetti F, Kingswood C. Review Panel of the ERSLAMTF. European Respiratory Society guidelines for the diagnosis and management of lymphangioleiomyomatosis. *European Respiratory Journal: Official Journal of the European Society for Clinical Respiratory Physiology* 2010;35: 14–26.
137. McCormack FX, Inoue Y, Moss J, Singer LG, Strange C, Nakata K, Barker AF, Chapman JT, Brantly ML, Stocks JM, Brown KK, Lynch JP, 3rd, Goldberg HJ, Young LR, Kinder BW, Downey GP, Sullivan EJ, Colby TV, McKay RT, Cohen MM, Korbee L, Taveira-DaSilva AM, Lee HS, Krischer JP, Trapnell BC, National Institutes of Health Rare Lung Diseases C, Group MT. Efficacy and safety of sirolimus in lymphangioleiomyomatosis. *New England Journal of Medicine* 2011;364: 1595–606.
138. Jeong YJ, Kim KI, Seo IJ, Lee CH, Lee KN, Kim KN, Kim JS, Kwon WJ. Eosinophilic lung diseases: A clinical, radiologic, and pathologic overview. *Radiographics: A Review Publication of the Radiological Society of North America, Inc* 2007;27: 617–37; discussion 37–9.
139. Solomon J, Schwarz M. Drug-, toxin-, and radiation therapy-induced eosinophilic pneumonia. *Seminars in Respiratory and Critical Care Medicine* 2006;27: 192–7.
140. Allen J. Acute eosinophilic pneumonia. *Seminars in Respiratory and Critical Care Medicine* 2006;27: 142–7.
141. Marchand E, Cordier JF. Idiopathic chronic eosinophilic pneumonia. *Seminars in Respiratory and Critical Care Medicine* 2006;27: 134–41.
142. Vijayan VK. Tropical pulmonary eosinophilia: Pathogenesis, diagnosis and management. *Current Opinion in Pulmonary Medicine* 2007;13: 428–33.
143. Agarwal R. Allergic bronchopulmonary aspergillosis. *Chest* 2009;135: 805–26.
144. Patterson K, Strek ME. Allergic bronchopulmonary aspergillosis. *Proceedings of the American Thoracic Society* 2010;7: 237–44.
145. Bosken CH, Myers JL, Greenberger PA, Katzenstein AL. Pathologic features of allergic bronchopulmonary aspergillosis. *American Journal of Surgical Pathology* 1988;12: 216–22.
146. Stevens DA, Schwartz HJ, Lee JY, Moskovitz BL, Jerome DC, Catanzaro A, Bamberger DM, Weinmann AJ, Tuazon CU, Judson MA, Platts-Mills TA, DeGraff AC, Jr. A randomized trial of itraconazole in allergic bronchopulmonary aspergillosis. *New England Journal of Medicine* 2000;342: 756–62.
147. Conron M, Beynon HL. Churg-Strauss syndrome. *Thorax* 2000;55: 870–7.
148. Hellmich B, Csernok E, Gross WL. Proinflammatory cytokines and autoimmunity in Churg-Strauss syndrome. *Annals of the New York Academy of Sciences* 2005;1051: 121–31.
149. Schmitt WH, Csernok E, Kobayashi S, Klinkenborg A, Reinhold-Keller E, Gross WL. Churg-Strauss syndrome: Serum markers of lymphocyte activation and endothelial damage. *Arthritis and Rheumatism* 1998;41: 445–52.
150. Zwerina J, Axmann R, Jatzwauk M, Sahinbegovic E, Polzer K, Schett G. Pathogenesis of Churg-Strauss syndrome: Recent insights. *Autoimmunity* 2009;42: 376–9.
151. Vaglio A, Martorana D, Maggiore U, Grasselli C, Zanetti A, Pesci A, Garini G, Manganelli P, Bottero P, Tumiati B, Sinico RA, Savi M, Buzio C, Neri TM, Secondary and Primary Vasculitis Study Group. HLA-DRB4 as a genetic risk factor for Churg-Strauss syndrome. *Arthritis and Rheumatism* 2007;56: 3159–66.
152. Sheikh J, Weller PF. Clinical overview of hypereosinophilic syndromes. *Immunology and Allergy Clinics of North America* 2007;27: 333–55.
153. Katz U, Shoenfeld Y. Pulmonary eosinophilia. *Clinical Reviews in Allergy & Immunology* 2008;34: 367–71.

154. Ackerman SJ, Bochner BS. Mechanisms of eosinophilia in the pathogenesis of hypereosinophilic disorders. *Immunology and Allergy Clinics of North America* 2007;27: 357–75.
155. Huizar I, Kavuru MS. Alveolar proteinosis syndrome: Pathogenesis, diagnosis, and management. *Current Opinion in Pulmonary Medicine* 2009;15: 491–8.
156. Borie R, Danel C, Debray MP, Taille C, Dombret MC, Aubier M, Epaud R, Crestani B. Pulmonary alveolar proteinosis. *European Respiratory Review: An Official Journal of the European Respiratory Society* 2011;20: 98–107.
157. Seymour JF, Presneill JJ. Pulmonary alveolar proteinosis: Progress in the first 44 years. *American Journal of Respiratory and Critical Care Medicine* 2002;166: 215–35.
158. Trapnell BC, Carey BC, Uchida K, Suzuki T. Pulmonary alveolar proteinosis, a primary immunodeficiency of impaired GM-CSF stimulation of macrophages. *Current Opinion in Immunology* 2009;21: 514–21.
159. Briens E, Delaval P, Mairesse MP, Valeyre D, Wallaert B, Lazor R, Cordier JF, Groupe D'etudes Et de Recherche Sur Les Maladies Orphelines P. Pulmonary alveolar proteinosis. *Revue de Maladies Respiratoires* 2002;19: 166–82.
160. Beccaria M, Luisetti M, Rodi G, Corsico A, Zoia MC, Colato S, Pochetti P, Braschi A, Pozzi E, Cerveri I. Long-term durable benefit after whole lung lavage in pulmonary alveolar proteinosis. *European Respiratory Journal: Official Journal of the European Society for Clinical Respiratory Physiology* 2004;23: 526–31.
161. Kavuru MS, Sullivan EJ, Piccin R, Thomassen MJ, Stoller JK. Exogenous granulocyte-macrophage colony-stimulating factor administration for pulmonary alveolar proteinosis. *American Journal of Respiratory and Critical Care Medicine* 2000;161: 1143–8.
162. Venkateshiah SB, Yan TD, Bonfield TL, Thomassen MJ, Meziane M, Czich C, Kavuru MS. An open-label trial of granulocyte macrophage colony stimulating factor therapy for moderate symptomatic pulmonary alveolar proteinosis. *Chest* 2006;130: 227–37.
163. Tazawa R, Trapnell BC, Inoue Y, Arai T, Takada T, Nasuhara Y, Hizawa N, Kasahara Y, Tatsumi K, Hojo M, Ishii H, Yokoba M, Tanaka N, Yamaguchi E, Eda R, Tsuchihashi Y, Morimoto K, Akira M, Terada M, Otsuka J, Ebina M, Kaneko C, Nukiwa T, Krischer JP, Akazawa K, Nakata K. Inhaled granulocyte/macrophage-colony stimulating factor as therapy for pulmonary alveolar proteinosis. *American Journal of Respiratory and Critical Care Medicine* 2010;181: 1345–54.
164. Seymour JF, Dunn AR, Vincent JM, Presneill JJ, Pain MC. Efficacy of granulocyte-macrophage colony-stimulating factor in acquired alveolar proteinosis. *New England Journal of Medicine* 1996;335: 1924–5.

# 11

# Lung cancer

CHRISTIAN COUTURE

Introduction 207
Risk factors 207
Epidemiology 209
Semeiology 209
Histopathologic classification 210
Molecular events involved in the development of lung cancer 212
    Diagnosis and staging 213
    Treatment and prognosis 217
References 220

## Introduction

Cancer results from the uncontrolled proliferation of a single cell that eventually forms a tumor, which initially invades its organ of origin. The tumor can then locally spread to nearby and even to distant organs, forming metastases and from there ultimately cause death. The mechanism by which a single cell gives rise to a cancerous tumor results from the interplay of different genetic and environmental factors. More than 95% of lung cancers are carcinomas because they stem from epithelial cells. In about 90% of cases, this results from the exposure of bronchial and alveolar epithelial cells to the carcinogens contained in cigarette smoke. The most common symptoms of lung cancer are cough, dyspnea (shortness of breath), hemoptysis (coughing up blood), and weight loss. Lung cancer is diagnosed on a biopsy examined under a microscope by a pathologist. The treatment and prognosis depend on the histological type and extent of tumor spread at diagnosis as well as the general condition of the patient. Current treatments for lung cancer include surgery, radiotherapy, conventional chemotherapy, targeted therapy, and immunotherapy. Even with treatment, lung cancer has a poor prognosis, the survival rate at 5 years reaching only 15%. This chapter describes the risk factors, epidemiology, semeiology, histopathological classification, diagnosis, staging, treatment, and prognosis of lung cancer.

## Risk factors

Smoking is by far the main risk factor. It is responsible for 90% of all lung cancers [1]. Cigarette smoke contains many carcinogens, the main one being benzopyrene [2]. The risk of dying of lung cancer is 20 times higher in active smokers than nonsmokers [3]. This risk is not only modulated mainly by the duration of smoking but also by the average cigarette consumption, age of initiation of smoking, time since smoking cessation, type of smoked product, and type of inhalation (deep vs. superficial). Secondary smoking also increases the risk of developing lung cancer by 20%–25% [4]. After quitting smoking the risk of developing lung cancer diminishes rapidly in the first 5 years after which the risk continues to decrease more slowly to go back, after 20 years, very close to that of a nonsmoker but an excess risk still persists throughout life thereafter [5,6]. Figure 11.1 illustrates the cumulative risk of death by lung cancer in smokers, nonsmokers, and ex-smokers quitting at various ages [7].

Radon exposure is the second cause of lung cancer after smoking and the first among nonsmokers [8]. It is an odorless, colorless radioactive gas derived from the natural decay of radium, itself derived from the decay of uranium found in Earth's crust.

The occupational exposure to asbestos and many other substances can also cause lung cancer. Although the proportion of lung cancers that these carcinogens cause is generally low, it is nevertheless important in populations of exposed workers. For most of these substances, a certain degree of synergy with smoking has also been described [4,9].

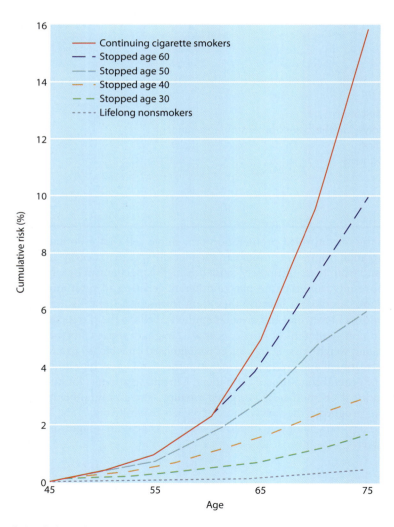

Figure 11.1 Risk of death from lung cancer in smokers, ex-smokers, and nonsmokers. (Reproduced from Peto R et al. *BMJ*, 321, 2000.).

## Epidemiology

Lung cancer was uncommon before the era of tobacco smoking. However, it has reached epidemic proportions with the industrialization of cigarette production to the point that it is the leading cause of cancer death in the United States and Canada as in many other countries, both in men and in women. The first robust epidemiological evidence linking smoking and lung cancer was published in 1956 [10]. Several countries then gradually adopted health and legislative measures to reduce smoking. In countries such as England, Holland, Belgium, Finland, Australia, New Zealand, United States, Singapore, Sweden, Denmark, Italy, and Canada, where these measures managed to reduce smoking rates, lung cancer mortality has started to decrease proportionally in the following 20–30 years. Figure 11.2 illustrates this tendency in the United States, showing that the rate of lung cancer mortality in a population is a reflection of smoking in this population 20–30 years earlier.

In some Eastern European countries such as Hungary and Poland or Southern Europe such as Spain and Portugal, smoking and lung cancer mortality rates are still high. In emerging countries such as China and India, lung cancer mortality is expected to significantly increase in the coming years due to adoption of mass cigarette smoking [11].

In the United States, the overall 5-year survival is 15%, 17% in women, and 13% in men. In men, there has been a decline in the lung cancer mortality rate since the mid-1980s; in women, this decline began only in the 2000s, both reflecting the respective gender-specific declines in tobacco smoking 20–30 years earlier [12].

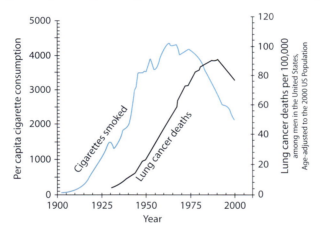

Figure 11.2 Relation of smoking and lung cancer death rate.

## Semeiology

Signs and symptoms in lung cancer patients are numerous but well described [13]. The most frequent at diagnosis are dyspnea, hemoptysis, cough, wheezing, chest or abdominal pain, dysphonia (voice hoarseness), digital clubbing, dysphagia, and signs of systemic disease such as fatigue, weight loss, and loss of appetite [14]. It is noteworthy that about 10% of lung cancer patients have no symptoms at diagnosis. It is typically found incidentally on chest radiography done for another reason.

Signs and symptoms due to local tumor growth include dyspnea and pneumonia following airway obstruction. A tumor can also bleed in the lungs, causing hemoptysis. It can eventually cause a pleural effusion by invading the visceral pleura or chest or back pain by extension to the chest wall or vertebrae.

The invasion or compression of mediastinal structures may be responsible for the following signs and symptoms:

- Recurrent laryngeal nerve: voice hoarseness
- Phrenic nerve: diaphragm muscle paralysis

- Sympathetic nerves: Claude–Bernard–Horner syndrome (myosis, eyelid ptosis, and facial anhidrosis)
- Superior vena cava: superior vena cava syndrome
- Pericardium: pericardial effusion and cardiac tamponade
- Heart: cardiac arrhythmias, heart failure
- Esophagus: dysphagia, bronchoesophageal fistula

Distant metastases become manifest by their direct effect on the affected organ. The most common sites of lung cancer metastases are the brain, bones, adrenal glands, the contralateral lung, liver, pericardium, and kidneys [15].

In addition to the above described manifestations explained by a local effect caused by the primary tumor or its metastases, there are also endocrine syndromes caused by the uninhibited secretion of substances by tumor cells. The best known endocrine syndromes are hyponatremia from the syndrome of inappropriate antidiuretic hormone secretion (SIADH) and Cushing's syndrome from production of adrenocorticotropic hormone (ACTH).

Finally, lung cancer may manifest as a paraneoplastic syndrome explained neither by the direct effect of the primary tumor or its metastases nor by an endocrine secretion. The best known include dermatomyositis/polymyositis, digital clubbing, transverse myelitis, myasthenia gravis, peripheral neuropathy, and encephalopathy.

## Histopathologic classification

The 2015 World Health Organization (WHO) classification of lung tumors lists 88 different histopathologic types of lung tumors [11]. Clinically speaking, a simple dichotomous classification is still today very much useful to physicians involved in the care of lung cancer patients: small cell and non-small cell lung cancer based on the the size and appearance of tumor cells under the microscope. Non-small cell lung carcinomas are generally either adenocarcinomas or squamous cell carcinomas. Approximately 50% of lung cancers are adenocarcinomas, 20% squamous cell carcinomas, and 17% small cell carcinomas [16]. The rest regroups various tumors that are beyond the scope of this chapter. Macroscopic and microscopic appearance of these main types of lung cancer are presented in Figures 11.3 through 11.5.

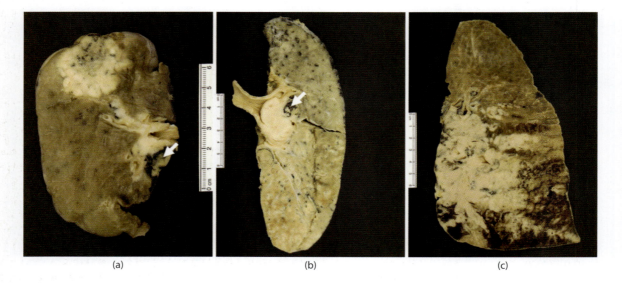

Figure 11.3 Macroscopic appearance of the main histologic types of lung cancer. **(a)** Adenocarcinoma in a pulmonary lobectomy specimen with peripheral tumor invading the pleura and with peribronchial lymph node metastasis (arrow). **(b)** Squamous cell carcinoma in a pneumonectomy specimen with central tumor invading the mainstem bronchus, with obstructive pneumonia and peribronchial lymph node metastasis (arrow). **(c)** Small cell carcinoma in an autopsy lung with central tumor diffusely invading the lung.

Histopathologic classification 211

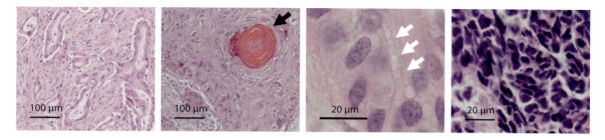

Figure 11.4 Salient features of the three main histologic types of lung cancer. Left to right: gland formation in adenocarcinoma, keratinization (black arrow), and intercellular bridges (white arrows) in squamous cell carcinoma, and scant cytoplasm, high nucleocytoplasmic ratio, and dark chromatin in small cell carcinoma.

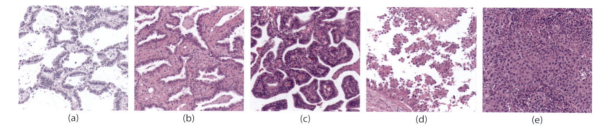

Figure 11.5 The five histologic patterns of lung adenocarcinoma according to the 2015 World Health Organization classification. (a) Lepidic. (b) Acinary. (c) Papillary. (d) Micropapillary. (e) Solid.

Small cell carcinoma is characterized by small tumor cells with scant cytoplasm and a nucleus with dark and uniform chromatin without prominent nucleoli. The nuclei are often crowded, giving the impression that they are molded on each other (nuclear molding). Small cell carcinomas typically have a central location because they arise from neuroendocrine cells of the epithelial lining of the first or second order bronchi. These tumors have neurosecretory granules (see Chapter 1) that may contain substances causing the neuroendocrine secretion syndromes described in the previous section of this chapter, including SIADH, hypercalcemia and Cushing's syndrome. The biological behavior of small cell carcinoma is aggressive. At diagnosis, it typically already forms a hilar mass with hilar or mediastinal lymph node metastases and is accompanied by distant metastases in two-thirds of cases.

Non-small cell lung carcinomas as a group differ histologically from small cell carcinoma by their larger cell size attributable to their more abundant cytoplasm. Tumor cells often have a nucleus with one or more prominent nucleoli. Adenocarcinoma is characterized by mucin production and/or any proportion of five histologic patterns (lepidic, acinar, papillary, micropapillary, or solid). Its preferential location is peripheral because it is thought to originate from alveolar pneumocytes. The lepidic pattern of adenocarcinoma respects the preexisting alveolar architecture and was formely named bronchoalveolar carcinoma. It presents radiologically as a ground glass opacity reminiscent of a pneumonic infiltrate rather than a tumor. Squamous cell carcinoma is characterized by the production of keratin or the formation of intercellular bridges. It derives from the basal cells of the bronchial lining. It is usually located centrally and is more likely than other types of lung cancer to become necrotic in its center and form a cavitary lesion.

In a clinical setting, the distinction between adenocarcinoma and squamous cell carcinoma may not always be easy by conventional histology either because the tumor is poorly differentiated or because the biopsy sample taken from the patient's tumor is small. Special stains can be used in this situation. Adenocarcinomas are typically positive for mucin stains like Alcian Blue and Mucicarmine and display a thyroid transcription factor (TTF)-1(+) p40(−) immunophenotype. Conversely, squamous cell carcinomas are negative for mucin stains and display a TTF-1(−) p40(+) immunophenotype (see Figure 11.6).

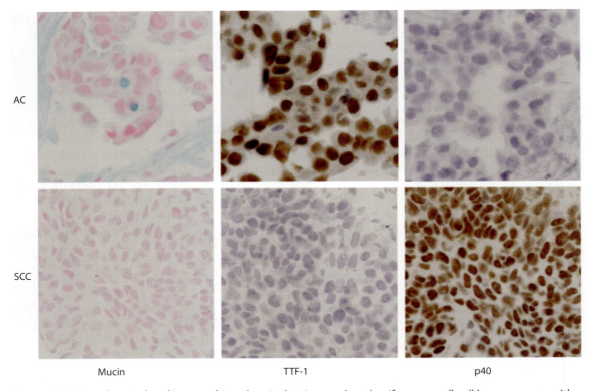

Figure 11.6 Histochemical and immunohistochemical stains used to classify non-small cell lung cancer as either adenocarcinoma or squamous cell carcinoma. Adenocarcinomas (AC; upper panel) are typically positive for mucin stains like Alcian Blue and display a TTF-1(+) p40(–) immunophenotype. Conversely, squamous cell carcinomas (SCC; lower panel) are negative for mucin stains and display a TTF-1(–) p40(+) immunophenotype.

It is important to realize that not all lung tumors are from the lung as it is a frequent metastatic site for primary tumors from other organs, particularly breast, colon, kidney, and melanoma of the skin. As mentioned in the previous section of this chapter, lung cancer itself frequently metastasizes to the brain, bone, adrenal glands, contralateral lung, liver, kidney, and pericardium. Thus, lung cancer is frequently diagnosed on a biopsy obtained from a metastatic site such as liver and conversely pulmonary metastases from other organs such as breast are often diagnosed on a lung biopsy. Once again, special stains can be helpful to clarify if the tumor cells found on a biopsy taken from a given organ represent a primary or a metastasis.

## Molecular events involved in the development of lung cancer

Molecular events are frequently involved in the development of lung cancer and vary in part according to histological type. Small cell carcinoma frequently has mutations in the RB1 and p53 genes. Squamous cell carcinoma also has a high rate of mutations in the p53 gene and expression of the protein encoded by the tumor suppressor gene RB1 is abolished in 15%. The inhibitor of cyclin-dependent kinase p16 (INKa) is inactivated in 65% of squamous cell carcinomas. Many allelic losses at loci containing tumor suppressor genes are also observed (3p, 9p, and 17p). Epidermal growth factor receptor (EGFR) is overexpressed in 80% although its gene is rarely mutated. Finally, however, HER-2/neu is highly expressed in 30% of these tumors without gene amplification as in breast cancer. For adenocarcinomas, aside from the aforementioned mutations of squamous cell carcinoma, several other mutations, usually mutually exclusive, represent promising targets for a whole range of recently developed specific therapies called targeted therapies. KRAS mutations are present in the tumors of 5% of nonsmokers and 30% of smokers.

They predict aggressive behavior. Currently, the most interesting mutations from a therapeutic point of view are those in the EGFR gene (15%–20%) and the anaplastic lymphoma kinase (ALK) gene rearrangements (2%) Many tumors express the surface protein programmed death ligand 1 (PD-L1), which binds to its receptor PD-1 on immune cells. This ligand–receptor interaction allows tumor cells to escape cytotoxic immune response. Immunotherapy aims at restoring the capacity of the immune system to destroy tumor cells by blocking this interaction using therapeutic antibodies directed against PD-L1 or PD-1. (see "Treatment and Prognosis" on page 217).

## Diagnosis and staging

In a patient with symptoms suggestive of lung cancer, it is important in order to eventually determine the appropriate treatment and prognosis to first prove the diagnosis of lung cancer on biopsies examined under a microscope by a pathologist and to determine the stage (extent) of the disease. Establishing the diagnosis and staging is done by questioning and examining the patient and performing diagnostic tests.

For lung cancer, the tumor node and metastases (TNM) staging system is the most widely used. In this staging system, the letter T refers to the extent of the primary **T**umor; the letter N refers to involvement of locoregional lymph **N**odes by tumor, and the letter M to **M**etastases, that is the spread of the tumor to distant organs. Each of these T, N, and M descpritors is first evaluated separately and then grouped into stages I, II, III, or IV. The current criteria used to determine the TNM stage of lung cancer [17] are presented in Tables 11.1 and 11.2.

Table 11.1 T, N, and M descriptors for the eighth edition of the tumor, node, and metastases (TNM) classification for lung cancer

| T: Primary tumor | |
|---|---|
| Tx | Primary tumor cannot be assessed or tumor proven by presence of malignant cells in sputum or bronchial washings but not visualized by imaging or bronchoscopy |
| T0 | No evidence of primary tumor |
| Tis | Carcinoma *in situ* |
| T1 | Tumor ≤3 cm in greatest dimension surrounded by lung or visceral pleura without bronchoscopic evidence of invasion more proximal than the lobar bronchus (i.e., not in the main bronchus)[a] |
| T1a(mi) | Minimally invasive adenocarcinoma[b] |
| T1a | Tumor ≤1 cm in greatest dimension[a] |
| T1b | Tumor >1 cm but ≤2 cm in greatest dimension[a] |
| T1c | Tumor >2 cm but ≤3 cm in greatest dimension[a] |
| T2 | Tumor >3 cm but ≤5 cm or tumor with any of the following features[c]:<br>• Involves main bronchus regardless of distance from the carina but without involvementof the carina<br>• Invades visceral pleura<br>• Associated with atelectasis or obstructive pneumonitis that extends to the hilar region, involving part or all of the lung |
| T2a | Tumor >3 cm but ≤4 cm in greatest dimension |
| T2b | Tumor >4 cm but ≤5 cm in greatest dimension |
| T3 | Tumor >5 cm but ≤7 cm in greatest dimension or associated with separate tumor nodule(s) in the same lobe as the primary tumor or directly invades any of the following structures:<br>• Chest wall (including the parietal pleura and superior sulcus tumors), phrenic nerve and parietal pericardium |

*(Continued)*

Table 11.1 (*Continued*) T, N, and M descriptors for the eighth edition of the tumor, node, and metastases (TNM) classification for lung cancer

| | |
|---|---|
| **T: Primary tumor** | |
| T4 | Tumor >7 cm in greatest dimension or associated with separate tumor nodule(s) in a different ipsilateral lobe to that of the primary tumor or invades any of the following structures:<br>• Diaphragm, mediastinum, heart, great vessels, trachea, recurrent laryngeal nerve, esophagus, vertebral body, and carina |
| **N: Regional lymph node involvement** | |
| Nx | Regional lymph nodes cannot be assessed |
| N0 | No regional lymph node metastasis |
| N1 | Metastasis in ipsilateral peribronchial and/or ipsilateral hilar lymph nodes and intrapulmonary nodes, including involvement by direct extension |
| N2 | Metastasis in ipsilateral mediastinal and/or subcarinal lymph node(s) |
| N3 | Metastasis in contralateral mediastinal, contralateral hilar, ipsilateral or contralateral scalene, or supraclavicular lymph node(s) |
| **M: Distant metastasis** | |
| M0 | No distant metastasis |
| M1 | Distant metastasis present |
| M1a | Separate tumor nodule(s) in a contralateral lobe; tumor with pleural or pericardial nodule(s) or malignant pleural or pericardial effusion[d] |
| M1b | Single extrathoracic metastasis[e] |
| M1c | Multiple extrathoracic metastases in one or more organs |

[a] The uncommon superficial spreading tumor of any size with its invasive component limited to the bronchial wall, which may extend proximal to the main bronchus, is also classified as T1a.
[b] Solitary adenocarcinoma, ≤3 cm with a predominately lepidic pattern and ≤5 mm invasion in any one focus.
[c] T2 tumors with these features are classified as T2a if ≤4 cm in greatest dimension or if size cannot be determined, and T2b if >4 cm but 5 cm in greatest dimension.
[d] Most pleural (pericardial) effusions with lung cancer are due to tumor. In a few patients, however, multiple microscopic examinations of pleural (pericardial) fluid are negative for tumor and the fluid is nonbloody and not an exudate. When these elements and clinical judgment dictate that the effusion is not related to the tumor, the effusion should be excluded as a staging descriptor.
[e] This includes involvement of a single distant (nonregional) lymph node.

Table 11.2 Stage groupings for the eighth edition of the TNM classification for lung cancer

| | | | |
|---|---|---|---|
| Occult carcinoma | TX | N0 | M0 |
| Stage 0 | Tis | N0 | M0 |
| Stage IA1 | T1a(mi) | N0 | M0 |
|  | T1a | N0 | M0 |
| Stage IA2 | T1b | N0 | M0 |
| Stage IA3 | T1c | N0 | M0 |
| Stage IB | T2a | N0 | M0 |
| Stage IIA | T2b | N0 | M0 |
| Stage IIB | T1a–c | N1 | M0 |
|  | T2a | N1 | M0 |
|  | T2b | N1 | M0 |
|  | T3 | N0 | M0 |

(*Continued*)

Table 11.2 (*Continued*) Stage groupings for the eighth edition of the TNM classification for lung cancer

| Stage IIIA | T1a–c | N2 | M0 |
|---|---|---|---|
|  | T2a–b | N2 | M0 |
|  | T3 | N1 | M0 |
|  | T4 | N0 | M0 |
|  | T4 | N1 | M0 |
| Stage IIIB | T1a–c | N3 | M0 |
|  | T2a–b | N3 | M0 |
|  | **T3** | N2 | M0 |
|  | T4 | N2 | M0 |
| Stage IIIC | T3 | N3 | M0 |
|  | T4 | N3 | M0 |
| Stage IVA | Any T | Any N | M1a |
|  | Any T | Any N | M1b |
| Stage IVB | Any T | Any N | M1c |

TNM, tumor, node, and metastasis; Tis, carcinoma *in situ*; T1a(mi), minimally invasive adenocarcinoma

The main tests to assess the primary tumor are chest radiography, computed tomography (CT), and bronchoscopy (see Figures 11.7 and 11.8).

Chest radiography is the basic examination. It is often used to detect the primary lung tumor or indirect manifestations such as atelectasis or pneumonia caused by obstruction of a bronchus, pleural effusion, or manifestations of lymph node metastases such as widening of the mediastinum or paralysis of the diaphragm. Chest CT allows one to assess the relationship of the tumor to the surrounding anatomic structures more precisely. It can also be very helpful to guide needle biopsies of otherwise inaccessible peripheral tumors or drainage of pleural effusions. Magnetic resonance imaging (MRI) provides an even greater level of

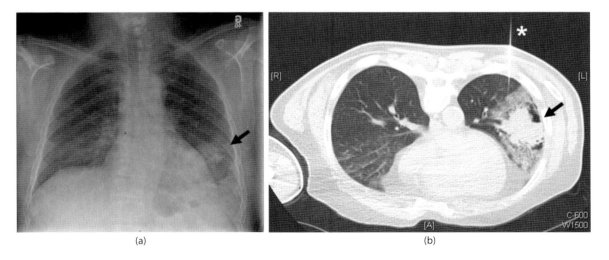

Figure 11.7 Radiology of lung cancer. **(a)** Chest radiography is a cheap and readily available exam to investigate patients with signs and symptoms suspicious of lung cancer. Here, it shows a tumor in the left lower lobe (arrow). **(b)** Chest computed tomography (CT) is used to evaluate in more details the extent of lung cancer. Here it is also used to guide a needle biopsy (asterisk) of a tumor in the left lower lobe (arrow).

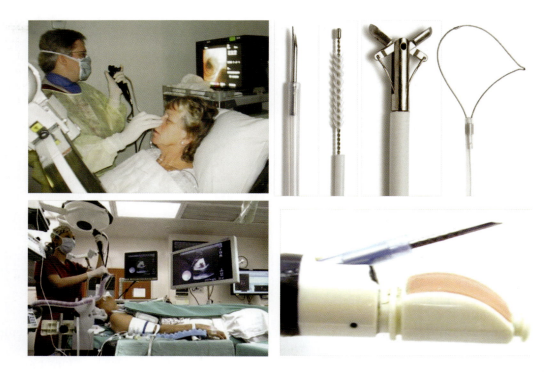

Figure 11.8 Bronchoscopy. Upper panel: Conventional bronchoscopy. A flexible bronchoscope equipped with a camera and a light source introduced into the patient's airways allows direct visualization of the bronchi. A channel in the bronchoscope also allows the passage of instruments to biopsy tumors directly visible in the bronchial lumen (left to right): needle, brush, forceps, and electrocautery snare. Lower panel: Endobronchial ultrasound (EBUS) bronchoscopy. A flexible bronchoscope equipped with an ultrasound probe and a retractable needle (right) introduced in the patient's airways allows ultrasound visualization and transbronchial needle aspiration of peribronchial anatomic structures of interest not visible by conventional bronchoscopy, especially mediastinal lymph nodes.

resolution than CT but this is only necessary for a minority of cases, for example, if there is suspicion that the tumor invades an anatomical structure whose resection would be problematic or even contraindicated, such as the heart, esophagus, a nerve, or a vertebra.

Bronchoscopy allows us to visualize the bronchial tree by inserting an instrument called a bronchoscope into the airways via the nose or mouth. This instrument is equipped with a light source and a camera to visualize in real time the lining of the trachea and bronchi. This instrument also allows biopsy and cytologic sampling (aspiration of bronchial secretions, bronchial brushing, and bronchoalveolar lavage). Bronchoscopy is especially useful for biopsies of central tumors, although peripheral tumors even those not directly visible may be sampled by bronchoalveolar lavage.

The main examination for metastases in regional lymph nodes and distant metastases is positron emission tomography (PET). This examination is based on the detection of positron annihilation in metabolically active tissues capturing and accumulating a deoxyglucose tracer labeled with a radioactive isotope of fluorine. Thus PET detects metabolically active tissues. This is important because inflammatory lesions may be metabolically active and mistaken for a tumor on PET. Also, despite its usefulness, PET does not replace histologic or cytologic documentation of cancer by biopsy. For mediastinal lymph nodes, the traditional biopsy technique, mediastinoscopy, is a surgical procedure performed under general anesthesia during which mediastinal lymph nodes are sampled through an incision above the sternal notch. This invasive procedure has been widely replaced in recent years by endobronchial ultrasound (EBUS) bronchoscopy because it provides the same results without the need for general anesthesia and it can be done on an outpatient basis. It is very similar to bronchoscopy. The instrument used is still a flexible bronchoscope equipped with an ultrasound probe that allows visualization through bronchial walls of mediastinal lymph node that can also be sampled with a retractable needle. Similarly, esophageal endoscopic ultrasound (EUS) works on the same principle but it gives access to different mediastinal lymph nodes and even to the adrenal glands. Mediastinoscopy, EBUS and EUS can thus confirm or rule out the presence of cancer cells in lymph nodes identified as suspicious of tumor involvement by PET. Other tests may be necessary to search for distant metastases, according to the patient's symptoms. Liver and adrenal metastases can be visualized by surface ultrasound or abdominal CT scan, which can also be used to guide a needle biopsy. Bone metastases can be visualized by bone scan if PET is not accessible. Brain metastases can be visualized by brain CT or MRI.

## Treatment and prognosis

The treatment of lung cancer depends mainly on three factors: (1) the histologic type of the tumor, (2) the TNM stage of the tumor, and (3) the patient's condition. Surgery, conventional chemotherapy, radiotherapy, targeted therapy, and immunotherapy are the therapeutic approaches currently available.

Once the investigation has confirmed the diagnosis of cancer, CT and PET scans are used to determine if the tumor is localized enough to be surgically resected or if it exceeds the extent beyond which it can not be cured by surgery. Currently, this threshold is at stage IIIA and only for cancer non-small cell lung cancer. Surgery for small cell lung cancer is reserved for rare cases of very early stage tumors. Moreover, even if the tumor is resectable given its histologic type and TNM stage, it is still necessary that the patient be medically fit enough to tolerate lung surgery. In particular, respiratory function tests and ventilation/perfusion (V/Q) scintigraphy can predict whether a patient's respiratory reserve will make him or her a candidate for the surgery by calculating the remaining functional lung volumes after the proposed surgery to remove the tumor. With an insufficient lung reserve (predicted forced expiratory volume [FEV] in 1 second of 800 mL or less), resection may be limited or even contraindicated. Similarly, a $VO_2$ max of less than 10 mL $O_2$/kg/min for exercise testing on a cycle ergometer is a predictor of postoperative complications usually making a patient nonoperable.

If the tumor is resectable and the patient is operable, the volume and extent of the surgical resection are variable: tumorectomy (tumor only), wedge resection (a small portion of a lung lobe), segmentectomy (an anatomic segment of a lung lobe), lobectomy or bilobectomy (one or two lobes), or pneumonectomy (a whole lung). In patients who are able to tolerate it, lobectomy remains the standard treatment for lung non-small cell lung cancer because it is associated with less recurrence than more limited resection (tumorectomy, wedge resection, and segmentectomy). These can, however, be acceptable for patients with poorer pulmonary reserve. All these surgical resections can be performed by thoracotomy, but the thoracoscopic approach is preferred whenever possible as it gives the same oncologic results while being less invasive, better tolerated and enabling faster patient recovery and shorter hospital stay [18].

Conventional chemotherapy in combination with radiotherapy is the standard treatment of small cell carcinoma [19]. Chemotherapy is also used in the treatment of metastatic non-small cell lung cancer. Chemotherapy agents are usually given in combination and according to histological type. For small cell carcinoma, a combination of cisplatin and etoposide is usually used. For non-small cell carcinoma, cisplatin or carboplatin is often used in combination with gemcitabine, paclitaxel, docetaxel, or vinorelbine. This chemotherapy may be given after surgery (adjuvant chemotherapy) or before (neoadjuvant chemotherapy) in order to improve the chance of cure in patients with stage II or III tumors [20].

Radiation therapy is often used in combination with chemotherapy. It can be used with curative intent for unresectable non-small cell lung cancer. This curative radiotherapy, often administered in high doses over a short period of time is called continuous hyperfractionated accelerated radiotherapy (CHART). In small

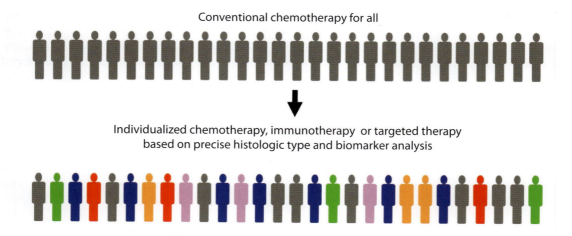

Figure 11.9 The paradigm shift in the treatment of metastatic non-small cell lung cancer.

cell carcinoma, chest radiation is indicated only when the disease is confined to a hemithorax. These patients also undergo prophylactic cerebral irradiation (PCI). Irradiation of smaller doses may also be administered as a palliative treatment. This does not require prior histologic confirmation of cancer, unlike other treatments. Finally, a localized form of radiation therapy, brachytherapy can be administered locally when an inoperable tumor is obstructing a bronchus [21].

Targeted therapies for lung cancer are still in their infancy but they have already changed the paradigm of uniform conventional chemotherapy, for all patients with metastatic non-small cell lung cancer to one in which individualized chemotherapy, immunotherapy or targeted therapy is selected based on the precise histologic type of a tumor and biomarker analysis (see Figure 11.9).

These therapies result in general in better response to treatment, longer survival, and less toxicity because they specifically target abnormal proteins produced by gene mutations present solely in cancer cells rather than imprecisely targeting all dividing cells, cancerous and normal, as in conventional chemotherapy. One crucial corollary is that tumors have to be tested for these mutations prior to deciding upon treatment because only patients with tumors harboring these specific mutated genes benefit from targeted therapy and at the same time do not respond to conventional chemotherapy. On the contrary, patients with tumors showing no mutations will benefit from conventional chemotherapy but not targeted therapy. Figure 11.10 illustrates the first two targeted therapies widely used in the treatment of metastatic lung cancer and for which tumors are currently tested: small inhibitor molecules for EGFR and ALK mutations and anti-PD-1 immunotherapy for programmed death-ligand (PDL)-1 expression by tumor cells [22,23].

Several other detectable and actionable lung cancer mutations in the UR2 sarcoma virus oncogene homolog 1 (ROS1), rearranged during transfection (RET), B rapidly accelerated fibrosarcoma (BRAF), mesenchymal–epithelial transition factor (MET), and Kirsten retrovirus-associated DNA sequences (KRAS) genes are to further expand targeted therapy options. Given the ever increasing number of potential targets to be tested, international guidelines are moving toward testing platforms allowing the simultaneous evaluation of multiple genes like massively parallel sequencing, also called next-generation sequencing, whether it be on traditional tissue biopsies or so-called "liquid" biopsies, using the tumor nucleic acids found in traces in blood, urine, and saliva [24].

Despite these new treatments, lung cancer prognosis is generally poor with an approximate overall 5-year survival rate of only 15%. This is essentially due to the late stage at which lung cancer is diagnosed

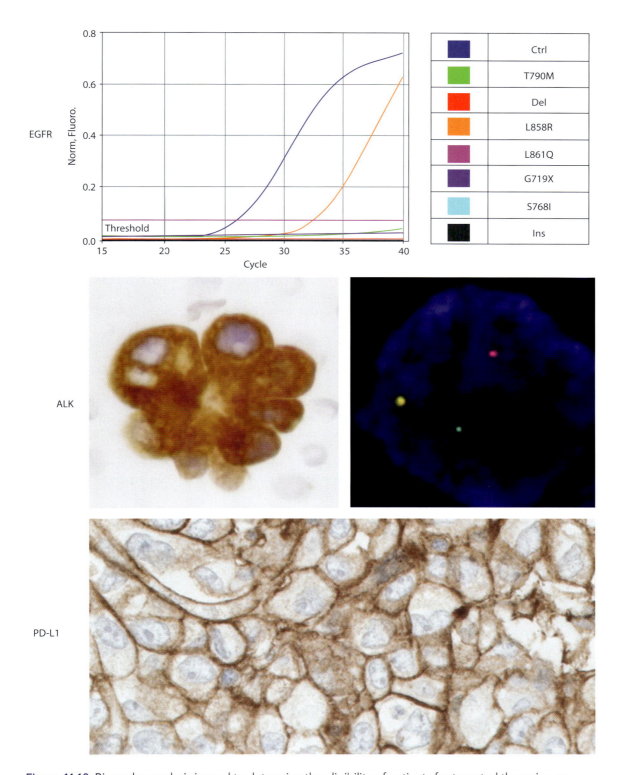

Figure 11.10 Biomarker analysis is used to determine the eligibility of patients for targeted therapies, or immunotherapy instead of conventional chemotherapy in metastatic non-small cell lung cancer. Upper panel: EGFR gene mutational analysis by the polymerase chain reaction positive for L858R activating mutation predicting sensitivity to erlotinib and gefitinib. Middle panel: ALK gene rearrangement detected by expression of ALK protein by immunohistochemistry (left) and confirmed by ALK gene break-apart by fluorescent *in situ* hybridization (right) predicting sensitivity to crizotinib. Lower panel: Strong diffuse membranous PD-L1 expression detected by immunohistochemistry predicting sensitivity to anti-PD-1 antibody pembrolizumab.

in the majority of patients, when curative surgery in not possible anymore. Because large-scale systematic screening studies have not yet managed to clearly translate into improved survival as in screening programs for breast, prostate, and colon cancer, lung cancer screening is therefore not recommended yet although recent data suggest that screening with low dose CT may reduce lung cancer mortality [25]. At a populational level, primary prevention aiming at tobacco smoking reduction via regulatory measures clearly has to be pursued.

# References

1. Biesalski HK, Bueno de Mesquita B, Chesson A, Chytil F, Grimble R, Hermus RJ, Köhrle J, Lotan R, Norpoth K, Pastorino U, Thurnham D. European consensus statement on lung cancer: Risk factors and prevention. Lung cancer panel. *CA Cancer J Clin* 1998; 48:167–176.
2. Hecht S. Tobacco carcinogens, their biomarkers and tobacco-induced cancer. *Nat Rev Cancer* 2003; 3:733–744. Review. Erratum in: *Nat Rev Cancer* 2004; 4:84.
3. Brennan P, Hainaut P, Boffetta P. Genetics of lung cancer susceptibility. *Lancet Oncol* 2011; 12:399–408.
4. Boffetta P, Trichopoulos D. Cancer of the lung, larynx, pleura. In: *Textbook of Cancer Epidemiology*, Adami HO, Hunter D Trichopoulos D, eds., Oxford: Oxford University Press, 2008, pp. 248–280.
5. IARC Working Group on the Evaluation of Carcinogenic Risks to Humans. Tobacco smoke and involuntary smoking. *IARC Monogr Eval Carcinog Risks Hum* 2004; 83:1–1438.
6. Alberg AJ, Samet JM. Epidemiology of lung cancer. *Chest* 2003; 123:21S–49S.
7. Peto R, Darby S, Deo H, Silcocks P, Whitley E, Doll R. Smoking, smoking cessation, and lung cancer in the UK since 1950: Combination of national statistics with two case-control studies. *BMJ* 2000; 321:323–329.
8. Catelinois O, Rogel A, Laurier D, Billon S, Hemon D, Verger P, Tirmarche M. Lung cancer attributable to indoor radon exposure in France: Impact on the risk models and uncertainty analysis. *Environ Health Perspect* 2006; 114:1361–1366.
9. O'Reilly KM, Mclaughlin AM, Beckett WS, Sime PJ. Asbestos-related lung disease. *Am Fam Physician* 2007; 75:683–688.
10. Doll R, Hill AB. Lung cancer and other causes of death in relation to smoking: A second report on the mortality of British doctors. *Brit Med J* 1956; 2:1071–1081.
11. Travis WD, Brambilla E, Burke AP, Marx A, Nicholson AG, eds. *WHO Classification of Tumours of Lung, Pleura, Thymus and Heart.* 4th ed. Lyon: IARC, 2015.
12. Siegel RL, Miller KD, Jemal A. Cancer statistics. *CA Cancer J Clin* 2016; 66:7–30.
13. Colby TV, Koss M, Travis WD. *Tumors of the Lower Respiratory Tract.* 3rd ed. Washington, DC: Armed Forces Institute of Pathology, 1995.
14. Hamilton W, Peters TJ, Round A, Sharp D. What are the clinical features of lung cancer before the diagnosis is made? A population based case-control study. *Thorax* 2005; 60:1059–1065.
15. Greene FL. *AJCC Cancer Staging Manual.* Berlin: Springer-Verlag, 2002.
16. Travis WD, Travis LB, Devesa SS. Lung cancer. *Cancer* 1995; 75:191–202. Erratum in: *Cancer* 1995; 75: 2979.
17. Goldstraw P, Chansky K, Crowley J, Rami-Porta R, Asamura H, Eberhardt WE, Nicholson AG, Groome P, Mitchell A, Bolejack V; International Association for the Study of Lung Cancer Staging and Pronostic Factors Committee, Advisory Boards, and Participating Institutions. The IASLC lung cancer staging project: Proposals for revision of the TNM stage groupings in the forthcoming (eighth) edition of the TNM classification of for lung cancer. *J Thorac Oncol* 2016; 11:39–51.

18. Villamizar NR, Darrabie MD, Burfeind WR, Petersen RP, Onaitis MW, Toloza E, Harpole DH, D'Amico TA. Thoracoscopic lobectomy is associated with lower morbidity compared with thoracotomy. *J Thorac Cardiovasc Surg* 2009; 138:419–425.
19. Hann CL, Rudin CM. Management of small-cell lung cancer: Incremental changes but hope for the future. *Oncology (Williston Park)* 2008; 22:1486–1492.
20. Besse B, Le Chevalier T. Adjuvant or induction cisplatin-based chemotherapy for operable lung cancer. *Oncology (Williston Park)* 2009; 23:520–527.
21. Klopp AH, Eapen GA, Komaki RR. Endobronchial brachytherapy: An effective option for palliation of malignant bronchial obstruction. *Clin Lung Cancer* 2006; 8:203–207.
22. Lindeman NI, Cagle PT, Beasley MB, Chitale DA, Dacic S, Giaconne G, Jenkins RB, Kwiatkowski DJ, Saldivar JS, Squire J, Thunnissen E, Ladanyi M. Molecular testing guideline for selection of lung cancer EGFR and ALK tyrosine kinase inhibitors: Guideline from the College of American Pathologists, International Association for the Study of Lung Cancer, and Association for Molecular Pathology. *Arch Pathol Lab Med* 2013; 137:828–860.
23. Herbst RS, Baas P, Kim DW, Felip E, Perez-Garcia JL, Han JY, Molina J, Kim JH, Arvis CD, Ahn MJ, Majem M, Fidler MJ, de Castro G Jr, Garrido M, Lubiniecki GM, Shentu Y, Im E, Dolled-Filhart M, Garon EB. Pembrolizumab versus docetaxel for previously treated, PD-L1-positive, advanced non-small-cell lung cancer (KEYNOTE-010): A randomized trial. *Lancet* 2016; 387:1540–1550.
24. Draft for the 2016 revised molecular testing guideline for selection of lung cancer EGFR and ALK tyrosine kinase inhibitors: Guideline from the College of American Pathologists, *International Association for the Study of Lung Cancer, and Association for Molecular Pathology* (www.iaslc.org).
25. The National Lung Screening Trial Research Team, Aberle DR, Adams AM, Berg CD, Black WC, Clapp JD, Fagerstrom RM, Gareen IF, Gatsonis C, Marcus PM, Sicks JD. Reduced lung-cancer mortality with low-dose computed tomographic screening. *N Engl J Med* 2011; 365:395–409.

# 12

# Occupational respiratory diseases

LOUIS-PHILIPPE BOULET and MARC DESMEULES

| | |
|---|---:|
| Introduction | 224 |
| Pneumoconiosis | 224 |
|     Epidemiology and prevalence | 225 |
|     Asbestosis | 225 |
|         Etiology | 225 |
|         Pathogenesis of asbestosis | 226 |
|         Clinical picture | 226 |
|     Silicosis | 228 |
|         Etiology | 228 |
|         Pathogenesis of silicosis | 228 |
|         Clinical picture | 228 |
|     Siderosis | 230 |
|         Etiology and pathogenesis | 230 |
|         Clinical picture | 230 |
|     Berylliosis | 230 |
|         Etiology and pathogenesis | 230 |
|         Clinical features | 231 |
| Occupational asthma | 231 |
|     Introduction | 231 |
|     Etiology | 231 |
|     Pathogenesis | 231 |
| Hypersensitivity pneumonitis (Extrinsic allergic alveolitis) | 236 |
| Workplace induced COPD/industrial chronic bronchitis | 237 |
|     Occupational infections | 238 |
|     Cancers of occupational origin | 238 |
| Acute inhalation accidents | 238 |
|     Acute bronchopneumopathies from irritant gas exposures | 238 |
|     Metal fumes fever | 239 |
|     Organic dust toxic syndrome (dust fever) | 239 |
|     Asphyxiations | 240 |
| Conclusion | 241 |
| References | 241 |

## Introduction

Occupational respiratory diseases attributable to exposure to various agents encountered at the workplace include a large variety of conditions characterized by the development of airway obstruction (e.g., asthma) or a disease predominant in the pulmonary parenchyma, often inducing a "restrictive syndrome," with a reduction of lung volumes (e.g., asbestosis/silicosis) [1–3]. A preexisting condition such as asthma or chronic obstructive pulmonary disease (COPD) can also worsen following exposures at the workplace, or be a cofactor in the development of a disease (e.g., asbestosis and lung cancer). Respiratory problems associated with work are a major cause of disability, work absenteeism, and mortality. The specific prevalence of these problems changes with time and is difficult to establish. We estimate that about 50% of all diseases acquired at the workplace are affecting the respiratory system.

Generally, the causal relationship between a given disease and an occupational exposure is established according to various factors that could include (1) the allergenic potential of substances involved, (2) the temporal relationship and the duration of exposure, (3) the dose–response effect, (4) radiologic features, (5) lung function tests, and (6) various laboratory tests. A classification of occupational respiratory diseases is provided in Table 12.1.

## Pneumoconiosis

Pneumoconiosis is defined as a chronic respiratory disease caused by the inhalation of metallic or mineral particles [4]. Many years of exposure are usually necessarily before developing the first signs of disease. The various mineral dusts retained in the bronchial tree will activate some chronic inflammatory mechanisms over the time and provoke major changes in tissue morphology. The intensity of those changes will vary according to the nature of the particles and their fibrogenic potential, the ability to induce a pulmonary fibrosis characterized by a deposition of collagen, and some other constituents of the extracellular matrix at the level of the lung parenchyma.

Table 12.1 Classification of occupational respiratory diseases

**Pneumoconiosis (caused by inorganic dust)**
- Fibrosing e.g., silicosis, asbestosis
- With no significant fibrosis e.g., siderosis
- Chronic granulomatous inflammation e.g., berylliosis

**Occupational asthma and related conditions**
- Occupational asthma with a latency period (i.e., caused by occupational sensitizers)
- Occupational asthma without a latency period
- Asthma aggravated by exposure at work
- Organic dust toxic syndromes (e.g., byssinosis)

**Hypersensitivity pneumonitis (extrinsic allergic alveolitis)**

**Industrial chronic bronchitis**

**Occupational infections**

**Cancers of occupational origin**

**Acute inhalation accidents**
- Acute bronchopneumopathies caused by irritant gases
- Metal fever
- Mycotoxicosis (*ODTS: organic dust toxic syndrome*)
- Asphyxia

When mineral particles are inhaled, a large part of those is eliminated by the mucociliary system of the airways which brings these particles to the pharynx to be swallowed. Other defense mechanisms include phagocytosis of particles by alveolar macrophages, although these last can be destroyed during this process, liberating therefore various inflammatory mediators. Some of these particles will remain in the lower airways and will even sometimes penetrate in the interstitium as well as at the level of pleural space. We can distinguish three main categories of pneumoconiosis:

1. *Fibrosing pneumoconiosis.* These are the most common and are caused by bioreactive dusts with a fibrogenic potential. Silicosis, asbestosis and other silicatosis (e.g., talc, mica, and vermiculite), and pneumoconiosis caused by hard metals and abrasives such as carborundum belong to this category.
2. *Pneumoconiosis with no or minimal fibrosing potential.* These pneumoconiosis, also called "overload" pneumoconiosis, result from the accumulation of dust in the lung interstitium without fibrosing response. Many types of dust, such as iron oxide (siderosis), carbon, graphite, barium, tin, aluminum, antimony, are associated with this category of pneumoconiosis.
3. *Chronic granulomatosis.* Berylliosis is an example. Berylliosis stimulates a lymphocytic immune response ("late response" type), which results in the formation of granulomas with cellular inflammation in the damaged organs.

## Epidemiology and prevalence

Measures aiming at improving hygiene at the workplace are increasingly established and allow reducing the level of exposure to iron oxide (siderosis), carbon, graphite, barium, tin, aluminum, antimony, and bioreactive dusts. These measures are more commonly applied by large enterprises, which have better resources in regard to the workplace hygiene. However, there are still significant problems in many of these, workers being exposed to high concentrations of mineral particles, particularly to silica, for example, during sandblasting. If we take into account the increased risk of bronchial cancers associated with asbestosis and silicosis, the excess mortality adds to the important socio-economic burden associated with these diseases.

## Asbestosis

### Etiology

We design by the name of "asbestosis" a group of complex hydrated silicates in a fibrous state. They include two main families: serpentine asbestosis and amphiboles [5].

- *Serpentine asbestosis—Chrysotile* (white asbestosis): these long fibers are flexible, resistant to fire and have been used in the production of asbestosis textiles. This form of asbestosis was often found in mining industry in Quebec since 1878, where chrysotile constitutes more than 90% of industrial asbestosis.
- *Amphiboles asbestosis:* this group includes five varieties of rigid fibers that are easy to break but have an excellent resistance to acids. They include anthophyllite, amosite, crocidolite, actinolite, and tremolite.

These forms of asbestosis share many common properties: they are resistant to stretching, friction, heat (500°C), corrosion and chemical inertia while they have a weak electric conductivity. Industrial applications of asbestosis have been multiplied during the twentieth century with an increased progression during World War II. The world tonnage achieved a plateau around 1977 and decreased significantly since then. Prolonged exposure to asbestosis can cause many pathologies (Table 12.2).

## Pathogenesis of asbestosis

The biologic reactivity of asbestosis is conditioned in part by the dimension of the fibers and their surface properties. For similar exposures, amphiboles have a greater pathogenic potency than chrysotile. Mechanisms of elimination of particles in the lung are more efficient in getting rid of chrysotile than amphiboles. The number of fibers that resist phagocytosis by alveolar macrophages and are retained in the pulmonary interstitium close to the respiratory bronchioles play an important role in this disease. These fibers stimulate the production of free oxygen and nitrogen radicals (reactive oxygen species [ROS] and reactive nitrogen species [RNS]). This oxidative stress causes a persistent inflammatory response with the production of cytokines, chemokines, growth factors as well as pro-inflammatory factors. These various mediators activate transcription factors, particularly the mitogen-activated protein kinases (MAPK), leading to a fibro-proliferative response of fibroblasts [6,7]. The production of fibronectin is stimulated by adjacent macrophages rich in transcription growth factor (TGF-β). An increased deposition of extracellular matrix and synthesis of collagen type I and II, with a reduction of collagen degradation can be observed. The lung parenchyma is progressively infiltrated by fibrous tissue which is nonfunctional. These complex mechanisms involve over many years and are shown schematically in Figure 12.1.

## Clinical picture

Asbestosis is a pneumoconiosis characterized by a progressive interstitial pneumonia associated with a prolonged and usually intense exposure to asbestosis at work. These patients can remain asymptomatic during many years and the first manifestation of the disease can develop after more than 20 years after the beginning of the occupational exposure.

Table 12.2 Main diseases associated with a long-term exposure to asbestosis

1. Asbestosis—diffuse interstitial pulmonary fibrosis
2. Hyaline and calcified pleural plaques
3. Benign pleurisy
4. Pleural mesothelioma
5. Lung cancer

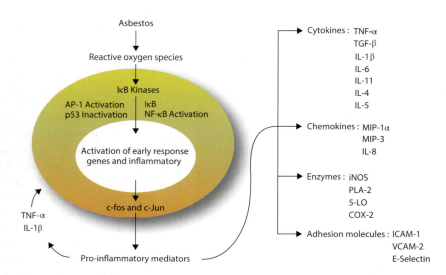

Figure 12.1 Schematic representation of mechanisms leading to the development of asbestosis. (Adapted from Manning, C.B. et al. 2002.)

At the clinical level, a progressive effort-induced dyspnea constitutes the main symptom. The development of fine crackles rales on chest auscultation is a physical sign of the disease. Chest tomodensitometry is a more sensitive test to detect the first signs of pulmonary fibrosis. The presence of hyaline calcified or pleural plaques, or pleural thickening associated with round-shaped atelectasis, help to differentiate asbestosis from other forms of pulmonary fibrosis (Figure 12.2). At the functional level, asbestosis induces progressively a restrictive syndrome with a reduction of lung volumes. The pulmonary function tests usually show this progressive reduction in lung volumes and a fall in the carbon monoxide (CO) diffusion capacity as well as a reduction in lung compliance, without significant bronchial obstruction. The pleural plaques have generally low or minimal effect on lung function: indeed, the benign pleural plaques (hyalines or calcified, pleural thickening, and round-shaped atelectasis) have a minimal effect on pulmonary function and their clinical prognosis is excellent in opposition to the lung fibrosis associated with asbestosis.

The diagnosis of lung asbestosis will be made following a history of prolonged exposure to asbestosis in the presence of lung infiltrations suggestive of this disease on chest radiograph, or more precisely on chest tomodensitometry, the presence of crackle rales on chest auscultation, and the presence of a restrictive syndrome [9]. If a biopsy specimen is available, the diagnosis can be done with a microscopic analysis of the tissue showing the presence of an interstitial fibrosis and some asbestos bodies. The free fibers are usually difficult to demonstrate by the usual optic microscopy technics, and mineralogical analysis ultramicroscopy can help to characterize the nature, number, and length of the mineral fibers and of the ferruginous bodies retained in the pulmonary tissue. This technique has brought precious information in cases where occupational exposure is difficult to establish.

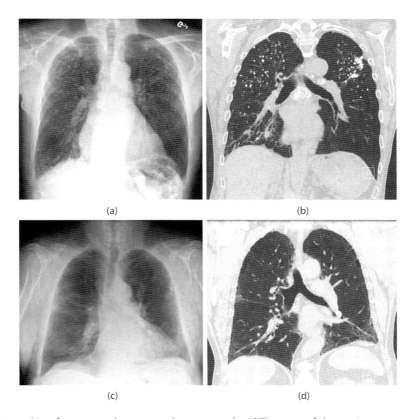

Figures 12.2 Examples of x-rays and computed tomography (CT) scans of the main pneumoconiosis.
(**a**) Chest radiograph of a patient with silicosis. (**b**) Tomodensitometry showing typical silicosis lesions.
(**c**) Chest radiograph of a patient with asbestosis. (**d**) Tomodensitometry showing early stages of asbestosis.

There is no cure for asbestosis and finally it can continue to develop even after cessation of exposure. Cessation of work can help to reduce the exposure to additional mineral fibers but not necessarily influence the evolution toward complications such as respiratory insufficiency. The risk of lung cancer increases with the exposure to asbestosis and this problem is amplified by smoking. The mortality associated with lung cancer in patients with asbestosis is between 30% and 50%. Only preventative measures targeting a reduction of exposure to dust, as well as smoking, may allow reduction of the frequency of this disease.

## Silicosis

### Etiology

Silicosis (silicon dioxide [$SiO_2$]) is the most abundant substance in the earth's crust in free state or combined in the form of silicates. Free silica can be found in the crystalline form (quartz, cristobalite, and tridymite) or amorphous form (diatomaceous earth). Silicosis is caused by the inhalation of free crystalline silica [10]. At the natural state, it is contained in variable quantities in the rock: about 30% in granite, 40% in slate, and 100% in sandstone. The drilling work in mines, tunnels, and quarries is carried out with the use of finely powdered pure silica; glass and ceramics industry and sandblast cleaning are some examples of professional contexts associated with silicosis.

### Pathogenesis of silicosis

Silicosis results from a chronic inflammatory process secondary to the prolonged inhalation of silica crystals similar to what is happening in asbestosis [11,12]. This reaction is conditioned by the number of particles, the type of silica, its surface properties, and the presence or not of other types of dust. Recently fragmented silica crystals, as in the sandblasting process, show more marked biological activity.

The alveolar macrophage plays a role in the onset of the pathologic process (Figure 12.3). Phagocytosis of silica particles activates the alveolar macrophage and can destroy this last, therefore releasing various oxidants and cytokines as well as particles that will perpetuate the inflammatory cycle. Many mediators of oxidative stress and from the initial inflammatory response are common in asbestosis and silicosis. The activated macrophage attracts inflammatory cells (T-lymphocytes, neutrophils, and mast cells) and stimulates the deposition of collagen by the fibroblasts.

Microscopic examination shows initially some reticulin foyers, surrounding macrophages loaded with silica particles, showing a birefringent appearance under polarized light. At the stage of the simple silicosis, this lesion evolves towards the formation of classic nodules of 2–6 mm of diameter, made of a center of concentrated collagen fibers and hyaline material surrounded by macrophages, lymphocytes, and plasma cells. At the stage of conglomerated silicosis, the number and volume of these nodules increase, leading to the formation of conglomerated fibrotic masses, paracicatricial emphysematous areas contributing to the destruction of the parenchyma, and increasing the loss of pulmonary function associated with silicosis. Once the process has begun, it perpetuates itself even after cessation of exposure. Some markers of autoimmune diseases can then appear in silicosis and bring some complications. The non-invasive search (e.g., in the sputum) for predictive markers of persistence of the fibrotic process could probably help predict the clinical outcomes according to some initial research work, but their value remains to be determined [13].

### Clinical picture

Silicosis is characterized by hyaline nodular fibrosis caused by prolonged inhalation of high concentrations of crystalline silica dust. According to the context, there are three clinical forms:

- **Classic silicosis.** The first radiologic signs often appear 20 years after the beginning of exposure. This is the most common form of silicosis and the content in silica of the inhaled dust is moderate, often less than 30%.

**Effects of silica on cellular responses**

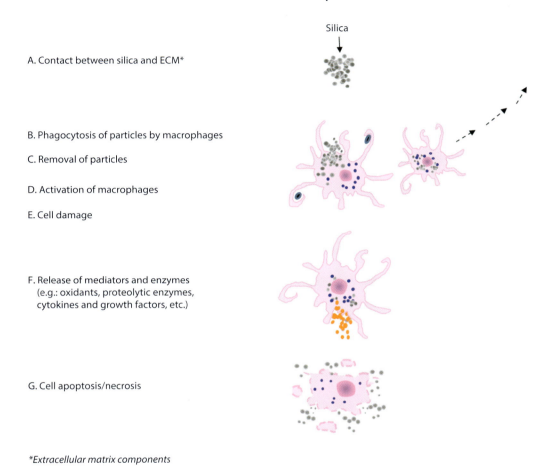

A. Contact between silica and ECM*

B. Phagocytosis of particles by macrophages
C. Removal of particles
D. Activation of macrophages
E. Cell damage

F. Release of mediators and enzymes
(e.g.: oxidants, proteolytic enzymes, cytokines and growth factors, etc.)

G. Cell apoptosis/necrosis

*Extracellular matrix components

Figure 12.3 Effects of silica on cellular responses.

- **Accelerated silicosis.** The diagnosis is usually made between 1 and 10 years from the beginning of the exposure and the disease evolves more rapidly. The content in silica at the workplace is generally high, for example, in sandblasting workers.
- **Acute silicosis.** This form is quite rare but can appear after exposure of only a few months to massive concentrations of silica. The evolution is very rapid and fibrotic lesions do not have the time to develop. The tissue response is accompanied by an alveolar filling by desquamated cells and a proteinaceous exudates called silicoproteinosis. Patients quickly evolve toward to cachexia and respiratory failure.

Patients suffering from simple silicosis can remain asymptomatic for a prolonged time period and the physical examination is usually normal. Radiologic abnormalities constitute the only manifestation of the disease. We can observe the presence of micronodules of 1–10 mm of diameter predominating in the upper half of the lungs. Hilar and mediastinal hypertrophy adenopathies are sometimes calcified, forming the classical "egg shell" pattern often found. In conglomerated silicosis, the fibrous masses are often bilateral and induce a distortion of lung hilae and bronchovascular structures. Chest tomodensitometry is more sensitive to detect small opacities of low profusion, the first sign of conglomerates and paracicatricial emphysema.

At this stage, respiratory symptoms develop; shortness of breath is frequent. Cough and sputum production are also common but their significance is often uncertain in the presence of smoking. Pulmonary function tests often show a mixture of obstructive and restrictive abnormalities, which could lead to respiratory insufficiency. Once the disease has developed, no treatment can allow modification of the outcomes of silicosis, which could be associated to many complications (see Table 12.3).

## Siderosis

### Etiology and pathogenesis

Inhalation of high quantities of mineral dusts can lead to their accumulation in the lung and produce abnormal chest radiographs without, however, inducing an inflammatory response or a fibrosis of the lung parenchyma. These inert dusts include iron oxide, graphite, carbon, slate, aluminum, antimony and barium. Siderosis is caused by the deposition of iron oxide in the lung [14]. Iron miners, polishers, and foundry workers are at risk. The most frequent source is linked to arc welding. On anatomical examination, the lung is of red color and shows rusty macules of about 1–4 mm of diameter. On microscopy, we can observe perivascular and peribronchiolar accumulation of brownish pigment and some ferruginous bodies centered on a black iron oxide particle.

### Clinical picture

In welders, the disease can develop more than 20 years after the beginning of exposure. It usually does not cause any specific sign or symptom. We can note on the chest radiograph some small round shape opacities of about 0.5–3 mm on both lungs without any conglomerate. The lung function remains normal. Contrary to silicosis, the radiologic features can regress after withdrawal from exposure. A contribution of such exposure to the development of lung cancer in iron miners of Lorraine has been suggested, although this has not been demonstrated in other contexts.

## Berylliosis

### Etiology and pathogenesis

Beryllium is a metal with quite remarkable properties. It is very light and very hard; it increases considerably the mechanical resistance of alloys with copper, aluminum, and magnesium. It conducts heat and electricity very well; it is not magnetizable and not detectable by radars. It is therefore commonly used in defense industries and aeronautics. Its use is relatively dangerous due to its intense sensitizing power in humans [15]. Inhalation of beryllium particles, even a low dose, can induce a cellular immune response causing the accumulation of

Table 12.3 Main complications of silicosis

*Respiratory insufficiency:* Often in conglomerated silicosis.
*Tuberculosis:* Relationship has been well established for a long time; 25% of accelerated silicosis develops mycobacterium infection: 50% to mycobacterium tuberculosis and 50% to atypical mycobacteria.
*Caplan syndrome:* Silicosis associated with rheumatoid polyarthritis leading to the development of necrotic pulmonary nodules.
*Collagen diseases:* Increase in the frequency of scleroderma (Erasmus syndrome) and disseminated lupus erythematous.
*Bronchial cancer:* The risk of a lung cancer is increased although less than in asbestosis.

CD4 T-lymphocytes in the lung. It can induce a progressive interstitial infiltrate with monocytes, noncaseating granuloma formation, and fibrosis. Individual susceptibility to develop berylliosis is increased in workers with HLA-DPB1 (Glu69) major histocompatibility complex alteration [16].

### Clinical features

The duration of exposure to beryllium required to initiate this sensitizing process can vary between 3 months and 30 years. The blood test looking at the proliferation of lymphocytes in contact with beryllium sulfate allows detection of such sensitization with a sensitivity about 80% and a specificity of 97% [17,18]. Clinical, radiological, and histopathological features are similar to those of sarcoidosis and can involve many organs. The most frequent symptoms include asthenia, fatigue, and dyspnea and are therefore nonspecific. On radiograph, we can observe hilar and mediastinal adenopathies as well as granulomatous nodular lesions. Evolution is relatively slow over many years. The lesions can regress under immunosuppressive treatment with corticosteroids.

When a patient is suspected to have chronic beryllium disease (CBD), the following are major criteria for such diagnosis:

1. A history of any beryllium exposure
2. A positive blood or bronchoalveolar lavage (BAL) beryllium lymphocyte proliferation test (BeLPT) [19]

## Occupational asthma

### Introduction

Occupational asthma can be defined as the development of a variable airway obstruction and hyperresponsiveness induced by a specific workplace exposure [20]. It is a clinical entity with still uncertain nosological limits in the medical literature. This lack of certainty in regard to its definition is in part due to the high frequency of asthma in the general population. It also results from its heterogeneity in a context of occupational exposures (high and low molecular weight substances [HMW, LMW]), the presence or absence of a latency period and in the variability of the etiopathogenic mechanisms—mediated by allergy or from non-immunoglobulin E (IgE) mechanisms, eosinophilic inflammation versus neutrophilic, and so on.

In places such as in the province of Quebec, occupational asthma is defined as asthma caused by a substance to which the workers are exposed at the workplace. This definition excludes asthmatics whose exacerbation of symptoms occurs from exposure to nonspecific irritants at work. This final form of asthma should also be distinguished from the irritant-induced asthma, which results from acute exposure to a toxic or strong respiratory irritant substance, its initial report being defined as reactive airways dysfunction syndrome (RADS). Irritant-induced asthma can occur after acute or repeated inhalation of such toxic/highly irritant substances (e.g., acids, ammonia) [21]. We can find the main types of workplace asthma in Table 12.4.

### Etiology

More than 450 substances can induce occupational asthma and this number keeps increasing. We can find the updated list of those substances on specialized internet sites, such as Asmapro or Haz-map. These different substances belong to the categories mentioned in Tables 12.5 and 12.6. Table 12.7 shows some of the main causes of occupational asthma in Quebec, as an example.

### Pathogenesis

Occupational asthma can result from immune or nonimmune mechanisms. In the case of immune mechanisms, this type of asthma appears generally after a latency period of variable duration between the

Table 12.4 Asthma related to work

**Occupational asthma**
*With a latency period*
    Allergic: mainly due to high molecular weight or low molecular weight sensitizers (e.g., flour, seafood, and acid anhydrides)
    Nonallergic: mainly caused by low molecular weight substances for which mechanism is undetermined (e.g., diisocyanates)
*Without latency period*
    Airway hyperresponsiveness caused by acute airway damage. (Chemical bronchitis with secondary hyperresponsiveness initially described as reactive airway dysfunction syndrome.)
*Work aggravated asthma*
    Preexisting asthma exacerbated by the contact of nonspecific irritants or other triggers (exercise, cold air) at work

Table 12.5 Categories of agents which can cause occupational asthma

**Chemical agents**
- **Acrylates.** e.g., methyl cyanoacrylate
- **Metals.** e.g., platinum salts, chromium
- **Aldehydes.** e.g., gluteraldehyde
- **Amines**. e.g., ethylenediamine
- **Anydride acids**. e.g., phthalic anhydride (epoxy)
- **Cleaning products**. e.g., chloramine
- **Isocyanates**. e.g., TDI, MDI, HDI, IPDI
- **Plastics**. e.g., polyvinyl chloride
- **Products from pyrolysis**. e.g., colophony
- **Fungicides**. e.g., chlorothalonil
- **Others**. e.g., persulfate (hairstyle), dyes

**Biological agents**
- **Animal proteins.** e.g., animal danders
- **Proteins from seafood.** e.g., lobsters
- **Enzymes.** e.g., amylase (flour)
- **Insects.** e.g., spruce budworm
- **Plants.** e.g., cereal grains, flour
- **Vegetal gums.** e.g., guar
- **Wood dust.** e.g., cedar, exotic woods (mahogany, etc.)
- **Molds.** e.g., *Aspergillus*

HDI, hexamethylene diisocyanate; IPDI, isophorone diisocyanate; MDI, methylenediphenyl diisocyanate; TDI, toluene diisocyanate.

beginning of exposure and the onset of symptoms. In general, we consider HMW agents to act through the production of antibodies such as IgE as common allergens [22,23]. Atopic subjects have a slight increase in the risk of developing this type of asthma following the exposure to this type of agents. For LMW agents such isocyanates, the development mechanisms of asthma are uncertain. Some show sensitizing properties but others are irritants. Isocyanates can cause a RADS following inhalation accidents while in many other

Table 12.6 Categories of agents according to molecular weight and type of work

| Low molecular weight agents | Type of work |
| --- | --- |
| Isocyanates | Painters, isolation industries, and plastics |
| Wood | Carpenters, cabinetmakers, and primary industry |
| Anhydrides | Plastic industry |
| Amines | Manufacture of lacquers, varnishes |
| Soldering Flux (organic acids in colophony) | Electronic industry |
| Chloramine T | Cleaning |
| Dyes | Textile industry |
| Persulphate | Hairdressers |
| Fomaldehyde, glutaraldehyde | Hospital staff |
| Acrylates | Adhesive industry, health care workers |
| Drugs | Pharmaceutical industry, hospital staff |
| Metals | Welders, electric plating, and metal refining |
| **High molecular weight agents** | **Type of work** |
| Cereals | Bakers |
| Animal antigens | Animal technician, veterinary |
| Enzymes | Cleaning industry, pharmaceutical, and bakers |
| Gums | Carpet industry, pharmaceutical |
| Latex | Health care providers |
| Seafood | Seafood processing |

*Note:* See internet sites *Asmapro* or *Haz-map* for a complete list.

Table 12.7 Main causes of occupational asthma in Quebec (1986–1999)

| Agents | Total | Frequency (%) |
| --- | --- | --- |
| Isocyanates | 201 | 25.2 |
| Flour | 128 | 16.1 |
| Wood dust | 79 | 9.9 |
| Seafood | 68 | 8.5 |
| Metals (welding) | 51 | 6.4 |
| Cereals (grains) | 41 | 5.1 |
| Epoxy resins, adhesives | 40 | 5.0 |
| Animal (danders) | 38 | 4.8 |
| Psyllium, drugs | 29 | 3.6 |
| Latex | 27 | 3.4 |
| Hairdressing | 12 | 1.5 |
| Others | 83 | 10.4 |
| **Total** | **797** | **100.0** |

cases, they will also cause an occupational asthma after a prolonged exposure to lower concentrations of these substances. In case of LMW substances, IgE does not seem usually involved, although some workers can develop such antibodies. IgG can sometimes be involved but their role is uncertain. Sensitizing subjects could present asthmatic responses even at low concentration of these agents; it is therefore of major importance to stop the exposure when the diagnosis is established.

Sensitized subjects could develop various types of asthmatic responses following exposure to offending agents (Figure 12.4):

- Immediate response: fall in expiratory flows within 1 hour following exposure
- Late response: fall in expiratory flows between 2 and 8 hours following exposure
- Mixed response: it combines the last two types of response
- Atypical response: late response without recovery from an initial fall in expiratory flows

Bronchial biopsies of workers with occupational asthma do not usually differ from those found in nonoccupational asthma: they usually show evidence of inflammation and remodeling. With isocyanates and red cedar, the airways can show a predominant lymphocytic response. T-cells show a CD8 phenotype and produce cytokines such as interferon-γ and interleukin (IL)-5 [24]. These agents can also act in activating nervous sensory receptors to release substance P and other neuropeptides although the role of these agents in the physiopathology of this type of asthma remains to be explored. Neuropeptides can cause a cough, airway smooth muscle contraction, and promote the production of bronchial secretion (Figure 12.5). In the case of RADS, it seems to be a sequelae of "chemical bronchitis" with marked epithelial desquamation and intense

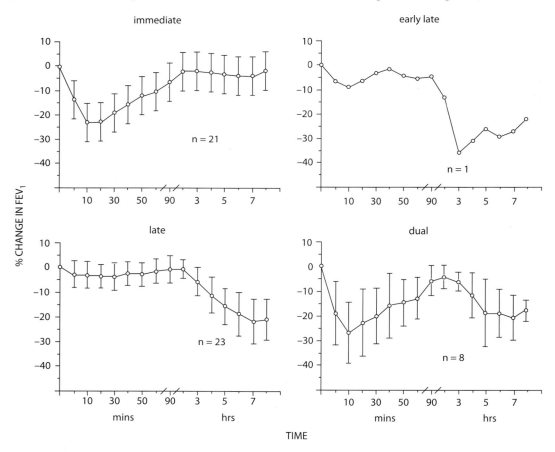

**Figure 12.4** Specific bronchial provocation tests. Mean ± SD or individual values of the % change in $FEV_1$ (on the ordinate) as a function of time since exposure (on the abscissa) for the four typical patterns of reactions. The number of subjects for each pattern is shown. (From Bernstein, I.L. et al., *Asthma in the Workplace*, Marcel Dekker, 1993; Cartier, A, Malo, J.L., *Chapter XII—Occupational Challenge Tests*).

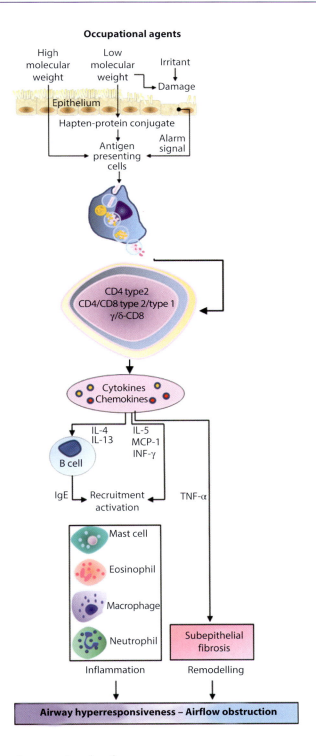

Figure 12.5 Mechanisms of occupational asthma.

airway remodeling process with the accumulation of collagen in the bronchial wall. After withdrawal from work, those affected by this process can still show residual signs of airway inflammation and remodeling although to a lesser degree [25–27].

The investigation of asthma in the workplace is summarized in Figure 12.6. This may vary from a region/country to another however. Withdrawal from exposure to the sensitizing agent could lead to a complete or partial remission of symptoms and lung function abnormalities. The treatment of occupational asthma is identical to that of nonoccupational asthma (Figure 12.7).

## Hypersensitivity pneumonitis (Extrinsic allergic alevolitis)

This disease has been described in Chapter 10. Its pathophysiology is similar whatever the etiologic factor. More than 300 agents have been suspected to cause a development of allergic alveolitis. Many are found in the workplace [28]. Farmer's lung, a common form of alveolitis and other various conditions summarized in Table 12.8. The description of the physiopathology of this disease can be found in Chapter 10.

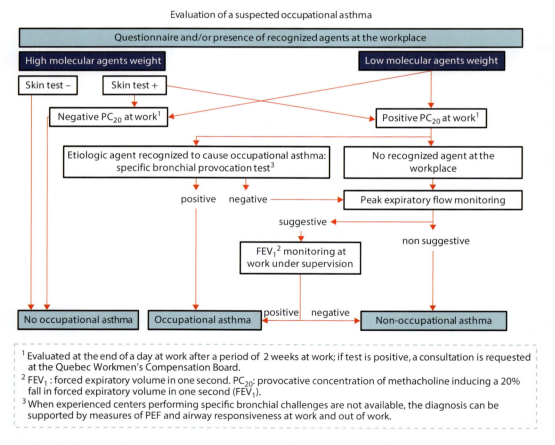

Figure 12.6 Evaluation of a suspected occupational asthma. (Courtesy of J.L. Malo et al.)

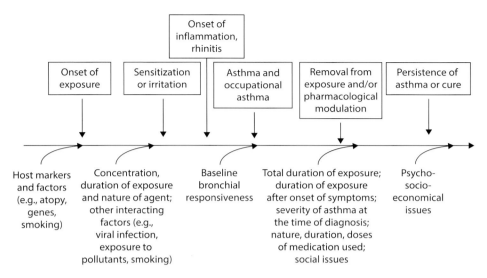

Figure 12.7 Natural history of asthma and occupational asthma. (From Malo, J.L. and Chan-Yeung, M., *Can Respir J.*, 14, 407–413, 2007).

Table 12.8 Examples of agents which can cause an occupational alveolitis

| Biological agents | Localization/type of work |
|---|---|
| Thermophilic actinomycetes (e.g., *Saccharopolyspora*) | Moldy hay, grain, and silage (farmers) |
| Birds proteins | Birf fanciers |
| *Thermoactinomyces sacchari*, *Thermoactinomyces vulgaris* | Sugar cane production |
| *Aspergillus*, *Scopulariopsis brevicaulis* | Smoking plantation |
| Mold spores, thermophilic actinomycetes | Mushroom production |
| Various molds on wood | Sawmill workers |
| *Bacillus subtilis* | Detergent industry |
| **Chemical agents** | **Localization/type of work** |
| Isocyanates (MDI, TDI, HDI) | Automobile painters, plastic industry |
| Phtalic anhydride | Epoxy resins |
| Industrial lubricants | Equipment operators |

MDI, methylenediphenyl diisocyanate; TDI, toluene diisocyanate.

## Workplace induced COPD/industrial chronic bronchitis

Occupational COPD is a syndrome that may develop in the course of various diseases such as asthma, chronic bronchitis, emphysema, or bronchiectasis. Its etiology is multifactorial and is identified based on epidemiologic, clinical, radiologic, or functional criteria. Airflow limitation can result from different factors: chronic inflammation of the bronchial mucosa, bronchial secretions, bronchoconstriction, and bronchoalveolar remodeling. Smoking is a predominant cause but other types of exposures can be involved. The association of bronchial ailments with some types of work leading to marked exposure to organic and inorganic dusts has been reported since the nineteenth century. Up to 10%–15% of COPD would result from occupational exposure.

Airway obstruction increases according to the intensity of dust exposure and associated with symptoms of chronic bronchitis and an accelerated decline in lung function [29,30]. In various groups of mining workers (coal, gold, etc.) airway obstruction increases according to dust levels independently of the development of pneumoconiosis [31]. In Quebec, studies by Martin et al. in aluminum industries showed an excess of obstructive diseases in workers of potrooms in the aluminum industry [32]. Occupational bronchitis can be found in miners, foundry workers, welders, aluminum industry workers (potrooms), and grain workers (elevators, longshoremen, and farmers). As smoking is very common in these workers, sometimes it is difficult to determine if the problem is caused by smoking or workplace exposure.

## Occupational infections

Some types of work bring a risk of infections for the workers. Infection can originate from a sick animal or human, or be transmitted from biological products that are handled. The main types of workers at risk are health care workers (physicians, dentists, nurses, technicians, hospital employees, home elderly, etc.), veterinarians, animal technicians, biologists, and laboratory technicians. Infections include mainly tuberculosis, tularemia, and deep mycosis (histoplamosis, blastomycosis).

## Cancers of occupational origin

There are more than 300 workplace substances with a carcinogenic potential. The main ones are found in Table 12.9. Despite pessimistic predictions of epidemiologists, less than 10% of respiratory cancers are of occupational origin, 85% being caused by smoking, and 5% being associated with other cancers. However, the problem remains a concern for the future.

No specific chemical or morphological characteristic can distinguish bronchial cancers of occupational origin from those caused by smoking. Quantification of mineral particles in the lung tissue can help to establish a causal link with some types of occupational exposures. See Chapter 11 for the pathogenesis of cancer.

## Acute inhalation accidents

## Acute bronchopneumopathies from irritant gas exposures

Inhalation of toxic gas can cause variable clinical pictures, sometimes difficult to classify in a coherent category. We can observe a transient irritation of the bronchial tree, asphyxia, acute pulmonary edema, bronchiolitis, systemic response, and mycotoxicosis.

Table 12.9 Substances with can cause or contribute to cancer

**Established link with bronchial occupational cancer**
- Asbestosis
- Arsenic
- Chromium and chromate
- Hydrocarbons derived from coal (coke, tar, and mineral oils)
- Ionizing radiations: radon, gamma rays

**Suspected agents, nonproved**
- Beryllium
- Cadmium
- Formaldehyde
- Silica (with silicosis)

Some gases are very reactive (Table 12.10) and able to induce chemical inflammatory reaction of the bronchial mucosa [33,34]. Intoxication with weak doses can simply cause bronchial irritation with a transient cough, while massive exposure may result in hemorrhagic pulmonary edema. Corrosive gas, very soluble, can cause its main effects on the proximal airways (larynx, trachea). Less soluble gases can penetrate more deeply in the lung and affect bronchioles and parenchyma more intensely. For the irritant gases, the intensity of exposure and solubility of the gas in the water are the main factors determining severity of the picture and the site of damage. During a fire, inhalation by the victims or firemen of large quantities of smoke can cause extensive damage to the bronchial tree. Combustion and degradation of various materials by heat (plastics, resins, coatings, etc.) release many irritant products.

Gases such as sulfuric anhydride ($SO_2$) and chlorine can provoke an intense inflammatory response and have a suffocating potential. $SO_2$ can combine with water to cause the formation of sulfurous acid and sulfuric acid. Chlorine is an oxidant that liberates nascent oxygen. These agents can cause an extensive chemical burn to the respiratory tree. The treatment includes humidity, oxygen, corticosteroids, and ventilator support if necessary in addition to antibiotics.

## Metal fumes fever

This febrile syndrome of limited evolution has been described in 1832 by Thackrah in a brass foundry. It is caused by inhalation of metallic vapors such as zinc or brass, mainly during the welding of galvanized metals [35]. Symptoms occur mostly on Monday (tachyphylaxis can be observed, with a reduction of the response in the following days) and appear 4–6 hours after inhalation. In the evening, the patient can present various malaises: myalgia, fever at 38–39°C, hoarseness, cough, chest tightness, and dyspnea often described as an influenza-like episode. This syndrome can disappear spontaneously in 24 hours. Chest auscultation and radiograph are generally normal. We can observe a transient reduction in vital capacity (VC) and $D_LCO$. In regard to the involved mechanisms, it is believed that zinc oxide acts directly on the alveolar macrophage and stimulates the liberation of cytokines (tumor necrosis factor [TNF]-α, IL-1) which mediates an acute inflammatory response.

## Organic dust toxic syndrome (dust fever)

The inhalation of organic dust can cause a febrile syndrome with chills, malaise, myalgia, headache, cough, and dyspnea [36–38]. This syndrome is usually called mycotoxicosis or organic dust toxic syndrome (ODTS). It constitutes the most frequent problem caused by inhalation of organic dust in the agricultural world. These particles come from hay or cereals contaminated by mushrooms and actinomycetes, wood particles, and can be found, for example, in confined environments in the pork industry. Inhalation of dust is generally massive being about 10 times higher than what could be causing an extrinsic allergic alveolitis [39]. We generally observe fever, lleucocytosis, and sometimes, on chest auscultation, crackling rales or wheezing. Pulmonary radiograph is generally normal. During its acute phase, lung function tests can show restrictive abnormalities. The BAL can show an increase in neutrophils and large quantities of fungal spores. The evolution usually results in a spontaneous recovery without sequelae.

Table 12.10 Corrosive gases and irritants

**Very soluble corrosive gases:**
Ammonia ($NH_3$), sulfuric anhydride ($SO_2$), chlorine ($Cl_2$), Chlorhydric acid (HCl), zinc chloride (ZnCL), acroleine, etc.

**Less soluble irritant gases:**
Nitrogen oxyte (NO, $N_2O_3$, and $NO_2$), ozone ($O_3$), phosgene ($COCl_2$), ethylene oxide ($C_2H_4O$), toluene isocyanate, aldehydes, etc.

## Asphyxiations

Asphyxia is an acute clinical process that induces hypoxia or anoxia, a defect in oxygenation of cells of the organism. There are two types of asphyxiant gases: simple and bioactive. Simple asphyxiant products such as nitrogen, $CO_2$, methane, and anesthetic gases remove oxygen from inhaled air. They do not have a specific toxicity. They cause a fall in the inspired $PO_2$ and arterial hemoglobin desaturation. If the individual survives, asphyxia can leave some sequelae, neurological mainly, according to its duration, to the severity of hypoxia and extension of tissue damage.

Bioactive asphyxia products are gases with a specific toxicity that can interfere with cell respiration by mechanisms indicated in Table 12.11.

Intoxication with CO represents a common form of asphyxia [40]. CO is produced by the incomplete combustion of fuel from automobiles, defective domestic heating systems, camping heating, or industry. Affinity of hemoglobin for CO is 200 times stronger than oxygen. Carboxyhemoglobin is a stable compound, which sequesters hemoglobin, and reduces its capacity to transport oxygen in causing an anemic hypoxemia. In the arterial blood, we observe a reduced $SaO_2$, associated with a normal $pO_2$. CO interferes also with the release of oxygen in the tissue, increasing the affinity of residual hemoglobin for oxygen (shift to the left of the $O_2$ dissociation curve). Finally, there is also a certain direct toxic effect on cells (e.g., nervous system). The normal carboxyhemoglobin level is less than 2%, while in smokers it can vary between 5% and 10%. In over 20%, we can observe of progressive clinical manifestations (Table 12.12).

Carboxyhemoglobin dissociates slowly and its half-life is about 4 hours. This half-life ($T_{1/2}$) can be reduced in providing oxygen or in using hyperbaric chamber.

Table 12.11 Mechanisms of action of bioactive asphyxiant gases

| Gases | Mechanisms |
|---|---|
| Carbon monoxide (CO) | Carboxyhemoglobin |
| Cyanide (HCN, $C_2N_2$) | Cytochrome oxidase paralysis |
| Hydrogene sulfide ($H_2S$) | Cytochrome oxidase paralysis |
|  | Respiratory irritant—Neurotoxic |

Table 12.12 Clinical presentation of carbon monoxide intoxication

| %HbCO | Symptoms |
|---|---|
| 5%–10% | Increased angina in patient with coronary disease, impairment of vigilance |
| 20% | Pulsating temporal headaches, cutaneous vasodilation, and effort dyspnea |
| 30% | Severe headaches, irritability, impaired judgment, impaired vision, nausea, and vomiting |
| 40%–50% | Syncope, confusion, collapsus, and cherry red coloration of tissues due to the presence of carboxyhemoglobin |
| 50%–60% | Coma, convulsions, Cheyne–Stokes breathing, respiratory insufficiency, and death |
| >80% | Rapid death |

## Conclusion

In conclusion, multiple agents present at the workplace can induce a variety of pulmonary diseases. We should always question the possibility that they have an occupational origin. Multiple mechanisms are involved as we have shown and could affect mainly the bronchial tree or lung parenchyma or other thoracic structures. A respiratory and environmental questionnaire associated with a physical examination and some blood tests (e.g., precipitins against various agents causing an alveolitis, lymphocytic proliferation test in berryliosis), in addition to lung function tests, and radiologic exams can in most cases lead to the identification of the disease and its causal factor.

## References

1. Morgan WC, Seaton A. *Occupational Lung Diseases*. Philadelphia, PA, London, Toronto: W.B. Saunders, 1975. 391 p.
2. Hendrick D, Burge P, Beckett WS, Churg A. *Occupational Disorders of the Lung*. London: W.B. Saunders, 2002 May 15. 638 p.
3. Meyer JD, Holt DL, Cherry NM, McDonald JC. SWORD '98: Surveillance of work-related and occupational respiratory disease in the UK. *Occup Med (Lond)*. 1999; 49(8): 485–489.
4. Weill H, Jones RN, Parkes WR. Silicosis and related diseases. In: Parkes WR, ed. *Occupational Lung Disorders*. London: Butterworth Heinemann, 1994. 285 p.
5. Craighead JE, Mossman BT. The pathogenesis of asbestos-associated diseases. *N Engl J Med*. 1982; 306(24): 1446–1455.
6. Robledo R, Mossman B. Cellular and molecular mechanisms of asbestos-induced fibrosis. *B J Cell Physiol*. 1999; 180(2): 158–166.
7. Manning, C.B. et al. Diseases caused by asbestos: Mechanisms of injury and disease development. *Int Immunopharmacol* 2002; 2(2–3): 191–200.
8. O'Reilly KM, Mclaughlin AM, Beckett WS, Sime PJ. Asbestos-related lung disease. *Am Fam Physician*. 2007; 75(5): 683–688.
9. Henderson DW, Jones ML, De Klerk N et al. The diagnosis and attribution of asbestos-related diseases in an Australian context: Report of the Adelaide Workshop on Asbestos-Related Diseases. October 6–7, 2000. *Int J Occup Environ Health*. 2004; 10(1): 40–46.
10. Cohen RA, Patel A, Green FH. Lung disease caused by exposure to coal mine and silica dust. *Semin Respir Crit Care Med*. 2008; 29(6): 651–661.
11. Rimal, B. et al. Basic pathogenetic mechanisms in silicosis: Current understanding. *Curr Opin Pulm Med* 2005; 11: 169–173.
12. Otsuki T, Maeda M, Murakami S et al. Immunological effects of silica and asbestos. *Cell Mol Immunol*. 2007; 4(4): 261–268.
13. Prince P, Boulay ME, Pagé N et al. Induced sputum markers of fibrosis and decline in pulmonary function in asbestosis and silicosis: A pilot study. *Int J Tuberc Lung Dis*. 2008; 12(7): 813–819.
14. Nemery B. Metal toxicity and the respiratory tract. *Eur Respir J*. 1990; 3(2): 202–219.
15. Samuel G, Maier LA. Immunology of chronic beryllium disease. *Curr Opin Allergy Clin Immunol*. 2008; 8: 126–134.
16. Sato H, Spagnolo P, Silveira L et al. BTNL2 allele associations with chronic beryllium disease in HLA-DPB1*Glu69-negative individuals. *Tissue Antigens*. 2007; 70(6): 480–486.
17. Stange AW, Furman FJ, Hilmas DE. The beryllium lymphocyte proliferation test: Relevant issues in beryllium health surveillance. *Am J Ind Med*. 2004; 46(5): 453–462.
18. Stange AW, Hilmas DE, Furman FJ. Possible health risks from low level exposure to beryllium. *Toxicology*. 1996; 111(1–3): 213–224.

19. Balmes JR, Abraham JL, Dweik RA et al. An official American Thoracic Society statement: Diagnosis and management of beryllium sensitivity and chronic beryllium disease. *Am J Respir Crit Care Med.* 2014; 190:e34.
20. Bernstein L, Chan-Yeung M, Malo J-L, Bernstein D (eds.). *Definition of Occupational Asthma.* Asthma in the Workplace. New York, NY: Marcel Dekker, 1993. 1 p.
21. Gautrin D, Boulet LP, Boutet M et al. Is the reactive airways dysfunction syndrome (RADS) a variant of occupational asthma? *J Allergy Clin Immunol.* 1994; 93: 12.
22. Maestrelli P, Boschetto P, Fabbri LM, Mapp CE. Mechanisms of occupational asthma. *J Allergy Clin Immunol.* 2009; 123(3): 531–542.
23. Cartier A, Malo JL. *Chapter XII—Occupational Challenge Tests.* 236 p.
24. Mamessier E, Milhe F, Guillot C et al. T-cell activation in occupational asthma and rhinitis. *Allergy.* 2007; 62(2): 162–169.
25. Sumi Y, Foley S, Daigle S et al. Structural changes and airway remodelling in occupational asthma at a mean interval of 14 years after cessation of exposure. *Clin Exp Allergy.* 2007; 37(12): 1781–1787.
26. Malo JL, Chan-Yeung M. Asthma in the workplace: A Canadian contribution and perspective. *Can Respir J.* 2007 Oct; 14(7): 407–413.
27. Boulet LP, Boutet M, Laviolette M et al. Airway inflammation after removal from the causal agents in occupational asthma due to high and low molecular weight agents. *Eur Respir J.* 1994; 7: 1567.
28. Girard M, Lacasse Y, Cormier Y. Hypersensitivity pneumonitis. *Allergy.* 2009; 64(3): 322–334.
29. Rushton L. Occupational causes of chronic obstructive pulmonary disease. *Rev Environ Health.* 2007; 22(3): 195–212.
30. Sunyer J, Zock JP, Kromhout H et al. Lung function decline, chronic bronchitis, and occupational exposures in young adults. *Am J Respir Crit Care Med.* 2005; 172: 1139–1145.
31. Naidoo RN, Robins TG, Seixas N et al. Differential respirable dust related lung function effects between current and former South African coal miners. *Int Arch Occup Environ Health.* 2005; 78(4): 293–302.
32. Chan-Yeung M, Wong R, MacLean L et al. Epidemiologic health study of workers in an aluminum smelter in British Columbia. Effects on the respiratory system. *Am Rev Respir Dis.* 1983; 127(4): 465–469.
33. Boulet LP, Bowie D. Acute occupational respiratory diseases. *European Respir Mon.* 1999; 11: 320–346.
34. Kampa M, Castanas E. Human health effects of air pollution. *Environ Pollut.* 2008; 151(2): 362–367.
35. Kaye P, Young H, O'sullivan I. Metal fume fever: A case report and review of the literature. *Emerg Med J.* 2002; 19(3): 268–269.
36. Laplante JJ, Dalphin JC, Piarroux R et al. Pathologies respiratoires en milieu agricole: A review. *Rev Prat.* 2007 Jun 15; 57: 56–59.
37. Seifert SA, Von Essen S, Jacobitz K et al. Organic dust toxic syndrome: A review. *J Toxicol Clin Toxicol.* 2003; 41: 185–193.
38. Von Essen S, Robbins RA, Thompson AB, Rennard SI. Organic dust toxic syndrome: An acute febrile reaction to organic dust exposure distinct from hypersensitivity pneumonitis. *J Toxicol Clin Toxicol.* 1990; 28: 389–420.
39. Malmberg P, Rask-Andersen A, Rosenhall L. Exposure to microorganisms associated with allergic alveolitis and febrile reactions to mold dust in farmers. *Chest.* 1993; 103: 1202–1209.
40. Weaver LK. Clinical practice. Carbon monoxide poisoning. *N Engl J Med.* 2009 Mar 19; 360(12): 1217–1225.

# 13

# Diseases of the pleura

JEAN DESLAURIERS

| | |
|---|---|
| Introduction | 244 |
| Anatomy of the pleural membranes and pleural space | 244 |
| Physiology of the pleural space | 245 |
|     Intrapleural pressures | 245 |
|     Pleural fluid | 245 |
| Pneumothorax | 246 |
|     Terminology | 246 |
| Spontaneous pneumothoraces | 247 |
|     Pathogenesis, diagnosis, and evaluation | 247 |
|         Primary spontaneous pneumothorax | 247 |
|         Secondary spontaneous pneumothorax | 248 |
|         Pneumothorax associated with AIDS | 248 |
|         Catamenial pneumothorax | 249 |
|     Physiological changes associated with pneumothoraces | 249 |
|         Uncomplicated and simple pneumothoraces | 249 |
|         Tension pneumothoraces | 249 |
|         Resorption of air from the pleural space | 249 |
| Treatment | 250 |
| Pleural effusions | 250 |
|     Pathophysiology | 250 |
|     Investigation, diagnosis, and pathogenesis | 251 |
| Neoplastic and paraneoplastic pleural effusions | 252 |
| Empyema | 253 |
|     Terminology and pathophysiology | 253 |
|     Categorizing risk for poor outcome | 254 |
|     Treatment | 254 |
| Conclusion | 256 |
| References | 256 |

## Introduction

Diseases of the pleura or of the pleural space are fairly common and, although their treatment may appear to be simple, their pathogenesis is often very complex [1,2]. Pleural effusions, for instance, can be secondary to a variety of intrathoracic, intraabdominal, or systemic disorders.

For patients presenting with a pleural disorder, careful recording of clinical history, complete physical examination, and imaging of the pleural space should always be the first line of investigation. When necessary, however, more invasive techniques such as thoracentesis, percutaneous pleural biopsy, and videothoracoscopy or videothoracoscopy (VATS) [3,4] can also be done allowing for a positive diagnosis to be documented in over 95% of cases.

A clear understanding of the anatomy and physiology of the pleural space as well as of the pathophysiology involved in disease processes such as pneumothoraces, pleural effusions, and empyemas greatly facilitates the selection of appropriate therapies.

## Anatomy of the pleural membranes and pleural space

The pleura is made of two serosal membranes, one covering the lung (the visceral pleura) and one covering the inner chest wall and medial surface of the mediastinum (the parietal pleura) [5]. The transition between parietal and visceral pleurae is at the pulmonary hilum. At this level, the reflection covers the constituents of the hilum, except inferiorly, where it extends down to the diaphragm through the inferior pulmonary ligament. The pleural space is the space delimited by these two membranes. Under normal conditions, the pleural space contains a small amount of fluid (0.1–0.2 mL/kg) that functions mainly as a lubricator and facilitator of proper lung movements during the various phases of respiration.

The visceral pleura covers the entire surface of the lung and extends deep into the interlobar fissures. It is thin, transparent, and tightly adherent, via elastic fibers, to the underlying lung surface. The parietal pleura can be divided into costal, mediastinal, and diaphragmatic pleurae, the transition between each segment being at the level of the pleural sinuses. The attachment of the parietal pleura to the chest wall is through a fibrous layer known as the endothoracic fascia (Figure 13.1).

The visceral pleura is devoid of somatic innervation and is thus insensitive. In contrast, the parietal pleura is innervated through a rich network of somatic, sympathetic, and parasympathetic fibers. At the level of the costal pleura, these fibers travel with the intercostal nerves while at the level of the diaphragm, they travel with the phrenic nerves.

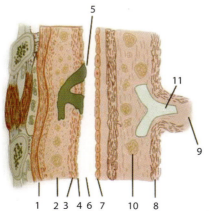

Figure 13.1 Layers of the parietal and visceral pleurae.

The pleural space is on the boundary of two lymphatic systems, both of which play a major role in the removal of fluid, cells, and foreign particles from the pleural space. In the subpleural space of the visceral pleura, large lymphatic capillaries form a meshed network that drains into the pulmonary lymphatic system. These capillaries are more abundant over the lower lobes and are connected to the deep pulmonary plexuses located in the interlobular and peribronchial spaces. This particular arrangement explains why bronchogenic carcinomas located in one pulmonary segment can drain into the lymphatics of a neighboring segment (cross over). This phenomenon mainly occurs at the level of the lower lobes.

The lymphatic drainage of the parietal pleura is more elaborate, with direct communication between the pleural space and the parietal pleural lymphatic channels. These communications, called stomata (see Figure 13.1) are 2–6 μm in diameter and predominate over the lower portions of the mediastinal, diaphragmatic, and costal pleura. They have endoluminal valves and drain into a network of submesothelial lymphatic lacunae. The stomata play an important role in the resorption of fluid and removal of proteins, particles, and cells from the pleural space.

## Physiology of the pleural space

### Intrapleural pressures

Pressures within the pleural space are proportional to those being developed within the lungs. When the lung volume is at functional residual capacity, the elastic forces of the lung and thorax are in equilibrium and the pleural pressure varies between −2 and −5 cm of water. As the lung volume increases to vital capacity during inspiration, the pleural pressure becomes progressively more negative and reaches −25 to −35 cm of water. In any condition in which elastic recoil of the lung is increased, such as can be observed in interstitial fibrosis, pulmonary edema, atelectasis, or after pulmonary resection, the pleural pressure will become more subatmospheric. The pleural pressure is not uniform around the lung surfaces being more negative at the apex (average of −7 to 9 cm of water) than at the base (average of 0 to −2 cm of water) in an upright subject.

### Pleural fluid

Pleural fluid is constantly secreted, mostly by filtration from the microvessels of the parietal pleura [6–10]. The composition of the normal pleural fluid is shown in Table 13.1. Its dynamic is based on the Starling equation (Figure 13.2), which states that the flow of fluid across the pleural space depends on the permeability coefficient of the pleural membranes, the difference in hydrostatic pressures across the pleural space,

Table 13.1 Composition of normal pleural fluid

Volume: 0.1–0.2 mL/Kg
Protein: 10–20 g/L
Albumin: 50%–70%
Glucose: As in plasma
Lactic dehydrogenase: <50% of plasma level
Cells/mm$^3$: 4,500
- Mesothelial cells: 3%
- Monocytes: 54%
- Lymphocytes: 10%
- Granulocytes: 4%
- Others: 29%

pH: 7.38 (mixed venous blood + 0.02)
Partial pressure of carbon dioxide (PaCO$_2$): 45 mmHg (same as in mixed venous blood)
Bicarbonate: 25 mmol/L (same as in mixed venous blood)

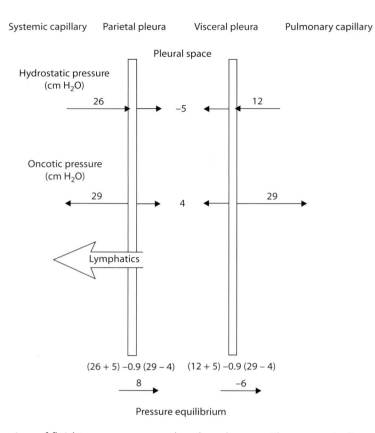

**Figure 13.2** Mechanism of fluid transport across the pleural space. The arrows indicate the direction of flow. Pressure equilibrium (Sterling equation) favors fluid filtration from the parietal pleura toward the visceral pleura where it is reabsorbed.

and the difference in osmotic pressures also across the pleural space. According to this equation, pressure equilibrium favors fluid filtration from the parietal pleura toward the visceral pleura where it is reabsorbed.

Recent studies have shown, however, that the resorption of pleural fluid may be through the lymphatic stomatas located in the parietal pleura rather than through the visceral pleura as suggested by the Starling equation.

# Pneumothorax

## Terminology

A pneumothorax is a pleural disorder characterized by the presence of air in the pleural space with secondary lung collapse. Pneumothoraces are usually classified as being spontaneous (primary or secondary) [11], traumatic, or iatrogenic (Table 13.2). Whereas primary spontaneous pneumothoraces occur in young patients without apparent lung disease, secondary pneumothoraces occur in patients with clinical or radiographic evidence of underlying lung disease, most often that of chronic obstructive pulmonary disease (COPD; Table 13.3).

Table 13.2 Classification of pneumothoraces

**Spontaneous**
Primary (normal individuals with apparently normal lungs)
Secondary (individuals with underlying lung disease)

- Chronic obstructive pulmonary disease
- Infectious lung disease
- Neoplastic lung disease
- Catamenial (associated with menstruation)
- Other lung diseases

**Posttraumatic** (blunt or penetrating injuries)
**Iatrogenic**

Table 13.3 Most important differences between primary and secondary pneumothoraces

|  | Primary | Secondary |
|---|---|---|
| Age | 15–40 | >40 |
| Gender | Mostly males | Mostly males |
| Smoking history | Often present | Generally present |
| Underlying lung disease | No | Yes |
| Body features | Tall and thin | Often have barrel chest |
| Main symptom | Chest pain | Dyspnea |
| Significant complications | Rare | Common and can be life threatening |
| Pathology | Apical vesicles (blebs) | Diffuse emphysema |
| Chances of recurrence after first episode | 10%–15% | 30%–50% |
| Chances of recurrence after second episode | 50% | >80% |

# Spontaneous pneumothoraces

## Pathogenesis, diagnosis, and evaluation

### Primary spontaneous pneumothorax

Primary spontaneous pneumothoraces are secondary to the rupture of small subpleural blebs (<2 cm) that themselves are the result of alveolar rupture with secondary air trapping between the elastic interna and externa of the visceral pleura. They are well demarcated from the normal adjacent lung parenchyma and are most commonly found at the apices of the upper lobes. Pathologically, they represent a variety of paraseptal emphysema. According to some authors, blebs are nearly always located at the lung apices of tall and thin individuals because these areas are the farthest from the hilum and thus could have suffered from some degree of ischemia during growth.

Primary spontaneous pneumothoraces can occur at rest or during exercise and they are most common in young men, usually <25 years of age. Chest pain is the usual symptom and its severity generally correlates with the degree of lung collapse. The diagnosis is best confirmed by erect postero-anterior chest radiograph although, on occasion, expiratory film may be useful to demonstrate a small pneumothorax that may have been missed on a standard film. Computed tomography (CT) scanning is, however, the better technique to estimate the size of the pneumothorax in addition to being useful in documenting the presence or absence of blebs or bullae in the adjacent lung parenchyma.

Complications associated with primary spontaneous pneumothoraces such as prolonged air leaks or failure of the lung to reexpand are uncommon. The risk of recurrence after a first episode is about 10%–15% while it is approximately 50% after a second episode. Most recurrences will occur within 2 years of the first episode and the majority are ipsilateral.

### Secondary spontaneous pneumothorax

Most individuals presenting with a secondary spontaneous pneumothorax [12] are males aged 45 or more and nearly all have an underlying pulmonary disorder, usually COPD (Table 13.4). In the vast majority of patients, dyspnea is the predominant symptom and it is often associated with some degree of hypoxia, hypercarbia, and respiratory acidosis. Because these patients have little or no respiratory reserve, a small pneumothorax is often poorly tolerated and can even be life threatening.

The diagnosis of secondary spontaneous pneumothoraces can be made on a standard postero-anterior chest radiograph although the radiograph can sometimes be difficult to interpret because of the presence of large bullae whose projection may be superimposed on that of the pneumothorax. In such cases, CT scanning may be necessary not only to demonstrate the presence of a pneumothorax but also to document the anatomy of the underlying bullous emphysema.

### Pneumothorax associated with AIDS

Several reports have described the association of spontaneous pneumothoraces with AIDS [13]. In these cases, the pneumothorax is in relation with the presence of cystic lesions usually located at the lung apices. These lesions consist of subpleural air spaces filled with an eosinophilic exudate, *Pneumocystis (jiroveci) carinii* organisms, fibrinous material, and macrophages. AIDS-related pneumothoraces may remain small and asymptomatic but, on occasion, their size will increase rapidly and they will become under tension, causing

Table 13.4 Common causes of secondary pneumothoraces

**Chronic obstructive pulmonary disease (COPD)**
- Emphysema
- Asthma

**Interstitial lung diseases**
- Pulmonary fibrosis
- Sarcoidosis

**Infectious lung diseases**
- Tuberculosis and other mycobacterial diseases
- Bacterial infections (necrotizing pneumonia, lung abscess)
- *Pneumocystis carinii* infections (AIDS)
- Mycotic infections

**Neoplastic lung diseases**
- Bronchogenic carcinomas
- Metastatic disease to the lung (lymphoma, sarcoma)

**Catamenial pneumothorax and pneumothorax secondary to pulmonary endometriosis**

**Others**
- Cystic fibrosis
- Collagen diseases, scleroderma
- Lymphangiomyomatosis

severe respiratory failure. In this population, synchronous bilateral pneumothoraces and bronchopleural fistulae are not uncommon, and there is also a high incidence of ipsilateral and contralateral recurrences.

### Catamenial pneumothorax

Pneumothoraces occurring within 48–72 hours after the onset of menstruations are called catamenial pneumothoraces [14]. Most occur on the right side, and they may be recurrent over several years before being diagnosed. They are usually small and patients consult for chest pain and dyspnea occurring at the beginning of their menstrual cycle.

The exact pathogenesis of catamenial pneumothoraces is still unknown but most experts think that air reaches the pleural space from the cervix and abdomen through congenital diaphragmatic defects. In some patients, catamenial pneumothoraces may also be caused by focal thoracic endometrial implants over the visceral pleura or in the lung, with air leakage occurring during menstruations.

## Physiological changes associated with pneumothoraces

### Uncomplicated and simple pneumothoraces

When a communication develops between lung and pleural space, the positive pressure of intra-alveolar air makes the air exit from the lung into the pleural space until there is no longer a difference between intrapleural and atmospheric pressures. Alveolar hypoventilation and hypoxemia, which can be observed in patients with >25% pneumothoraces, are in relation to a ventilation–perfusion mismatch. Pneumothoraces can also affect the mechanical properties of the lung and lead to significant reductions in lung compliance, vital capacity, total lung capacity, and functional residual capacity. In addition, the normal pleural pressure gradient between apex and base tends to disappear in patients with pneumothoraces.

### Tension pneumothoraces

During an episode of tension pneumothorax, a positive intrapleural pressure builds up during the expiration phase of the respiratory cycle because air continues to flow in the pleural space with no possibility of evacuation. This accumulation of air under positive pressure compresses the mediastinum and mediastinal structures with secondary decrease in venous return and ultimately in cardiac output. Mediastinal compression can also be associated with compression of the contralateral lung generating an additional decrease in oxygenation and cardiac output.

### Resorption of air from the pleural space

The pleural membranes are semipermeable structures through which gases can be reabsorbed by simple diffusion and equilibration and, in general, the rate of resorption is directly proportional to the quality of the pleural membrane. With a fibrotic pleura, for instance, the rate of resorption is lower than with a normal pleura. The rate of resorption is also proportional to the available surface area of the pleura and amount of gas contained in the pleural cavity. The greater the amount of gas, the longer it takes for reabsorption. In pneumothoraces, the pressure gradient between gas contained in the pleural space and pressures in the subpleural venous system is the driving force directing this diffusion process. In general, the resorption rate of a pneumothorax is approximately that of 1.25% of radiologic volume per day.

Each gas contained in the pleural space is reabsorbed independently of the others, resorption taking place gradually and in successive phases. During the first phase, there is equilibration of oxygen and carbon dioxide partial pressures and during the second phase, there is progressive resorption of the remaining intrapleural gases like nitrogen. Gradually, the intrapleural pressure recovers its normal negative pressure thus favoring lung reexpansion. The composition of gases in the pleural space can also vary and influence its rate of resorption. For example, oxygen is more diffusible and soluble than other gases, and thus its transfer from pleura to circulation is faster than that of carbon dioxide or nitrogen.

## Treatment

In individuals presenting with spontaneous primary pneumothoraces, air evacuation from the pleural space by simple aspiration or through conventional tube thoracostomy is indicated for patients with >20% pneumothoraces and for those with significant symptoms [15]. Definitive surgery may be indicated at the time of the first episode in patients with tension pneumothoraces, persistent air leakage (>4–5 days), pneumohemothoraces (occurs in approximately 5% of cases), and failure of the lung to reexpand. Recurrence is, however, the most common indication for surgery, which is usually recommended at the time of the second episode. The operative procedure which involves bleb resection and some form of mechanical pleurodesis (parietal pleurectomy or pleural abrasion) can be done through an axillary incision or more commonly through a thoracoscopic approach.

Most patients with secondary spontaneous pneumothoraces, especially those in relation to COPD, should initially be treated with tube thoracostomy because, in this population, even small pneumothoraces are poorly tolerated. If the pleural space is adequately drained, the lung will reexpand, the patient will stabilize, and treatment options can be further evaluated. Because of the significant incidence of prolonged air leaks, high risks of recurrence, and potential lethality of the condition, many surgeons now recommend that surgical intervention should be considered at the time of the first occurrence. The emergence of VATS has considerably changed the magnitude of operation which can now be done with low operative morbidity and mortality, even in high-risk cases [16].

Whenever possible, initial management of patients with AIDS-related pneumothoraces should be conservative because small pneumothoraces will often resolve with observation alone. Refractory or substantial pneumothoraces should, however, be drained. The most efficient method for managing pneumothoraces associated with prolonged air leaks or when they are recurrent is videothoracoscopic resection of the diseased site and mechanical pleurodesis. VATS talc poudrage can also be effective in controlling the disease.

Management of the first occurrence of a catamenial pneumothorax is similar to that of other types of pneumothoraces. Management of recurrences is more controversial and includes several options, such as the use of oral contraceptives or weak androgens to suppress ovulation, chemical pleurodesis, and mechanical pleurodesis. If a pregnancy is undesired or if the hormonal therapy is not working, tubal ligation should be considered.

## Pleural effusions

## Pathophysiology

Pleural effusions develop because of a disturbance in the normal mechanisms that move 5–10 L of fluid across the pleural space every day. Increased capillary permeability (inflammation, tumor implants), increased hydrostatic pressure (heart failure), reduced oncotic pressure (hypoalbuminemia), increased negative intrapleural pressure (atelectasis), and decreased lymphatic drainage (lymphatic obstruction) can all be the cause of a pleural effusion (Table 13.5).

Table 13.5 Mechanisms favoring the occurrence of a pleural effusion

| |
|---|
| Increased vascular hydrostatic pressure (heart failure) |
| Reduced vascular oncotic pressure (hypoalbuminemia) |
| Increased microvascular permeability (inflammation) |
| Impaired lymphatic drainage (neoplasm) |
| Increased negative pressure within the pleural space (atelectasis) |
| Transdiaphragmatic movement of fluid from the abdomen to the pleural space through microscopic diaphragmatic fenestrations (pancreatitis) |

## Investigation, diagnosis, and pathogenesis

The typical symptoms associated with pleural effusions are those of dyspnea, cough, and chest discomfort. The clinical setting in which a pleural effusion develops is an important consideration and, often, influences the approach to diagnosis. A patient who has a small effusion in conjunction with pneumonia, for instance, is likely to have a parapneumonic effusion. The same is true of a patient with known congestive heart failure who develops a right-sided pleural effusion or of a woman who develops a pleural effusion after having been treated for breast cancer and who is likely to have metastatic pleuritis.

Knowledge of the most common etiologies of pleural effusions is also helpful in establishing a proper diagnosis (Table 13.6). In North America, for example, the four more common causes of pleural effusions are congestive heart failure, bacterial pneumonia, malignant neoplasms, and pulmonary embolism. Similarly, the most common causes of malignant pleural effusions are lung cancer, breast cancer, and lymphoma.

Conventional imaging is the mainstay for the evaluation of patients with pleural effusions [17–19]. Small effusions (200–500 mL) will cause blunting of the costophrenic angle while larger effusions will produce the classic meniscus sign and massive effusions a complete opacification of the hemithorax. A lateral decubitus view is sometimes useful to determine if the effusion is free flowing or encapsulated. CT scanning facilitates the detection of small amounts of pleural fluid and is also helpful to detect loculated collections or to distinguish between a pleural lesion and a parenchymal process. Ultrasonography is complementary to CT in detecting small amounts of fluid (can detect 3–5 mL). Subpulmonic effusions are fluid collections located between the base of the lung and the diaphragm.

If the cause of the effusion is still undetermined after imaging, a thoracentesis should be performed usually under ultrasound guidance (Table 13.7). It is diagnostic in 50%–60% of cases, and higher yield can be obtained in processes such as empyemas (turbid or purulent fluid), hemothoraces (bloody fluid), and chylothoraces (clear milky fluid) (Table 13.8). Pleural fluid obtained by thoracentesis (approximately 50 mL in routine cases) should be sent for cytological examination, culture, and cell count. Approximately 60%–80% of patients with metastatic pleuritis will have a positive cytology in their pleural fluid.

Normal pleural fluid is clear and it has a low protein concentration (1.0–1.5 g/dL), <1500 nucleated cells/mm$^3$, glucose and lactate dehydrogenase (LDH) concentrations equal to those of serum, and a pH which is >7.62.

Pleural effusions are classified as exudates or transudates on the basis of their protein and LDH contents. An effusion is considered as an exudate if the protein pleural fluid-to-serum ratio is >0.5 and that of LDH >0.6. The pleural fluid concentration in glucose is also helpful because a level <60 mg/dL (or <50% of serum glucose concentration) is only observed in malignant or tuberculous effusions, parapneumonic effusions, and effusions associated with rheumatoid arthritis. Several authors have also reported that a pH of <7 in conjunction with a glucose level <60 mg/dL is indicative that a parapneumonic effusion is likely to progress to frank empyema.

Table 13.6 Most common causes of pleural effusions

**Transudates**
- Congestive heart failure, myxedema
- Cirrhosis of the liver
- Nephrotic syndrome, glomerulonephritis, and peritoneal dialysis
- Pulmonary embolism, sarcoidosis

**Exudates**
- Primary or secondary neoplasms, lymphomas
- Infections: bacterial (parapneumonic effusions), tuberculosis, viral, and fungal (rare)
- Gastrointestinal: pancreatitis, subphrenic abscess, and esophageal rupture
- Collagen diseases: rheumatoid arthritis, systemic lupus erythematosus, and Wegener granulomatosis
- Miscellaneous: trauma, radiation injury, and postoperative

Table 13.7 Analysis of pleural fluid obtained by thoracentesis

**Macroscopic aspect of the fluid**
- Bloody, turbid, purulent, and milky

**Cytological examination and cell count (white blood cells)**

**Culture and sensitivity**

**Biochemistry**
- pH, glucose, proteins, and LDH
- Amylase (elevated in cases of pancreatitis and esophageal perforation)
- Triglycerides (elevated (>110 mg/dL) in cases of chylothoraces)

LDH, lactate dehydrogenase.

Table 13.8 Tips to determine the cause of a pleural effusion

| Color of the fluid | Suggested diagnosis |
| --- | --- |
| Red (bloody) | Malignancy, pulmonary embolism, trauma, and tuberculosis |
| Yellow (straw color) | No specific diagnosis |
| Yellow (greenish color) | Infection |
| White (milky) | Chylothorax |
| Brown (chocolate sauce) | Anaerobic liver abscess |
| Black | Aspergillosis |
| **Characteristic of the fluid** | **Suggested diagnosis** |
| Viscous | Malignant mesothelioma (hyaluronic acid), chronic empyema |
| Purulent | Acute empyema |
| Turbid | Parapneumonic effusion, lipidic effusion |
| Debris | Rheumatoid arthritis |

Source: Modified from Al-Jahdali, H., Menzies, R.I., *Can J Diagn.*, 13, 105–113, 1996.

If the cause of the effusion is still unclear after thoracentesis, the patient should undergo a diagnostic thoracoscopy which allows direct access to 90%–100% of the surfaces of both visceral and parietal pleura. In experienced hands, thoracoscopy is a safe procedure with a diagnostic accuracy of 90%–100%. In addition, a pleurodesis can be done should it be necessary such as in cases of malignant pleural effusions.

## Neoplastic and paraneoplastic pleural effusions

A pleural effusion containing malignant cells is called a malignant pleural effusion [20–24]. These effusions result from the cumulative effects of increased capillary permeability secondary to tumor implants on pleural surfaces (increased fluid production) and impaired fluid resorption due to tumor invasion of the pleuro-mediastinal lymphatics (lymphatic obstruction; Table 13.9). Direct invasion of the parietal pleura by lung cancer or less commonly by primary pleural tumors is yet another mechanism that can increase fluid production. Through a combination of each of these mechanisms, several liters of fluid can accumulate in the pleural space, causing lung (ipsilateral and contralateral) as well as mediastinal (vena cava) compression. Ultimately, these compressions will cause loss of pulmonary function and decrease in cardiac output.

Although nearly all forms of malignant processes can be the cause of malignant pleural effusions, approximately two-thirds of these effusions are accounted for by lung cancer, breast cancer, and lymphomas. In approximately 15% of patients, the site of the primary will remain unknown, even after an extensive investigation.

Table 13.9 Interaction between the mechanisms that may result in pleural effusions in cancer patient

| Mechanism | Decreased lymphatic drainage | Increase in osmotic pressure | Increased permeability | Increased venous pressure |
|---|---|---|---|---|
| Pleural implants | + | + | + | − |
| Lymphatic metastasis | | | | |
| • Nodes | + | + | − | − |
| • Lymphangitis | + | + | − | − |
| Suspension of neoplastic cells | + | + | + | − |
| Other syndromes that may contribute | | | | |
| • Superior vena cava | + | + | − | + |
| • Heart failure | + | + | − | + |
| • Pericardial effusion | + | + | − | − |
| • Infection | + | + | + | − |
| • Mediastinal radiation | + | + | − | − |
| • Hypoalbuminemia | − | + | − | + |

*Source:* From Harper, G.R., *Clin Cancer Briefs.*, 1, 1, 1979; Roth, J.A. et al., *Thoracic Oncology*, W.B. Saunders, Philadelphia, PA, 1989.
+, contributes; −, does not contribute

Paraneoplastic pleural effusions are cancer-related effusions in which no malignant cells are found. In lung cancer, the significance of such effusions which are usually secondary to bronchial obstruction is that patients can still undergo complete and potentially curative resection.

The treatment of patients with initial or recurrent malignant pleural effusions can be complex. Given the limited survival of most of these individuals, it must provide expedient and effective relief of symptoms, minimize hospitalization time, and improve quality of life. The two techniques that are currently used to achieve these objectives are those of chemical pleurodesis (talc, doxycycline, and bleomycin) or the insertion of an intrapleural catheter, such as the PleurX catheter, which facilitates daily evacuation of the fluid that can be done at home.

## Empyema

Empyema thoracis is defined as a purulent pleural effusion [25–30]. Although the infection usually originates from the lung, it may have entered the pleural space through the chest wall or from sources below the diaphragm or in the mediastinum. Management depends on the cause of the empyema and clinical stage, the state of the underlying lung, the presence or absence on an associated bronchopleural fistula, and the patient's clinical and nutritional status.

## Terminology and pathophysiology

The American Thoracic Society recognizes three distinct stages in the formation of an empyema that are indicative of disease progression in the pleural space (Table 13.10). Early in the disease process (acute or exudative phase, stage 1), the pleural membranes are edematous and discharge a thin exudative fluid called a parapneumonic effusion. With early and vigorous treatment of the underlying pneumonia, most of these

Table 13.10 Stages in the evolution of an empyema

| Stage | Phase | Characteristics |
|---|---|---|
| 1 | Exudative (acute phase) | Edema of pleural membranes |
|   |   | Pleural fluid of low viscosity and containing few inflammatory cells |
| 2 | Fibrinopurulent (transition phase) | Important fibrin deposits over the pleural membranes |
|   |   | Pleural fluid becomes purulent |
| 3 | Organization (chronic phase) | Ingrowth of fibroblasts |
|   |   | Formation of a thick fibrous peel over the lung surface |

effusions will remain uninfected, and they will generally be associated with a good outcome. At this very early stage, the volume of pleural effusion is minimal, and the effusion is free flowing on lateral decubitus films.

If the disease process is allowed to continue, large amounts of fibrin will be deposited, mostly over the parietal pleura. The amount of pleural fluid will also increase significantly and it will become loculated. When the host reaction is eventually overwhelmed by the number and virulence of the inoculum, the pleural fluid becomes turbid or frankly purulent (fibrinopurulent phase, stage 2). If left undrained, these collections are associated with poor outcomes even if the pleura is still relatively intact and the lung could still be reexpanded.

Within 3–4 weeks or sometimes sooner, organization (stage 3) begins with massive ingrowth of fibroblasts and formation of collagen fibers over both parietal and visceral pleura. The lung, which at this stage is virtually functionless, is imprisoned within a thick fibrous peel and can no longer expand with tube drainage. Complications of the empyema can occur at any time during the evolution of the disease process although they are most likely to be seen during the organization phase (Table 13.11)

## Categorizing risk for poor outcome

The real difficulty in the management of patients with parapneumonic effusions is to distinguish between a noncomplicated, noninfected effusion, and a complicated one in which the empyema is pending or already present. Evaluating the risk for poor outcome and categorizing it (Table 13.12) is, therefore, important and should be based on three variables: pleural space anatomy, pleural fluid bacteriology, and pleural fluid biochemistry. The presence or absence of clinical symptoms, such as fever, chest pain, or systemic toxicity, is less important because these can be related to the underlying pneumonia as much as to the parapneumonic effusion.

Standard chest radiographs are useful, at least initially, to document the presence of a pleural effusion and to determine if the collection is free flowing or loculated (decubitus films). CT scanning is useful to assess the underlying lung as well as to determine the presence or absence of loculations, thickened parietal pleura, or trapped lung. Ultrasonography is perhaps the best imaging technique to demonstrate septations and loculations.

Biochemical analysis of the pleural fluid is important, specifically measurement of pH, glucose, and LDH values. If the pH of the pleural fluid is >7.3, the glucose concentration >60 mg/dL, and the LDH value <1000 IU/L parapneumonic effusions generally do not necessitate tube drainage. In contrast, pleural effusions with low fluid pH (<7.2) may represent an indication for tube drainage, especially if the effusion is large (half or more of the hemithorax). Low glucose concentration (<60 mg/dL) and high LDH contents (>1000 IU/L) may also be indicative of an impending empyema and these effusions generally necessitate tube drainage.

## Treatment

Empyema management depends on the clinical stage of disease, patient's clinical status, and risk for poor outcome (Figure 13.3). Patients with very low or low risk of poor outcome do not require tube drainage

Table 13.11 Possible complications of empyemas

- Bronchopleural fistula (spontaneous drainage of empyema in a bronchus)
- Empyema necessitatis (spontaneous drainage of empyema through the skin)
- Mediastinal abscess, subphrenic abscess
- Pericarditis
- Chest wall contraction and fibrothorax
- Pulmonary fibrosis

Table 13.12 Categorizing risk in patients with parapneumonic effusions

| Anatomy of the pleural effusion | Bacteriology of fluid | Biochemistry of fluid | Risk of poor outcome | Indication for drainage |
|---|---|---|---|---|
| Minimal and free flowing (<10 mm) | Unknown | Unknown | Very low | No |
| Small to moderate and free flowing (>10 mm) (<1/2 hemithorax) | Gram negative stain or culture | pH ≥7.2<br>Glucose >60 mg/dL<br>LDH <1,000 IU/L | Low | No |
| Larger free flowing (= 1/2 hemithorax) loculated effusion, acute parapneumonic effusion with thickened, and parietal pleura | Gram positive stain or culture | pH ≤7.1<br>Glucose <40 mg/dL<br>LDH >1,000 IU/L | Moderate | Yes |
| | Frank pus | pH <7.0 | High | Yes |

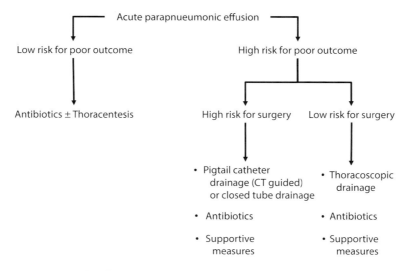

Figure 13.3 Suggested algorithm for managing parapneumonic effusions during the acute phase.

because the effusion will likely disappear (reabsorption by pleural membranes) with the resolution of the pneumonia. In those individuals, treatment consists primarily of antibiotic therapy with or without repeated thoracentesis. In patients with high or very high risk of poor outcome, removal of contaminated pleural fluid or of pus by closed tube drainage or by thoracoscopy is mandatory. The thoracoscopic approach is currently preferred being optimal to evacuate the pus, disrupt loculations, remove fibrin, reexpand the lung, and properly position one or two chest tubes in the most dependent portions of the space. In these patients, tube or thoracoscopic drainage results in improved survival, shortened hospital stay, lower incidence of complications of the empyema, and reduced need for second interventions.

## Conclusion

The pleura is a thin and permeable membrane covering the inner chest wall, mediastinum, diaphragm, and lung surfaces in continuity. Under normal physiological conditions, this arrangement creates a closed space (pleural space) in which exists a dynamic equilibrium between fluid transudation and resorption, explaining why there are only a few millimeters of fluid in the space at any given time. With perhaps the exception of primary malignant pleural neoplasms, all disease processes of the pleural space are secondary to one of two pathogenetic mechanisms: (1) disruption of the integrity of the pleural membranes with accumulation of foreign substances such as air, blood, pus, or lymph in the pleural space and (2) disruption of the process of normal fluid transudation/resorption resulting in the accumulation of fluid in the pleural space.

Since intrathoracic disorders involving the pleura or pleural space are not uncommon, a good understanding of these mechanisms is essential if one hopes to solve the clinical problems that can be encountered.

## References

1. Black LF. The pleural space and pleural fluid. *Mayo Clin Proc* 1972; 47: 493–506.
2. Sahn SA. State of the art. The pleura. *Am Rev Resp Dis* 1988; 138: 184–234.
3. Daniel TM. Diagnostic thoracoscopy for pleural disease. *Ann Thorac Surg* 1993; 56: 639–640.
4. Harris RJ, Kavuru MS, Rice TW, Kirby TJ. The diagnostic and therapeutic utility of thoracoscopy. A review. *Chest* 1995; 108: 828–841.
5. Wang NS. Anatomy of the pleura. *Clin Chest Med* 1998; 19: 229–240.
6. Agostini E, Zocchi L. Mechanical coupling and liquid exchanges in the pleural space. *Clin Chest Med* 1998; 19: 241–260.
7. Zocchi L. Physiology and pathophysiology of pleural fluid turnover. *Eur Resp J* 2002; 20: 1545–1558.
8. D'Angelo E, Loring SH, Gioia ME et al. Friction and lubrication of pleural tissue. *Respir Physiol Neurobiol* 2004; 142: 55–68.
9. Lai-Fook SJ. Pleural mechanics and fluid exchange. *Physiol Rev* 2004; 84: 385–410.
10. Mehran RJ, Deslauriers J. Anatomy and physiology of the pleural space. In *Pearson's Thoracic and Esophageal Surgery*. Patterson GA, Cooper JD, Deslauriers J et al. Editors. Philadelphia, PA: Churchill Livingstone-Elsevier, 2008, Chapter 82, pp. 1001–1007.
11. Sahn SA, Heffner JE. Spontaneous pneumothorax. *N Engl J Med* 2000; 342: 868–874.
12. Tanaka F, Itoh M, Esaki H et al. Secondary spontaneous pneumothorax. *Ann Thorac Surg* 1993; 55: 372–376.
13. Trachiotis GD, Vricella LA, Alyono D et al. Management of AIDS-related Pneumothorax. *Ann Thor Surg* 1996; 62: 1608–1613.
14. Carter EJ, Ettensohn DB. Catamenial pneumothorax. *Chest* 1990; 98: 713–716.
15. Baumann MH, Strange C, Heffner JE et al. Management of spontaneous pneumothorax. An American College of Chest Physicians Delphi consensus statement. *Chest* 2001; 119: 590–602.
16. Freixinet JL, Canalis E, Julia G et al. Axillary thoracotomy versus videothoracoscopy for the treatment of primary spontaneous pneumothorax. *Ann Thor Surg* 2004; 78: 417–420.

17. Bartter T, Santarelli R, Akers S, Pratter MR. The evaluation of pleural effusion. *Chest* 1994; 106: 1209–1214.
18. Al-Jahdali H, Menzies RI. How to diagnose pleural effusions. *Can J Diagn* 1996; 13: 105–113.
19. Smyrnios NA, Jeder PJ, Irwin RS. Pleural effusion in an asymptomatic patient: Spectrum and frequency of causes and management considerations. *Chest* 1990; 97: 192–196.
20. Harper GR. Pleural effusions in cancer. *Clin Cancer Briefs* 1979; 1: 1.
21. Roth JA, Ruckdeschel JC, Weisenberger TH, eds. *Thoracic Oncology.* Philadelphia, PA: WB Saunders, 1989.
22. Reeder LB. Malignant pleural effusions. *Curr Treat Options Oncol* 2001; 2: 93–96.
23. Antony VB, Loddenkemper R, Astoul P et al. Management of malignant pleural effusions. ERS/ATS statement. *Eur Respir J* 2001; 18: 402–419.
24. Putman JB. Malignant pleural effusions. *Surg Clin North Am* 2002; 82: 867–883.
25. Magovern CJ, Rusch VW. Parapneumonic and post-traumatic pleural space infections. *Chest Surg Clin North Am* 1994; 4: 561–582.
26. Bryant RE, Salmon CJ. Pleural empyema. *Clin Infect Dis* 1996; 22: 747–764.
27. Colice G, Curtis A, Deslauriers J et al. Medical and surgical treatment of parapneumonic effusions. An evidence-based guideline. *Chest* 2000; 82: 643–671.
28. De Hoyos A, Sundaresan S. Thoracic empyema. *Surg Clin North Am* 2002; 82: 643–671.
29. Roberts JR. Minimally invasive surgery in the treatment of empyema: Intraoperative decision making. *Ann Thorac Surg* 2003; 76: 225–230.
30. Light RW. Parapneumonic effusions and empyema. *Clin Chest Med* 1985; 6: 55–62.

# 14

# Cystic fibrosis (mucoviscidosis)

LARA BILODEAU

| | |
|---|---|
| Introduction | 259 |
| Pathophysiology | 260 |
| Structure and function of CFTR protein | 260 |
| Genetics | 261 |
| Classification of disease-causing mutations | 261 |
| Class I mutations: defect in CFTR protein synthesis | 261 |
| Class II mutations: defect in CFTR protein maturation with premature degradation | 261 |
| Class III mutations: defect in CFTR protein regulation | 261 |
| Class IV mutations: defect in CFTR protein conductance | 261 |
| Class V mutations: defect in CFTR protein transcription | 261 |
| Class VI mutations: accelerated CFTR protein degradation | 261 |
| Correlations between genotype and phenotype | 261 |
| Pathophysiology underlying respiratory tract malfunction | 263 |
| Regulation of airway surface liquid volume under normal conditions | 263 |
| Epithelial ion flux | 263 |
| Impaired bicarbonate secretion | 264 |
| Infection | 265 |
| Relevance to age | 265 |
| Diagnosis | 266 |
| Principles of therapeutic interventions | 266 |
| Conclusion and future perspectives | 267 |
| References | 267 |

## Introduction

Cystic fibrosis (CF), also called mucoviscidosis, is an autosomal recessive genetic disorder that mostly affects the lungs and gastrointestinal tract. In the Caucasian population, it is the most common genetically associated fatal disease. Classically, CF-associated clinical manifestations are those of thick and tenacious airway mucus accumulation, chronic bronchial infection, and exocrine pancreatic insufficiency-related malabsorption. In general, the symptoms become apparent early in life and in most cases, the diagnosis is made before the age of 2.

CF is caused by gene mutations leading to an absence or dysfunction of a protein called "cystic fibrosis transmembrane conductance regulator (CFTR)." This protein has an important role in epithelial transmembrane ion transport in different organs, most notably the lungs, pancreas, and intestines. In Canada, one of 25 individuals has a CFTR gene defect, and it is estimated that the incidence of CF is one per 3600 live births [1]. This incidence is distinctly lower in the Hispanic (1/9000) [2], the Asiatic (1/32,000) [3], and the African-American (1/15,000) [4] populations.

Although there are no curative therapies currently available, the life expectancy of individuals suffering from CF has gone up quite steadily over the past few decades. In Canada, for instance, CF median survival has risen from 24 years in 1982 to 51.8 years in 2014 [5]. As a result, the number of adults afflicted by CF is now higher than that of children. This increase in life expectancy relates to a more aggressive management of downstream consequences of disease, such as malnutrition and chronic bronchopulmonary infections, involvement of interdisciplinary treatment teams, and more common diagnosis of milder forms of disease [6]. In patients afflicted by CF, lung disease remains the main cause of disease-related morbidity and mortality.

## Pathophysiology

### Structure and function of CFTR protein

It is now well documented that the CFTR protein's main function is to conduct chloride across the epithelial apical membranes of several organs such as the upper and lower respiratory tracts, sweat glands, pancreatic ducts, biliary canaliculi, intestines, and vas deferens.

The CFTR protein belongs to a family of transmembrane conductance proteins called "adenosine triphosphate (ATP)-binding cassette (ABC) transporters." It contains 1480 amino acids and consists of five distinct domains including two transmembrane domains each having six segments, two nucleotide-binding domains (NBD1 and NBD2), and one regulatory domain (R) (Figure 14.1). The transmembrane domain segments act as chloride channels while NBD1 and NBD2 domains are involved in ATP hydrolysis, and R domain contains numerous phosphorylation sites [7]. In order to become activated, the CFTR protein requires phosphorylation of R domain sites by protein kinase A (PKA), which is itself regulated by cyclic adenosine monophosphate (AMP). Once phosphorylation has occurred, the opening and closing of epithelial chloride channels are regulated by ATP hydrolysis at the level of the nucleotides NBD1 and NBD2 domains. Chloride channel deactivation is done by phosphatase proteins at the level of the regulator domain [8–10].

In addition to acting as a chloride transport channel, the CFTR protein also plays a role in regulating other membrane channels such as the epithelial sodium channel (ENaC) where it acts as an inhibitor. It is also involved in the transport of bicarbonate ($HCO_3^-$) and proteins across epithelial cell membranes [11].

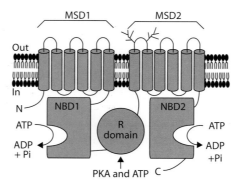

Figure 14.1 Structure of CFTR protein. MSD 1 and 2, membrane-spanning domains 1 and 2; NBD 1 and 2, nucleotide-binding domains 1 and 2; ATP, adenosine triphosphate; AMP, adenosine monophosphate; R domain, regulator domain; PKA, protein kinase A. (From Sheppard, D.N., Welsh, M.J., *Physiol Rev*, 79, s23–s45, 1999.)

# Genetics

The CF gene defect, which was first identified in 1989, is located on the long arm of chromosome 7 and it has 27 CFTR protein-coding exons. As of now, more than 2000 different CFTR mutations have been described [12], the most common being the *F508del* (lack of a phenylalanine residue at position 508 of CFTR) mutation, which is present in approximately 70% of CF chromosomes worldwide [13]. The majority of other mutations are rare with less than 10 mutations having an incidence of more than 1% [11]. The prevalence of mutations also varies significantly among different ethnic groups.

## Classification of disease-causing mutations

Mutations have been grouped into six different classes based on the mechanism by which they lead to CFTR dysfunction [14–16].

### Class I mutations: defect in CFTR protein synthesis

Class I mutations cause an interruption in protein CFTR synthesis through "premature stop codons." The end result of the process is an incomplete protein that is rapidly degraded in the cytoplasm.

### Class II mutations: defect in CFTR protein maturation with premature degradation

In Class II mutations, which include the *F508del* mutation, the CFTR protein is inadequately processed, the end result being the production of a "misfolded protein." The misfolded protein is identified as abnormal by the cell control mechanisms and, as such, is prematurely degraded within the endoplasmic reticulum.

### Class III mutations: defect in CFTR protein regulation

In Class III mutations, the CFTR protein reaches the cell apical membrane but does not respond to c-AMP or ATP stimulation. These mutations are located in the nucleotide-binding domains (Figure 14.2).

### Class IV mutations: defect in CFTR protein conductance

In Class IV mutations, the CFTR protein reaches the cell apical membrane and responds in normal fashion to stimulation. It has, however, abnormal conductance properties that translate into significant reductions in chloride transportation.

### Class V mutations: defect in CFTR protein transcription

In Class V mutations, the CFTR protein is normal but there are reduced numbers of transcripts due to a faulty transcription at the level of pre-RNA exon messengers.

### Class VI mutations: accelerated CFTR protein degradation

In Class VI mutations, the terminal part of the CFTR protein is lost but the efficiency of the chloride channel is preserved. The end result is defective CFTR stability at the cell surface and a protein that is being degraded in an accelerated fashion [16].

Recently, a more complex classification has been proposed, which takes into account that a single mutation can cause multiple defects. This new classification would include 31 classes: the six original classes and 26 of their combinations [16].

## Correlations between genotype and phenotype

The only cystic fibrosis clinical manifestation that correlates with CFTR genotype is exocrine pancreatic insufficiency. Class I, II, and III mutations, which are the commonest, are associated with significant

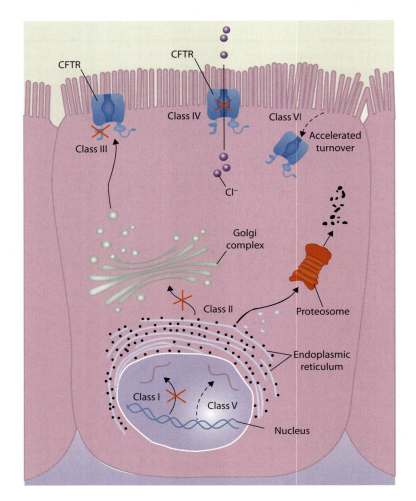

Figure 14.2 Classes of CFTR mutations. (From Rowe, S. et al., *N Engl J Med*, 352, 1992–2001, 2005.)

reductions in CFTR protein expression and function. Individuals afflicted by two mutations of these classes, both homozygotes and heterozygotes, will suffer from exocrine pancreatic insufficiency [17]. In contrast, class IV, V, and VI mutations are less severe so that an individual harboring one of them will usually have normal pancreatic function even when that mutation is associated with a class I, II, or III mutation [18]. In addition, cystic fibrosis patients harboring less severe mutations (classes IV, V, VI) will generally have a more favorable evolution from a respiratory standpoint when compared to those harboring two severe mutations (class I, II, III) [19]. One cannot assert, however, that individuals harboring two class I, II, or III CFTR mutations will automatically have a more severe form of disease. Indeed two people can harbor identical CFTR mutations but yet present different patterns of clinical evolution [20].

Disease evolution is thus influenced by other factors such as environment, tobacco smoke exposure, socioeconomic conditions, and response to treatment [21]. It is also likely that gene modifiers are having an impact on disease severity through mechanisms such as alterations in CFTR synthesis or modifications in infection susceptibility and inflammatory response [21,22].

## Pathophysiology underlying respiratory tract malfunction

Several hypotheses have been invoked to explain the link between CF lung disease and altered chloride transport [23]. One such hypothesis postulates that, in CF, the thin fluid layer covering the airway, the "airway surface liquid (ASL)" could be hypertonic due to increased sodium chloride concentration. This salt-rich fluid could generate dysfunction of salt-sensitive antimicrobial molecules with secondary increased susceptibility to infections [24,25]. This hypothesis has, however, never been confirmed and, indeed, other similar studies have shown that in CF, ASL is isotonic just as it is in normal lungs [26–28].

Another more accepted hypothesis, called the "ASL volume hypothesis," suggests that, in CF, ASL is volume depleted or dehydrated. Under normal conditions, ASL has two layers, the periciliary liquid layer and the mucus layer. The low-viscosity periciliary liquid layer creates a favorable environment for efficient ciliary function in addition to having a lubricating role to prevent mucus adherence to the surface epithelium. The mucus layer main function is to trap particles and microorganisms in order to facilitate their evacuation [29].

## Regulation of airway surface liquid volume under normal conditions

ASL volume is mostly regulated through an active ion transport mechanism that is present across the surface epithelium (Figure 14.3) [30,31]. Since the epithelial cells are water permeable, any change in sodium concentration on their surfaces will lead to passive water shift (osmotic gradient) with secondary changes in ASL volume. It is important to understand that for efficient mucociliary clearance, ASL volume should always be maintained at cilia height (7 μm).

If there is an excess of ASL, active sodium absorption will be enhanced through the ENaC and this will, in turn, cause transcellular water movement toward the epithelial surface layer (via aquaporines) as well as passive paracellular chloride movement in order to maintain electrochemical neutrality.

If, on the other hand, there is depletion of ASL, sodium absorption through ENaC will be inhibited and chloride will be secreted, mostly at the level of CFTR channels. This will secondarily generate passive sodium movement (electrochemical gradient) and more transcellular water movement onto the epithelial surface layer (osmotic gradient).

## Epithelial ion flux

In individuals suffering from CF, CFTR dysfunction will cause sodium hyperabsorption (loss of ENaC inhibition) and reduced chloride secretion [32–34]. The end result will be ASL depletion due to sodium

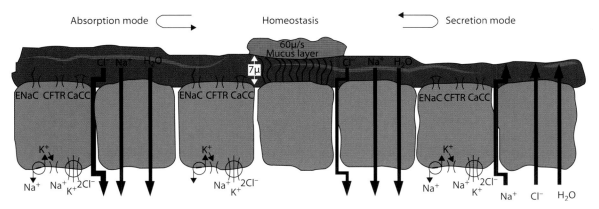

Figure 14.3 Regulation of airway surface liquid (ASL) volume in the respiratory tract through epithelial ion flux. (From Elkins, M.R., Bye, P.T., *Curr Opin Pulm Med*, 12, 445–452, 2006.)

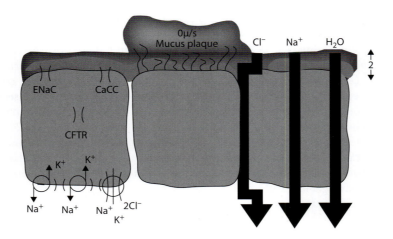

Figure 14.4 Respiratory epithelial ion flux in cystic fibrosis. (From Elkins, M.R., Bye, P.T., *Curr Opin Pulm Med*, 12, 445–452, 2006.)

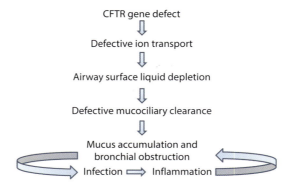

Figure 14.5 Cystic fibrosis pathophysiology. (From Ratjen, F.A., *Respir Care*, 54, 595–602, 2009.)

hyperabsorption, which cannot be compensated by chloride secretion. This ASL depletion is believed to cause increased mucus adherence onto the epithelial cell surface with secondary compromised mucociliary clearance (Figure 14.4).

## Impaired bicarbonate secretion

CFTR dysfunction also impairs bicarbonate secretion in the airways, leading to reduced ASL pH. It has been demonstrated in the CF pig model that acidic ASL decreases antibacterial activity, which can be restored by alkalinisation of airway surface [35]. In addition, bicarbonate play a role in maintaining hydration and normal viscosity of airway mucus [36].

As a consequence of CFTR dysfunction, thick and tenacious secretions will accumulate in the bronchi, creating mucus plugging and encouraging chronic bacterial infection. Pathogen accumulation will trigger the occurrence of an intense neutrophilic inflammatory reaction with the release of cytokines, proteinases, and free radicals [11,37], which will gradually lead to nonreversible airway epithelium damage and bronchiectasis. Neutrophil necrosis is also associated with DNA release, which increases mucus viscosity. At this stage, a vicious circle of mucus retention, bronchial obstruction, infection, and inflammation (Figure 14.5) will have been established.

The classic symptoms observed in patients with CF lung disease are those of chronic cough and increased sputum production. Over time, patients will also develop symptoms, such as shortness of breath, related to chronic obstructive pulmonary disease. Typically, patients will have recurring episodes of symptom exacerbation requiring systemic antibiotic therapy and, ultimately, they may go into respiratory failure that is the commonest cause of death in this population.

## Infection

Bacterial pulmonary infections are typical of CF lung disease and these infections generally begin at a very young age [38–40]. During childhood, most infections are caused by *Staphylococcus aureus*, followed by *Pseudomonas aeruginosa* and *Haemophilus influenza* [41–43]. Prevalence of *P. aeruginosa* infection increases with age. In Canada, about 45% of adult CF patients are chronically infected by this pathogen compared to 70% in the United States (Figure 14.6). Chronic infection by *P. aeruginosa* is associated with increased morbidity and mortality [44–45].

### Relevance to age

In order to survive in the respiratory tract of CF patients, *P. aeruginosa* has been able to develop strategies protecting it from both natural host defenses and antimicrobial agents. One possible strategy is that it can transform itself into a mucoid form (mucoid *P. aeruginosa*). This mucoid *P. aeruginosa* can secrete large amounts of

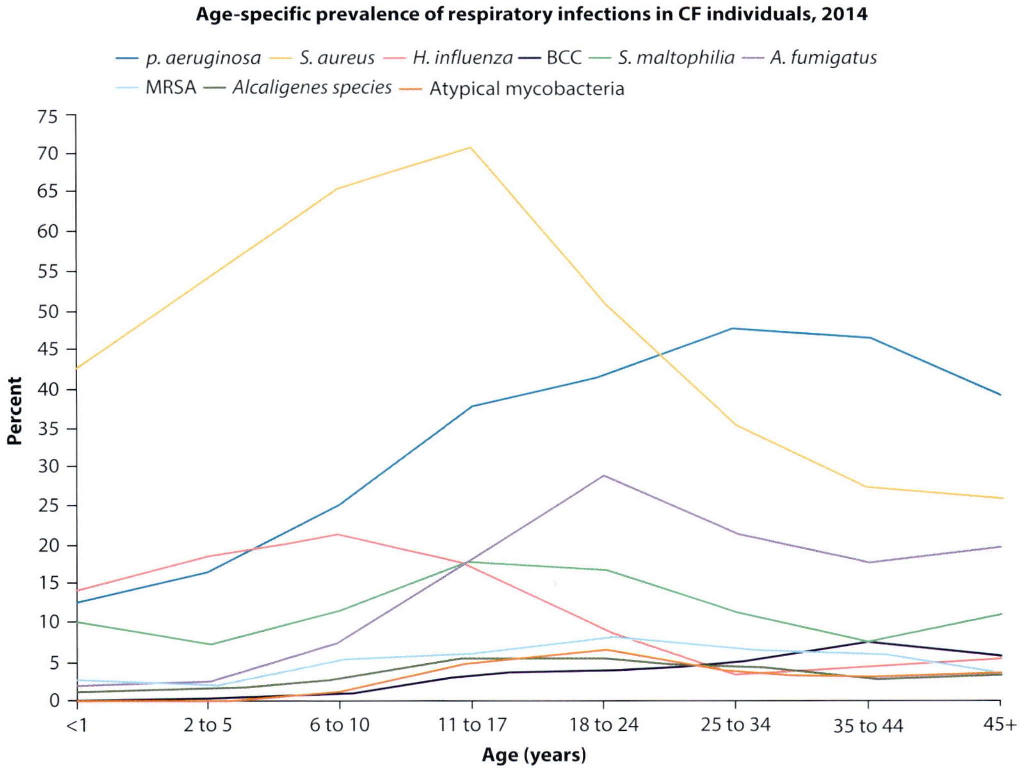

Figure 14.6 Prevalence of pulmonary infections in relation to patient age. (From The Canadian Cystic Fibrosis Registry, Annual Report 2014. www.fibrosekystique.ca.)

"exopolysaccharide alginate," a bacteria-coating substance that protects it from mucociliary clearance, immune host response, and antibiotics [46–48]. Another efficient survival mechanism relates to the production of "*P. aeruginosa* biofilms" [49]. According to this hypothesis, the bacteria initially multiply in microcolonies or biofilms. When the number of such microcolonies is large enough, they produce a capsular polysaccharide matrix that encapsulates them, thus preventing phagocytosis and antimicrobial agent penetration.

Other pathogens that can colonize the respiratory tract of CF patients include those of the *Burkholderia cepacia* species, which can be associated with accelerated decline in respiratory function. On occasion, patients infected with this species will have an associated very severe systemic reaction (cepacia syndrome), which can rapidly lead to patient death [50].

## Diagnosis

The diagnosis of CF relies on laboratory documentation of CFTR protein dysfunction or the presence of two CF-causing mutations associated with typical clinical manifestations, a history of CF in a sibling, or a positive newborn screening. Before the advent of newborn screening, the diagnosis of CF was essentially made on the basis of typical clinical symptoms such as those of chronic pulmonary or sinus infection, meconium ileus, failure to thrive, pancreatic failure, malnutrition, salt-depletion syndromes, and male infertility due to congenital absence of the vas deferens. Currently, most countries with high CF prevalence have implemented newborn screening programs that allow detection of the disease before the occurrence of clinical manifestations. The newborn screening consists of measuring the level of immunoreactive trypsinogen in the blood of newborns. An elevated level identifies newborns at risk of CF but it is not diagnostic. Therefore, additional evaluations such as sweat chloride testing or *CFTR* mutation detection must be done to confirm the diagnosis. Newborn screening protocols vary by center but the most frequently used method is measurement of immunoreactive trypsinogen followed by genetic testing [51].

Ever since it was validated in 1959, the sweat chloride test has become the gold standard to diagnose CF. The test consists of locally stimulating sweat secretion by pilocarpine iontophoresis. Once secretion has occurred, sweat is harvested and measurements of chloride concentration are obtained. A diagnosis of CF can be made when chloride sweat levels are equal to or greater than 60 mmol/L.

The diagnosis of CF can also be confirmed by the identification of two CF-causing mutations in each copy of the *CFTR* gene. Currently available tests allow for the detection of the commonest CF mutations that account for 90% of the mutations observed in the population. *CFTR* gene sequencing can be done to detect rare mutations [52].

## Principles of therapeutic interventions

There is currently no curative treatment for CF. Therapeutic strategies should therefore largely focus on prevention and management of disease-associated downstream consequences such as chronic pulmonary infections. This is best done by early and interdisciplinary management of such problems as well as patients being managed in specialized centers. Schematically, the basic principles of treatment should aim at preventing malnutrition, evacuating bronchial secretions, and treating efficiently bacterial infections.

The majority of CF patients have exocrine pancreatic insufficiency-associated malabsorption that can, in some cases, progress to severe malnutrition syndromes. In such cases, pancreatic enzymes, in the form of oral tablets, taken at every meal alleviate the problem. A nutritional regimen with hypercaloric diets and adequate daily hydration is also recommended to prevent malnutrition syndromes from occurring.

Active chest physiotherapy is very useful to help patients cough up thick and tenacious bronchial secretions and several techniques are available with comparable efficiency [53]. It is important, however, to adjust the use of physiotherapy techniques to patient needs. Medications can also be added as adjuvants to physiotherapy either to decrease bronchial secretion viscosity (mucolytic agents such as rhDNase) or improve ASL and airway rehydration (osmotic agents such as NaCl 7% solutions).

There are three important aspects to be considered when treating CF-associated respiratory infections and these include (1) early eradication of the bacteria P. aeruginosa, (2) treatment of chronic P. aeruginosa infection, and (3) treatment of acute respiratory exacerbations. When P. aeruginosa becomes apparent in bronchial secretions for the first time, it is usually sensitive to antibiotic treatment. At this stage, antibiotic treatment is indicated in order to eradicate it, thus avoiding chronic airway colonization. When treating chronic P. aeruginosa infection, long-term antibiotic nebulization treatment can be useful to prevent deterioration of pulmonary function, lower bacterial load and virulence, and control patient's symptomatology. To achieve this objective, the three most commonly used agents are tobramycin, colistin, and aztreonam. CF patients presenting with acute exacerbation of respiratory symptoms should be managed with systemic antibiotherapy [46].

## Conclusion and future perspectives

Ever since the discovery of the *CFTR* gene in 1989, our knowledge of CF pathophysiology has considerably improved. It has led to the development of new drugs targeting the underlying basic defect. These molecules are called CFTR potentiators and correctors. In the last few years, two of these drugs have become available to treat patients with specific mutations and several others are currently under investigation [54–55]. Research in the field of gene therapy has also made some progress recently. Such new and promising treatments could drastically change the management of CF patients in future years [56].

## References

1. Dupuis A, Hamilton D, Cole DEC et al. Cystic fibrosis birth rates in Canada: A decreasing trend since the onset of genetic testing. *J Pediatr* 2005; 147: 312–315.
2. Grebe TA, Seltzer WK, DeMarchi J et al. Genetic analysis of Hispanic individuals with cystic fibrosis. *Am J Med Genet* 1994; 54: 443–446.
3. Imalzumi Y. Incidence and mortality rates of cystic fibrosis in Japan, 1969–1992. *Am J Med Genet* 1995; 58: 161–168.
4. Hamosh A, Fitz-Simmons SC, Macek M Jr et al. Comparison of the clinical manifestations of cystic fibrosis in black and white patients. *J Pediatr* 1998; 132: 255–259.
5. Le Registre canadien sur la fibrose kystique, rapport annuel de 2014. www.fibrosekystique.ca.
6. Davis PB. Cystic fibrosis since 1938. *Am J Respir Crit Care Med* 2006; 173: 475–482.
7. Riordan JR, Rommens JM, Kerem B et al. Identification of the cystic fibrosis gene: Cloning and characterization of complementary DNA. *Science* 1989; 245: 1066–1073.
8. Sheppard DN, Welsh MJ. Structure and function of the CFTR chloride channel. *Physiol Rev* 1999; 79: s23–s45.
9. Akabas MH. Cystic fibrosis transmembrane conductance regulator. Structure and function of an epithelial chloride channel. *J Biol Chem* 2000; 275: 3729–3732.
10. Rowe SM, Miller S, Sorscher EH. Cystic fibrosis. *N Engl J Med* 2005; 352(19): 1992–2001.
11. Ratjen FA. Cystic fibrosis: Pathogenesis and future treatment strategies. *Respir Care* 2009; 54(5): 595–602.
12. The Cystic Fibrosis Mutation Database. http://www.genet.sickkids.on.ca/cftr.
13. Zielenski J, Tsui LC. Cystic fibrosis: Genotypic and phenotypic variations. *Annu Rev Genet* 1995; 29: 777–807.
14. Haardt M, Benharouga M, Lechardeur D et al. C-terminal truncations destabilize the cystic fibrosis transmembrane conductance regulator without impairing its biogenesis. A novel class of mutation. *J Biol Chem* 1999; 274: 21873–21877.
15. Rowntree RK, Harris A. The phenotypic consequences of CFTR mutations. *Annals of Human Genetics* 2003; 67: 471–485.
16. Veit G et al. From CFTR biology toward combinatorial pharmacotherapy: expanded classification of cystic fibrosis mutations. Molecular Biology of the Cell 2016; 27 :424-433.

17. Zielenski J. Genotype and phenotype in cystic fibrosis. *Respiration* 2000; 67: 177–233.
18. Koch C, Cuppens H, Rainisio et al. European Epidemiologic Registry of Cystic Fibrosis (ERCF): Comparison of major disease manifestations between patients with different classes of mutations. *Pediatr Pulmonol* 2001; 31: 1–12.
19. Mckone EF, Emerson SS, Edwards KL et al. Effect of genotype on phenotype and mortality in cystic fibrosis: A retrospective cohort study. *Lancet* 2003; 361: 11671–1676.
20. Kerem E, Corey M, Kerem BS et al. The relation between genotype and phenotype in cystic fibrosis--analysis of the most common mutation (delta F508). N Engl J Med 1990;323:1517-22.
21. Slieker MG, Sanders EA, Rijkers GT et al. Disease modifying genes in cystic fibrosis. *J Cyst Fibros* 2005; 4(Suppl 2): 7–13.
22. Sontag MK, Accurso FJ. Gene modifiers in pediatrics: Application to cystic fibrosis. *Adv Pediatr* 2004; 51: 5–36.
23. Donaldson SH, Boucher RC. Update on pathogenesis of cystic fibrosis lung disease. *Curr Opin Pulm Med* 2003; 9: 486–491.
24. Zabner J, Smith JJ, Karp PH et al. Loss of CFTR chloride channels alters salt absorption by cystic fibrosis airway epithelia in vitro. *Mol Cell* 1998; 2: 397–403.
25. Smith JJ, Travis SM, Greenberg EP et al. Cystic fibrosis airway epithelia fail to kill bacteria because of abnormal airway surface fluid. *Cell* 1996; 85: 229–236.
26. Jayaraman S, Song YL, Vetrivel L et al. Noninvasive in vivo fluorescence measurement of airway-surface liquid depth, salt concentration, and pH. *J Clin Invest* 2001; 107: 317–324.
27. Caldwell RAC, Grubb BR, Tarran R et al. In vivo airway surface liquid Cl-analysis with solid-state electrodes. *J Gen Physiol* 2002; 119: 3–14.
28. Knowles MR, Robinson JM, Wood RE et al. Ion composition of airway surface liquid of patients with cystic fibrosis as compared with normal and disease-control subjects. *J Clin Invest* 1997; 100: 2588–2595.
29. Tiddens HA, Donaldson SH, Rosenfeld M et al. Cystic fibrosis lung disease starts in the small airways: Can we treat it more effectively? *Pediatr Pulmonol* 2010; 45(2): 10–117.
30. Thelin WR, Boucher RC. The epithelium as a target for therapy in cystic fibrosis. *Curr Opin Pharmacol* 2007; 7(3): 290–295.
31. Elkins MR, Bye PT. Inhaled hypertonic saline as a therapy for cystic fibrosis. *Curr Opin Pulm Med* 2006; 12(6): 445–452.
32. Matsui H, Grubb BR, Tarran R et al. Evidence for periciliary liquid depletion, not abnormal ion composition, in the pathogenesis of cystic fibrosis airways disease. *Cell* 1998; 95: 1005–1015.
33. Tarran R, Grubb BR, Parsons D et al. The CF salt controversy: In-vivo observations and therapeutic approaches. *Mol Cell* 2001; 8: 149–158.
34. Kunzelmann K, Schreiber R, Nitschke R et al. Control of epithelial Na+ conductance by the cystic fibrosis transmembrane conductance regulator. *Pflugers Arch* 2000; 440: 193–201.
35. Pezzulo AA, Tang XX, Hoegger MJ, et al. Reduced airway surface pH impairs bacterial killing in the porcine cystic fibrosis lung. *Nature* 2012; 487: 109–13.
36 Gustafsson JK, Ermund A, Ambort D, et al. Bicarbonate and functional CFTR channel are required for proper mucin secretion and link cystic fibrosis with its mucus phenotype. J Exp Med 2012;209:1263–72.
37. Chimiel JF, Berger M, Konstan MW. The role of inflammation in the pathogenesis of CF lung disease. *Clin Rev Allergy Immunol* 2002; 23: 5–27.
38. Khan TZ, Wagener JS, Bost T et al. Early pulmonary inflammation in infants with cystic fibrosis. *Am J Respir Crit Care Med* 1995; 151: 1075–1022.
39. Muhlebach MS, Stewart PW, Leigh MW et al. Quantitation of inflammatory responses to bacteria in young cystic fibrosis and control patients. *Am J Respir Crit Care Med* 1999; 160: 186–191.

40. Balough K, McCubbin M, Weinberger M et al. The relationship between infection and inflammation in the early stages of lung disease from cystic fibrosis. *Pediatr Pulmonol* 1995; 20: 63–70.
41. Dakin CJ, Numa AH, Wang H, Morton JR et al. Inflammation, infection and pulmonary function in infants and young children with cystic fibrosis. *Am J Respir Crit Care Med* 2002; 165: 904–910.
42. Rosenfeld M, Gibson RL, McNamara S et al. Early pulmonary infection, inflammation and clinical outcomes in infants with cystic fibrosis. *Pediatr Pulmonol* 2001; 32: 356–366.
43. Amstrong DS, Grimwood K, Carlin JB et al. Lower airway inflammation in infants and young children with cystic fibrosis. *Cam J Respir Crit Care Med* 1997; 156: 1197–1204.
44. Emerson J, Rosenfeld M, McNamara S et al. *Pseudomonas aeruginosa* and other predictors of mortality and morbidity in young children with cystic fibrosis. *Pediatr Pulmonol* 2002; 34: 91–100.
45. Nixon GM, Armstrong DS, Carzino R et al. Clinical outcome after early *Pseudomonas aeruginosa* infection in cystic fibrosis. *J Pediatr* 2001; 138: 699–704.
46. Gibson RL, Burns JL, Ramsey BW. Pathophysiology and management of pulmonary infections in cystic fibrosis. *Am J Respir Crit Care Med* 2003; 168: 918–951.
47. Worltizsch D, Tarran R, Ulrick M et al. Effects of reduced mucus oxygen concentration in airway Pseudomonas infections of cystic fibrosis patients. *J Clin Invest* 2002; 109: 317–325.
48. Davies JC, Bilton D. Bugs, biofilms, and resistance in cystic fibrosis. *Respir Care* 2009; 54(5): 628–638.
49. Wagner VE, Iglewski BH. *P. aeruginosa* biofilms in CF infection. *Clin Rev Allergy Immunol* 2008; 35(3): 124–134.
50. Tablan OC, artone WJ, Doerhuk CF et al. Colonization of the respiratory tract with *Pseudomonas cepacia* in cystic fibrosis. Risk factors and outcomes. *Chest* 1987; 91 (4): 527–532.
51. Farrell PM, Rosenstein BJ, White TB et al. Guidelines for diagnosis of cystic fibrosis in newborns through older adults: Cystic Fibrosis Foundation consensus report. *J Pediatr* 2008; 153: s4–s14.
52. Flume PA, Robinson KA, O'sullivan BP et al. Cystic fibrosis pulmonary guidelines: Airway clearance therapies. *Respir Care* 2009; 54(4): 522–537.
53. Rosenfeld M, Sontag MK, Ren CL. Cystic Fibrosis Diagnosis and Newborn Screening. *Pediatr Clin N Am* 2016; 63: 599–615.
54. Ramsey BW, Davies J, Gerard McElvaney N et al. A CFTR potentiator in patients with cystic fibrosis and the G551D mutation. *N Engl J Med* 2011; 365: 1663–1672.
55. Wainwright CE, Elborn JS, Ramsey BW et al. Lumacaftor-ivacaftor in patients with cystic fibrosis homozygous for Phe508del CFTR. *N Engl J Med* 2015; 373: 220–231.
56. Ratjen F. New pulmonary therapies for cystic fibrosis. *Curr Opin Pulm Med* 2007; 13: 541–546.

# 15

# Bronchiectasis

LOUIS-PHILIPPE BOULET

| | |
|---|---|
| Introduction | 271 |
| Main etiologic factors | 272 |
| Other entities | 274 |
| Mechanisms of development of bronchiectasis | 275 |
| Clinical evaluation | 276 |
| Natural history of the disease | 277 |
| Basic principles of treatment | 277 |
| Conclusion | 279 |
| References | 279 |

## Introduction

We define the term "bronchiectasis" as a permanent widening (dilatation) of the bronchi, generally presenting clinically as a persistent cough with excessive phlegm production and recurrent respiratory infections. It can develop in one or many locations in the lungs. Bronchiectasis has been initially described by Laennec in 1819 as a "dilatation des bronches avec suppuration" meaning "bronchial dilation with production of purulent sputum" [1]. Bronchiectasis is often associated with recurrent respiratory infections, sometimes with unusual agents such as *Pseudomonas aeruginosa*. It is caused by a large number of disorders, but often results from a postinfectious inflammatory process (Table 15.1) [2].

The prevalence of bronchiectasis is not very well known and varies according to the region or country where studies have been done. A survey from the United States reports a prevalence of bronchiectasis of 4.2 for 100,000 individuals between the age of 18 and 34 and close to 272 for 100,000 individuals 75 years and above [3]. This prevalence indeed increases with age and is higher in women compared to men. It is variable according to the contributing conditions and remains to be defined for many of those. With the increased use of chest tomodensitometry, it has become obvious that this problem has been underdiagnosed. This entity has also often been confounded with chronic obstructive pulmonary disease (COPD) [4]. Radiological bronchiectasis without symptoms should, however, be differentiated, both in healthy subjects and in association with some pathologies, from those producing clinically significant symptoms, in order to provide appropriate treatment.

Bronchiectasis can be classified as cylindrical, varicose, saccular (cystic), or follicular, according to its appearance (Figure 15.1) [5,6]. Cylindrical bronchiectasis consists of a uniform dilatation of the bronchus. The term "varicose" means that it is more irregularly shaped, looking like a pearl necklace, while the cystic

Table 15.1 Etiology or risk factors of developing bronchiectasis

1. **Bronchial obstruction**
    a. Foreign body
    b. Obstructive neoplasm
    c. Infections (mycobacteria, etc.)
    d. Extrinsic airway compression (tumor, lymphadenopathy)
2. **Postinfectious**
    a. Postpneumonia
    b. Whooping cough
    c. Mycobacteria (*Mycobacterium tuberculosis, M. avium* complex)
    d. Measles
3. **Alterations of bronchial mucociliary defense mechanisms**
    a. Ciliary dyskinesia (primary or secondary)
    b. Kartagener syndrome
    c. Young's syndrome
4. **Immunodeficiency**
    a. Hypogammaglobulinemia
    b. HIV infection
    c. Neoplasm (including hematological diseases and myeloma)
    d. Connective tissue disease or inflammatory bowel disease
5. **Cystic fibrosis**
6. **Recurrent bronchial aspiration**
7. **Allergic bronchopulmonary aspergillosis**
8. **Rare diseases**
    a. Yellow nail syndrome
    b. Congenital cartilage development defect
        i. Mounier–Kuhn syndrome: Congenital tracheobronchomegaly
        ii. Ehlers-Danlos and Marfan syndrome: Disorder of connective tissue
    c. Williams–Campbell syndrome
    d. Bronchial atresia
    e. Diffuse panbronchiolitis (particularly in Japan)
9. **Other possible contributing causes**
    a. Gastroesophageal reflux disease (GERD)
    b. Pulmonary fibrosis (traction bronchiectasis)
    c. Sarcoidosis
    d. Postlung transplant
    e. Malnutrition and cachexia
    f. COPD/$\alpha$-1 antitrypsin deficiency

or saccular is round shaped. Finally, follicular bronchiectasis is characterized by the presence of lymphoid nodules in the bronchial wall, often found in diseases of the child. The clinical manifestations have no correlation with the pathological type of bronchiectasis [7].

## Main etiologic factors

There are many diseases leading to the development of bronchiectasis (Table 15.1). They can be associated with a localized process damaging the bronchi or to a systemic disease. With appropriate evaluation, their

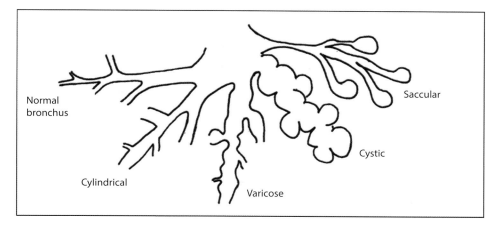

Figure 15.1 The various types of bronchiectasis.

etiology can be found in about half of the cases [8]. The most frequent causes are associated with bronchial obstruction, either intrinsic or extrinsic, with alterations of systemic or local lung defense mechanisms, often following respiratory infections, or in a context of systemic or multiorgan disease (Table 15.1).

The etiology of bronchiectasis is therefore unknown in about half of patients [9]. In a study from the United Kingdom on 150 adult patients with bronchiectasis, these abnormalities were considered to be associated with an immune defect ($n = 12$), cystic fibrosis ($n = 4$), Young's syndrome ($n = 5$), ciliary dysfunction ($n = 3$), bronchial aspiration ($n = 6$), diffuse panbronchiolitis ($n = 1$), congenital abnormality ($n = 1$), allergic bronchopulmonary aspergillosis ($n = 11$), rheumatoid arthritis ($n = 4$), and respiratory infection of childhood ($n = 44$), the cause being uncertain for the other patients. A more recent report from the European Bronchiectasis Network (EMBARC) found a cause of bronchiectasis in 60% of 1258 patients, the most common being postinfectious (20%), COPD (15%), rheumatic disorders (10%), and immunodeficiency (6%) [10].

Bronchiectasis can be limited to a lobe or widespread, the lower lobes being more often affected [11,12]. The "middle lobe syndrome," an entity frequently observed in the past, is attributed to the compression of the right middle lobe bronchus by lymph nodes, often secondary to a past tuberculous infection [13,14]. A similar compression of a bronchus could be found in the presence of a neoplasm or following atypical mycobacterial infections [15].

Obstructive causes of bronchiectasis include foreign body aspiration—mainly found in the right inferior lobe—obstructive endobronchial tumor, and respiratory infectious sequelae, particularly with bronchial stenosis [16]. It could also result from extrinsic compression by tumors or lymph nodes, as mentioned previously. This type of lesion is not always evident on chest radiograph and endoscopy is needed to detect the cause of obstruction [17].

Among the most frequent etiologies of bronchiectasis, we also find childhood respiratory infections such as pertussis, measles, influenza, adenovirus infections, or severe bronchiolitis. A bronchiolitis following a respiratory infection can be associated with structural damage and weakening of the bronchus, which favors bacterial colonization and chronic infection.

Chronic rhinosinusitis and primary ciliary dyskinesia are also frequently associated with bronchiectasis, particularly in patients with cystic fibrosis [18]. Nasal polyps are often found [19], and the analysis of secretions coming from the nose and sinus could reveal the presence of agents such as *Staphylococcus aureus*, *Haemophilus influenza*, and sometimes *Pseudomonas aeruginosa* [2,12,20].

In the presence of an alteration of body defense mechanisms, either systemic or acquired, or in the presence of congenital immunodeficiency associated with mucociliary dyskinesia, bronchiectasis is often a consequence of the difficulty to fight bronchial infection [21]. In primary mucociliary dyskinesia, there is a defect of the mucociliary system, with inefficient elimination of bronchial secretions that help keep the bronchial tree sterile [22]. Different types of structural abnormalities and/or ciliary function defects, and also the absence of ciliae, can lead to the development of bronchiectasis, but this problem is often associated with infections of other organs such as sinuses, and to infertility. Primary ciliary dyskinesia is an autosomal recessive disease of uncertain prevalence. It classically presents in childhood (although it is often identified only at a later age) as recurrent otitis media and sinusitis. Half of those patients will have dextrocardia. Young's syndrome is a rare subset of primary ciliary dyskinesia that presents as bronchiectasis, rhinosinusitis, and reduced fertility from azoospermia. Kartagener syndrome is characterized by dextrocardia, sinusitis, and bronchiectasis, mainly in lung bases and right middle lobe, as well as left middle lobe [23]. In primary dyskinesia, we find defects of the dynein arms, the site of adenosine triphosphatase (ATPase) activity, a structure necessary for the normal ciliary function in the bronchial epithelium [22,24]. This abnormality is also present at the level of the nasosinusal mucosa and these entities are therefore often diagnosed by nasal biopsy [25]. In this context, the measurement of nitric oxide (NO) usually brings low values in most patients [26].

When bronchiectasis is due to bronchial aspiration of material from the stomach, it is usually located in the inferior lobes. Another form of aspiration can be related to gastroesophageal reflux, with aspiration of gastric fluid, but the exact contribution of this problem in the development of bronchiectasis remains to be determined [27].

Allergic bronchopulmonary aspergillosis, an allergic response to *Aspergillus* colonizing the airways, can usually be found in asthmatic patients (sometimes in cystic fibrosis), the resulting chronic eosinophilic inflammatory process leading to the destruction of the bronchial wall and the development of central bronchiectasis [28]. It is important to make the diagnosis as proper treatment could improve symptoms and prevent further development of bronchiectasis. We also find the presence of antibodies against *Aspergillus* and high levels of immunoglobin E (IgE) associated to an intense bronchial and blood eosinophilia. Symptoms often include a cough productive of large volumes of thick phlegm, which may lead to a worsening of underlying asthma. Chest radiograph can show fleeting infiltrations. The usually central bronchiectasis are evident on chest computed tomography (CT).

Cystic fibrosis is an autosomal hereditary disease caused by a defect of the cystic fibrosis gene *cystic fibrosis transmembrane conductance regulator* (*CFTR*) localized on the long arm of chromosome 7q31.3 [29]. This disease affects 1 out of 2500 Caucasians and it is characterized by an increased chloride concentration in sweat, a pancreatic insufficiency, and progressive bronchiectasis mainly located in the upper lobes. In presence of manifestations such as clubbing, malnutrition, diabetes, exocrine pancreatic insufficiency, and a reduction of masculine fertility, the diagnosis should be considered. The mechanisms of development of bronchiectasis in this disease are associated with repeated infections in the context of an altered defense mechanism, related to the change in the physical properties of bronchial secretions, making them difficult to eliminate due to their increased viscosity and dehydration of the lining layer of airway fluid (see Chapter 14).

## Other entities

The presence of bronchiectasis has been increasingly recognized in patients with COPD, associated or not with a deficit in α-1 antitrypsin, following the increased use of chest tomodensitometry, with an estimated prevalence of 29%–50% of patients, particularly in those with frequent exacerbations of COPD [30,31]. In such cases, infections with Gram negative bacteria such as *P. aeruginosa* can be found [32,33]. There is certainly an overlap between COPD and bronchiectasis in some patients, sometimes called the "bronchiectasis–COPD overlap syndrome (BCOS)," although bronchiectasis can also be observed in the so-called "asthma–COPD overlap (ACO)." A study from the United Kingdom showed that 42.5% of patients with bronchiectasis had a diagnosis of asthma and 36.1% had a diagnosis of COPD [34]. This may however reflect the effect of bronchial dilatation on pulmonary function, although these obstructive diseases can also contribute to the development of bronchiectasis, possibly from associated respiratory infections/airway inflammatory processes.

Otherwise, bronchiectasis can be associated with multiple rare entities such as congenital diseases, general cachexia or fibrosing lung diseases (traction bronchiectasis), heart-lung or bone marrow transplant, and associated bronchiolitis [35].

Bronchiectasis has been found in 20%–35% of patients with rheumatoid arthritis, although at variable degrees [36,37]. Sjögren and Churg–Strauss syndromes [38,39] can be associated with bronchiectasis, following immunosuppression and traction phenomena caused by underlying fibrosis.

In the presence of hypogammaglobulinemia, repeated sinus and lung infections are usually documented since childhood, although respiratory infections may develop mostly in middle age. Finally, bronchiectasis may (although rarely) occur in hematological malignancies and myeloma, probably related to a deficit in immune function. HIV-related bronchiectasis seems to be related to recurrent infections, including those caused by mycobacteria.

The "yellow nail syndrome" is a rare condition associated with yellow nails, chronic respiratory disease, and pleural effusion from primary lymphedema. Mounier–Kuhn syndrome is a congenital disorder considered to be due to atrophy of elastic fibers of the trachea and main bronchi, leading to the dilatation of trachea (tracheobronchomegaly) and proximal bronchiectasis.

## Mechanisms of development of bronchiectasis

Bronchiectasis can be associated with a mild to moderate bronchial obstruction [40,41]. A "vicious circle" of bronchial damage of infectious origin or from other causes can develop in a subject genetically predisposed to be colonized by bacteria following a defect in mucociliary defense mechanisms. The persistence of bacteria in the airway causes a chronic inflammatory response that damages the bronchial wall. This could promote recurrent infections, with further damage to the airways (Figure 15.2).

A pathologic evaluation of 200 lung specimens with bronchiectasis has shown the presence of marked inflammation in the bronchial wall, particularly in small airways [42]. The zones of bronchial dilatation

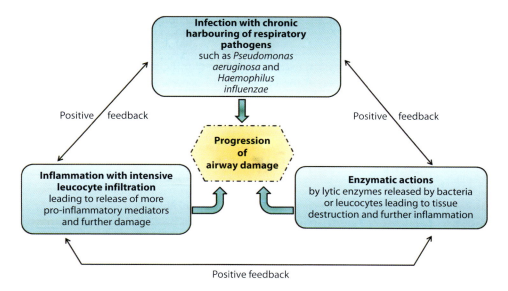

Figure 15.2 Clinical challenges in managing bronchiectasis. The pathogenesis of bronchiectasis showing the interactive pathogenic elements, namely infection, inflammation, and enzymatic actions. These interact to perpetuate the continued airway destruction in bronchiectasis. (Adapted from Tsang KW, Bilton D, *Respirology*, 14, 637–650, 2009.)

showed a loss of elastin and in the advanced form, a destruction of the airway muscle and bronchial cartilage. A variable fibrosis was noted as well as peribronchial and atelectatic changes. Follicular bronchiectasis is characterized by the presence of lymphoid follicles in the bronchial wall.

The inflammatory response associated with bronchiectasis is mostly neutrophilic [43]. The neutrophil is a cell producing enzymes such as proteases and elastases, involved in the destruction of the bronchial wall [44]. We can also find macrophages and lymphocytes, particularly T-lymphocytes, involved in the production of lymphoid follicles [45].

It is therefore probable that the three main elements interacting to produce bronchiectasis are the infectious, inflammatory, and enzymatic components (Figure 15.2) [46]. The association of these processes may cause a progressive destruction of the airways with the development of secondary bronchiectasis.

From 60% to 80% of patients with bronchiectasis are colonized by pathogenic microorganisms. A study of 89 patients with bronchiectasis over a period of 5 years showed initial colonization with *H. influenzae* in 47% of patients, 12% for *P. aeruginosa*, while there was no microorganism that could be identified in 21% of cases [47]. After a 5-year follow-up, 40% were colonized by *H. influenzae* and 18% with *Pseudomonas*. A correlation was noted between the presence of colonization by these agents and the severity of the disease. In general, it becomes almost impossible to eradicate the *Pseudomonas* despite repeated antibiotic treatment, and its proliferation brings exacerbations of variable frequency over time [48]. The persistence of these infections damages the various structural elements of the airways, particularly bronchial cilium [49].

In the presence of bronchiectasis, the inflammatory process could cause an alteration of local defense mechanisms and reduce elimination of secretions, therefore allowing the colonization with bacteria, notably following damage to the mucociliary apparatus [50]. An activation of T-lymphocytes, particularly of CD8 type, neutrophils, and macrophages can be observed [51,52].

Bronchial destruction could be promoted by a possible unopposed neutrophil elastase activity [53]. Neutrophils can also produce various mediators and cytokines, including leukotriene B4 (LTB4), interleukin-8 (IL-8), and tumor necrosis factor-alpha (TNF-α). LTB4 promotes neutrophil migration and degranulation. IL-1β mediates the inflammatory process and fibrosis, and TNF-α has a role in the elastolytic degradation of proteoglycans in the lung, interacting with IL-1 in the production of prostaglandins. IL-8 is a powerful chemoattractant, also inducing the activation of neutrophils [54]. However, increased sputum levels of human neutrophil peptides (alpha-defensins), which not only have antimicrobial properties but also impair neutrophil phagocytosis, have been found in patients with stable bronchiectasis [55].

In patients with bronchiectasis, adhesion molecules, involved in the migration of leukocytes in enflamed zones, can play a role in the persistence of the inflammatory process [56]. Finally, as discussed later, the destruction of the bronchial wall can result from the action of neutrophilic catalytic enzymes such as elastases or metalloproteinases, with a possible contribution of superoxide radicals [57]. Bacterial pathogens such as *Pseudomonas* can produce proteases, which cleave and disable CXCR1, reducing neutrophil recruitment and bacterial killing [58]. Contrary to this, antiproteases such as alpha-1 antitrypsin can restore CXCR1 and improve bacterial destruction. Furthermore, increased sputum viscosity can foster bacterial infections and bronchial damage.

Finally, a possible role of vitamin D deficiency in recurrent exacerbations of bronchiectasis was studied in 402 patients (50% were vitamin D deficient) with noncystic bronchiectasis over a period of 3 years [59]. Vitamin D-deficient patients had more sputum colonization with bacteria including *Pseudomonas*, more frequent respiratory symptoms and exacerbations, and increased sputum markers of neutrophil inflammation. More research is needed to confirm these observations and clarify the possible underlying mechanisms involved.

## Clinical evaluation

The diagnosis of bronchiectasis can be suspected clinically when large volumes of sputum are produced daily. Such chronic bronchorrhea of variable quantity, particularly in the nonsmokers, is associated with recurrent pulmonary infection. The diagnosis of bronchiectasis is confirmed by chest tomodensitometry, typically showing an increase in the internal diameter of the bronchus, which is superior to the adjacent pulmonary artery, and by an absence of reduction of the bronchial diameter at the periphery of the lung, with observable bronchi in the peripheral 2 cm of the lung [60] (Figure 15.3). In general, bronchial dilatation is observed in proximal bronchi after the fifth subdivision. Their topography can help suggest an etiology.

The quantity of bronchial secretions produced seems to be correlated with the decline in pulmonary function and quality of life [61]. A pleuritic chest pain can occur in 20%–30% of cases; hemoptysis is sometimes noted. According to the etiology, we can find an associated rhinosinusitis in about three out of four patients, dyspnea in two-thirds, and fatigue in about 75% [62]. Symptoms may have been present for many years at the time of diagnosis. On physical examination, crackling rales (crepitations) can be heard on chest auscultation, mostly basal and bilateral. Wheezing is also present in about one-fifth of patients while clubbing is rarely observed (but for cystic fibrosis).

Sinus radiograph or tomodensitometry can reveal an associated chronic rhinosinusitis. According to the suspicion of a specific etiology, some tests can be useful such as complete blood count, serum immunoglobulins (IgG, IgA, IgM, and IgE), evaluation of bronchial ciliary function, sweat test (cystic fibrosis), and dosage of rheumatoid factor, as well as different antibodies, skin prick test with *Aspergillus* and precipitins for this last, serum α1-antitrypsine or protein electrophoresis, bacterial culture, search for mycobacterial and fungal agents, and evaluation of response to antibiotics during a respiratory infection. Other more specialized tests are sometimes needed to confirm the diagnosis. Spirometry can reveal associated airway obstruction.

## Natural history of the disease

Pulmonary function of patients with bronchiectasis declines more rapidly with time than in normal subjects and we often observe the development of an obstructive syndrome of variable magnitude [63]. In regard to the clinical outcomes, there are four principal patterns [64]:

1. *Rapidly progressive bronchiectasis*: In general, these patients present with a rapid progression of the bronchiectasis with a development of bilateral cystic changes. These patients are usually young and have a marked bronchorrhea with systemic involvement.
2. *Slowly progressive bronchiectasis*: These patients have a slow progression of bronchiectasis over many decades with an increase in the frequency of exacerbations and an increasing volume of phlegm produced over time.
3. *Indolent disease*: Bronchiectasis often located in the right middle lobe, often asymptomatic and showing no progressive deterioration of the condition. This is probably a sequela of previous problem for which there is no residual inflammatory process.
4. *Hemoptysis*: Some patients have hemoptysis of variable quantities of blood as a main manifestation of their disease. This can require an intervention such as bronchial arterial embolization, and episodes of hemoptysis can be triggered by an underlying infection.

The prognosis of bronchiectasis has improved in the last decades, particularly for those associated with cystic fibrosis, but they remain a major cause of mortality, possibly up to 13% over a period of 5 years [65], particularly in the presence of hypoxemia, hypercapnia, or severe disease.

## Basic principles of treatment

There is generally no possible cure of bronchiectasis, but in some cases of localized bronchiectasis with repeated infections, a surgical intervention can be considered. We should pay attention, however, to the prevention and treatment of complications, particularly bronchial infections, for which respiratory

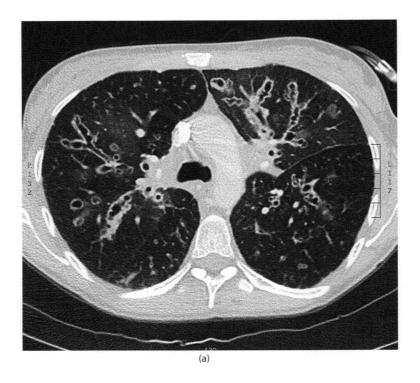
(a)

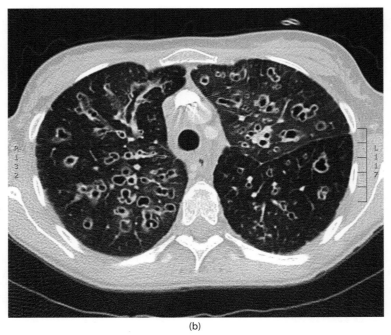
(b)

Figure 15.3 Chest tomodensitometry sections showing extensive bronchiectasis in a 26-year-old patient with cystic fibrosis.

physiotherapy and various techniques of elimination of bronchial secretions can be useful. A daily bronchial drainage can be facilitated by adequate hydration. Antibiotics are used to treat acute exacerbations and to prevent exacerbations in reducing the bacterial load [66]. In some cases, regular nebulization of antibiotics (tobramycin, colimycine, etc.) can be considered to maintain the number of bacteria at a minimum.

Bronchodilators and corticosteroids can be used in some patients, particularly in the presence of airway obstruction. Inhalation of mannitol has been proposed to promote phlegm production [67]; DNAse is a treatment often used in cystic fibrosis to decrease mucus viscosity and make secretions easier to eliminate. This latter treatment has no indication for other conditions associated with bronchiectasis [68]. The increase in viscosity is possibly due to the presence of polymers such deoxyribonucleic acid (DNA) coming from leukocytes. Pulmozyme (Dornase alfa) is a mucolytic agent made of recombinant human deoxyribonuclease I, which cleaves extracellular DNA to reduce mucus viscosity.

Contributing upper airway infectious processes should always be sought. Influenza and pneumococcal vaccines should be prescribed and treatment of baseline conditions is of course important.

## Conclusion

In conclusion, bronchiectasis is characterized by bronchial damage, secondary to an inflammatory process and generally postinfectious, which causes a permanent dilatation of the bronchi, making them less efficient in eliminating bronchial secretions. It is often associated with an obstructive syndrome of variable magnitude, but which can increase over time. The treatment of bronchiectasis consists mainly in the treatment and prevention of respiratory infections, respiratory physiotherapy, and in some cases of isolated bronchiectasis, surgical resection of the affected zone.

## References

1. Laennec RTH. In *A Treatise on Disease of the Chest, with Plates*. Translated from French of RTH Laennec, MD, with a preface and notes by John Forbes, MD. New York, NY: Hajner Publishing 1962. Originally published in London in 1821.
2. Morrissey BM. Pathogenesis of bronchiectasis. *Clin Chest Med* 2007; 28: 289–296.
3. Weycker D, Edelsberg J, Oster G, Tino G. Prevalence and economic burden of bronchiectasis. *Clin Pulm Med* 2005; 12: 205–209.
4. Tsang KW. Solutions for difficult diagnostic cases of acute exacerbations of chronic bronchitis. *Chemotherapy* 2001; 47 (Suppl. 4): S28–S38.
5. Reid L. Reduction in bronchial subdivisions in bronchiectasis. *Thorax* 1950; 5: 223–247.
6. Barker AF. Bronchiectasis. *N Engl J Med* 2002; 346: 1383–1393.
7. Cohen M, Sahn SA. Bronchiectasis in systemic diseases. *Chest* 1999; 116: 1063–1674.
8. Pasteur MC, Helliwell SM, Houghton SJ et al. An investigation into causative factors in patients with bronchiectasis. *Am J Respir Crit Care Med* 2000; 162: 277–284.
9. Pasteur MC, Helliwell SM, Houghton SJ et al. An investigation into causative factors in patients with bronchiectasis. *Am J Respir Crit Care Med* 2000; 162: 1277–1284.
10. Lonni S, Chalmers JD, Goeminne PC et al. Etiology of non-cystic fibrosis bronchiectasis in adults and its correlation to disease severity. *Ann Am Thorac Soc* 2015; 12: 1764.
11. King PT, Holdsworth SR, Freezer NJ et al. Characterisation of the onset and presenting clinical features of adult bronchiectasis. *Respir Med* 2006; 100: 2183–2189.
12. King PT. The pathophysiology of bronchiectasis. *Int J Chron Obstruct Pulmon Dis* 2009; 4: 411–419.
13. Graham EA, Burford TH, Mayer TH. Middle lobe syndrome. *Postgrad Med* 1948; 4: 29.
14. Albo RJ, Grimes OF. The middle lobe syndrome: A clinical study. *Dis Chest* 1966; 50: 509–518.

15. Bertelsen S, Struve-Christensen E, Aasted A et al. Isolated middle lobe atelectasis: Aetiology, pathogenesis, and treatment of the so-called middle lobe syndrome. *Thorax* 1980; 35: 449–452.
16. King PT, Holdsworth SR, Freezer NJ et al. Outcome in adult bronchiectasis. *J COPD* 2005; 2: 27–34.
17. Karakoc F, Cakir E, Ersu R et al. Late diagnosis of foreign body aspiration in children with chronic respiratory symptoms. *Int J Pediatr Otorhinolaryngol* 2007; 71: 241–246.
18. Robertson JM, Friedman EM, Rubin BK. Nasal and sinus disease in cystic fibrosis. *Paediatr Respir Rev* 2008; 9: 213–219.
19. Coste A, Gilain L, Roger G et al. Endoscopic and CT-scan evaluation of rhinosinusitis in cystic fibrosis. *Rhinology* 1995; 33: 152–156.
20. Wise SK, Kingdom TT, McKean L et al. Presence of fungus in sinus cultures of cystic fibrosis patients. *Am J Rhinol* 2005; 19: 47–51.
21. Verghese A, al-Samman M, Nabhan D et al. Bacterial bronchitis and bronchiectasis in human immunodeficiency virus infection. *Arch Intern Med* 1994; 154: 2086–2091.
22. Tsang KW, Tipoe GL, Zheng L. Ciliary assessment in bronchiectasis. *Respirology* 2000; 5: 91–98.
23. Tsang KW, Ip M, Ooi CG et al. Kartagener's syndrome: A re-visit with Chinese perspectives. *Respirology* 1998; 3: 107–112.
24. Omran H, Kobayashi D, Olbrich H et al. Ktu/PF13 is required for cytoplasmic pre-assembly of axonemal dyneins. *Nature* 2008; 456: 611–616.
25. Noone PG, Leigh MW, Sannuti A et al. Primary ciliary dyskinesia: Diagnostic and phenotypic features. *Am J Respir Crit Care Med* 2004; 169: 459–467.
26. Arnal JF, Flores P, Rami J et al. Nasal nitric oxide concentration in paranasal sinus inflammatory diseases. *Eur Respir J* 1999 Feb; 13 (2): 307–312.
27. Shi G, Bruley des Varannes S, Scarpignato C et al. Reflux related symptoms in patients with normal oesophageal exposure to acid. *Gut* 1995; 37: 457–464.
28. Agarwal R. Allergic bronchopulmonary aspergillosis. *Chest* 2009; 135: 805–826.
29. Tsui LC. Population analysis of the major mutation in cystic fibrosis. *Hum Genet* 1990; 85: 391.
30. Patel IS, Vlahos I, Wilkinson TM et al. Bronchiectasis, exacerbation indices, and inflammation in chronic obstructive pulmonary disease. *Am J Respir Crit Care Med* 2004; 170: 400–407.
31. O'Brien C, Guest PJ, Hill SL et al. Physiological and radiological characterisation of patients diagnosed with chronic obstructive pulmonary disease in primary care. *Thorax* 2000; 55: 635–642.
32. Eller J, Ede A, Schaberg T et al. Infective exacerbations of chronic bronchitis. Relation between bacteriologic etiology and lung function. *Chest* 1998; 113: 1542–1548.
33. Miravitlles M, Espinosa C, Fernandez-Laso E et al. Relationship between bacterial flora in sputum and functional impairment in patients with acute exacerbation of COPD. *Chest* 1999; 116: 40–46.
34. Quint JK, Millett ER, Joshi M et al. Changes in the incidence, prevalence and mortality of bronchiectasis in the UK from 2004 to 2013: A population based cohort study. *Eur Respir J* 2016; 47: 186–193.
35. Morehead RS. Bronchiectasis in bone marrow transplantation. *Thorax* 1997; 52: 392–393.
36. Cortet B, Flipo RM, Remy-Jardin M et al. Use of high resolution computed tomography of the lungs in patients with rheumatoid arthritis. *Ann Rheum Dis* 1995; 54: 815–819.
37. Hassan WU, Keaney NP, Holland CD et al. High resolution computed tomography of the lung in lifelong non-smoking patients with rheumatoid arthritis. *Ann Rheum Dis* 1995; 54: 308–310.
38. Larche MJ. A short review of the pathogenesis of Sjogren's syndrome. *Autoimmun Rev* 2006; 5: 132–135.
39. King P. Churg-Strauss syndrome and bronchiectasis. *Respir Med Extra* 2007; 3: 26–28.
40. Nicotra MB, Rivera M, Dale AM et al. Clinical, pathophysiologic, and microbiologic characterization of bronchiectasis in an aging cohort. *Chest* 1995; 108: 955–961.
41. Pasteur MC, Helliwell SM, Houghton SJ et al. An investigation into causative factors in patients with bronchiectasis. *Am J Respir Crit Care Med* 2000; 162: 1277–1284.
42. Whitwell F. A study of the pathology and pathogenesis of bronchiectasis. *Thorax* 1952; 7: 213–219.

43. Loukides S, Bouros D, Papatheodorou G et al. Exhaled $H_2O_2$ in steady-state bronchiectasis: Relationship with cellular composition in induced sputum, spirometry, and extent and severity of disease. *Chest* 2002; 121: 81–87.
44. Khair OA, Davies RJ, Devalia JL. Bacterial-induced release of inflammatory mediators by bronchial epithelial cells. *Eur Respir J* 1996; 9: 1913–1922.
45. Lapa e Silva JR, Guerreiro D, Noble B et al. Immunopathology of experimental bronchiectasis. *Am J Respir Cell Mol Biol* 1989; 1: 297–304.
46. Tsang KW, Bilton D. Clinical challenges in managing bronchiectasis. *Respirology* 2009 Jul; 14(5): 637–650.
47. King PT, Holdsworth SR, Freezer NJ et al. Microbiologic follow-up study in adult bronchiectasis. *Respir Med* 2007; 101: 1633–1638.
48. Ho PL, Lam WK, Ip MSM et al. The effects of Pseudomonas aeruginosa infection in clinical parameters in steady state bronchiectasis. *Chest* 1998; 114: 1623–1629.
49. Tsang KW, Rutman A, Kanthakumar K et al. *Haemophilus influenzae* infection of human respiratory mucosa in low concentrations of antibiotics. *Am Rev Respir Dis* 1993; 148: 201–207.
50. Prasad M, Tino G. Bronchiectasis: Part 1. Presentation and diagnosis. *J Respir Dis* 2007; 28: 545–554.
51. Zheng L, Shum H, Tipoe GL et al. Macrophages, neutrophils and tumour necrosis factor-alpha expression in bronchiectatic airways in vivo. *Respir Med* 2001; 95: 792–798.
52. Lapa e Silva JR, Guerreiro D et al. The immunological component of the cellular inflammatory infiltrate in bronchiectasis. *Thorax* 1989; 44: 668–673.
53. Chan SC, Leung VO, Ip MS et al. Shed syndecan-1 restricts neutrophil elastase from alpha1-antitrypsin in neutrophilic airway inflammation. *Am J Respir Cell Mol Biol* 2009; 41: 620.
54. Tsang KW, Ho PL, Lam WK et al. Inhaled fluticasone reduces sputum inflammatory indices in severe bronchiectasis. *Am J Respir Crit Care Med* 1998; 158: 723–727.
55. Voglis S, Quinn K, Tullis E et al. Human neutrophil peptides and phagocytic deficiency in bronchiectatic lungs. *Am J Respir Crit Care Med* 2009; 180: 159.
56. Zheng L, Tipoe G, Lam WK et al. Up-regulation of circulating adhesion molecules in bronchiectasis. *Eur Respir J* 2000; 16: 691–696.
57. Stockley RA. Neutrophils and protease/antiprotease imbalance. *Am J Respir Crit Care Med* 1999; 160: 49–52.
58. Hartl D, Latzin P, Hordijk P et al. Cleavage of CXCR1 on neutrophils disables bacterial killing in cystic fibrosis lung disease. *Nat Med* 2007; 13: 1423.
59. Chalmers JD, McHugh BJ, Docherty C et al. Vitamin-D deficiency is associated with chronic bacterial colonisation and disease severity in bronchiectasis. *Thorax* 2013; 68: 39.
60. McGuinness G, Naidich DP. CT of airways disease and bronchiectasis. *Radiol Clin North Am* 2002; 40: 1–19.
61. Martinez-Garcia MA, Perpina-Tordera M, Roman-Sanchez P et al. Quality-of-life determinants in patients with clinically stable bronchiectasis. *Chest* 2005; 128: 739–745.
62. Mal H, Rullon I, Mellot F et al. Immediate and long-term results of bronchial artery embolization for life-threatening hemoptysis. *Chest* 1999; 115: 996–1001.
63. Tsang KW, Bilton D. Clinical challenges in managing bronchiectasis. *Respirology* 2009; 14: 637–650.
64. King PT, Holdsworth SR, Freezer NJ et al. Outcome in adult bronchiectasis. *J COPD* 2005; 2: 27–34.
65. Keistinen T, Saynajakangas O, Tuuponen T et al. Bronchiectasis: An orphan disease with a poorly-understood prognosis. *Eur Respir J* 1997; 10: 2784–2787.
66. Evans DJ, Bara AI, Greenstone M. Prolonged antibiotics for purulent bronchiectasis. *Cochrane Database Syst Rev* 2003; 4: CD001392.
67. Daviskas E, Anderson SD, Eberl S et al. Inhalation of dry powder mannitol improves clearance of mucus in patients with ronchiectasis. *Am J Respir Crit Care Med* 1999; 159(6): 1843–1848.
68. O'Donnell AE, Barker AF, Ilowite JS et al. Treatment of idiopathic bronchiectasis with aerosolized recombinant human DNase I. rhDNase study group. *Chest* 1998; 113(5): 1329–1334.

# Index

## A

AAT, *see* Alpha-1 antitrypsin
Abnormal airway repair process, 81
Abnormal proteinase activity, 107
ABPA, *see* Allergic bronchopulmonary aspergillosis
Accelerated silicosis, 229
Acid-base equilibrium disturbance, carbon dioxide, 31
Acid–base status, carbon dioxide, 27–28
Acid homeostasis, carbon dioxide, 31
Acinus, 10
ACO, *see* Asthma–COPD overlap
Acquired form PALP, 196
Active chest physiotherapy, 266
Acute bronchopneumopathies, 238–239
Acute eosinophilic lung diseases, 194
Acute hypoxemia, 57
Acute inhalation accidents
  acute bronchopneumopathies from irritant gas exposures, 238–239
  asphyxiations, 240
  fever metals, 239
Acute interstitial pneumonia (AIP), 192

Acute respiratory distress syndrome (ARDS), 135, 137
Acute respiratory insufficiency
  hypercapnia treatment, 64
  hypercapnic respiratory insufficiency, 60
  hypoxemia treatment, 62
  hypoxemic respiratory insufficiency, 57
  mixed respiratory insufficiency, 60
  respiratory insufficiency, 56
  upper airways obstruction, 56
Acute silicosis, 229
Adaptive immunity, 106, 107
Adenocarcinomas, 211
Adenosine triphosphate (ATP)-binding cassette (ABC) transporters, 260
Adhesion molecules, bronchiectasis, 276
Affymetrix, 44
AHR, *see* Airway hyperresponsiveness
AIP, *see* Acute interstitial pneumonia
Air distribution network, respiratory system, 16
Airway eosinophilia, 77
Airway hyperresponsiveness (AHR), 75, 89–90
Airway inflammation, role of, 74, 75
Airway obstruction, 88, 102, 238
Airway remodeling, 80–83

Airways, dynamic compression of, 21
Airway surface liquid (ASL) volume, 263
Allele-specific extension reaction, 41
Allergic asthma, 77
  development of, 74
  model of, 84
Allergic bronchoconstriction, 84
Allergic bronchopulmonary aspergillosis (ABPA), 195, 274
Allergic march asthma, 74
Alpha-1-antichymotrypsin antiproteases, 110
Alpha-1 antitrypsin (AAT), 104
  deficiency, 184
Alveolar capillary exchange zones, 58
Alveolar hypoventilation, 58, 60
Alveolar hypoxia, 121
Alveolar macrophages, 77, 104, 105, 153, 158
Alveolar stage, lungs, 4
Alveolar ventilation, carbon dioxide, 26
Amphiboles, 226
Amphiboles asbestosis, 225
ANCA, *see* Antineutrophil cytoplasmic antibodies
Animal model system, 46, 48
Antigen-specific antibody, 35
Antineutrophil cytoplasmic antibodies (ANCA), 184

283

Antiproteinases, imbalance between proteinases and, 104
APAH, *see* Associated pulmonary hypertension
ARDS, *see* Acute respiratory distress syndrome
Asbestosis
  clinical picture, 226–228
  etiology, 225
  pathogenesis of, 226
ASL volume, *see* Airway surface liquid volume
Asphyxia, 240
Asphyxiations, 240
Aspirin-induced asthma, 86
Associated pulmonary hypertension (APAH), 124
Asthma, 33
  airway hyperresponsiveness, 89–90
  airway remodeling, 80–83
  aspirin-induced, 86
  characteristics of main categories, 72–73
  clinical expression of, 88
  definition and characteristics of, 68
  dendritic cells, 79
  epithelial cells, 79–80
  etiologic factors and phenotypes, 71
  genetic factors, 73
  main inflammatory cells playing role in, 77
  model of allergic, 84
  neurogenic mechanisms, 83
  nonallergic, 85
  pathogenesis of, 75
  physiologic changes in, 88–89
  prevention of, 90
  risk factors of, 70
  role of airway inflammation, 74, 75–76
  severe, 86–87
  T- and B-lymphocytes, 78
  therapeutic targets, 90–92
Asthma attacks, 86

Asthma–COPD overlap, (ACO), 88, 274
Autoantibodies, 107

**B**

Bacterial pathogens, bronchiectasis, 276
Bacterial pulmonary infections, 265
BAL, *see* Bronchoalveolar lavage
BALT, *see* Bronchus-associated lymphoid tissue
BALTs, *see* Bronchial associated lymphatic tissues
Basophils, 77
BCOS, *see* Bronchiectasis–COPD overlap syndrome
Berylliosis, 225, 230–231
Beryllium, 230
Besnier–Boeck–Schaumann disease, *see* Sarcoidosis
Bicarbonate system, pK of, 29
Bioactive asphyxiant gases, 240
Biomarker analysis, lung cancer, 219
Biopsies, interstitial lung diseases, 179
Black bands, 36
Blood distribution network, circulatory system, 16
B-lymphocytes, 78
B-lymphocyteslymphocyte, 107
Bone morphogenic protein receptor II (BMPR2), 124
Breathing (respiration), 164
  components of, 22
Breathing disorders, 164
Bronchi
  anatomy of, 5, 6
  histology of, 7, 8
Bronchial arteries, 11
Bronchial associated lymphatic tissues (BALTs), 107, 153
Bronchial biopsies, with occupational asthma, 234
Bronchial cartilage, 7

Bronchial epithelial cells, 81
Bronchial epithelium, 7
  cells of, 9
Bronchial glands, 7
Bronchial mucosa, 99
Bronchial thermoplasty, 92
Bronchiectasis, 271
  clinical challenges in, 275
  clinical evaluation, 276–277
  development mechanisms of, 275–276
  entities of, 274–275
  etiologic factors, 272–274
  history of, 277
  inflammatory process, 276
  treatment principles of, 277–279
Bronchiectasis–COPD overlap syndrome (BCOS), 274
Bronchioles, 5
  histology of, 10
Bronchoalveolar lavage (BAL), 35, 103, 179
  in hypersensitivity pneumonitis, 181
Bronchodilators, bronchiectasis, 279
Bronchopulmonary segments, 5
Bronchoscopy, lung cancer, 215, 216
Bronchus-associated lymphoid tissue (BALT), 12
Buffer concept, carbon dioxide, 29
Burkholderia cepacia, 266

**C**

Canalicular stage, lungs, 3
Cancers, occupational origin, 238
Carbamino group, 27
Carbamino-hemoglobin groups, 27
Carbon dioxide ($CO_2$)
  acid–base status, 27–28
  acid homeostasis, 31
  alveolar ventilation, 26
  buffer concept, 29
  Henderson–Hasselbalch equation, 30
  pH concept, 28–29
  pK, 29–30

Carbon monoxide (CO), intoxication, 240
Carboxyhemoglobin, 240
Cardio-respiratory system, functional anatomy, 16
Carina, 4
Carrington's disease, 194
Cas enzyme, 46
Cas9 system, 46
Cationic proteins, 84
Caucasian population, 259
CBD, *see* Chronic beryllium disease
CD4+ T-lymphocytes, 108
CD8+ T-lymphocytes, 108
Cellular immunity, 150–153
Cellular model system, 46, 48
Cellular respiration, respiratory mechanics, 24
Cellular senescence, 105
Central sleep apnea, 169–170
Centrilobular emphysema, lung with, 100
Centriole, 14
CF, *see* Cystic fibrosis
CF-associated respiratory infections, 267
CF gene defect, 261
CFTR, *see* Cystic fibrosis transmembrane conductance regulator
CHART, *see* Continuous hyperfractionated accelerated radiotherapy
Chemokines CXCL9/monokine, 109
Chemotaxis, 109
Chemotherapy, lung cancer, 217
Chest radiography, lung cancer, 215
Chest tomodensitometry bronchiectasis, 278
pulmonary fibrosis, 227
silicosis, 229
Cheyne–Stokes respiration, 170
Chlorine, 239
Chronic beryllium disease (CBD), 231
Chronic bronchitis, 98, 99

Chronic bronchorrhea, 276
Chronic eosinophilic lung diseases, 194–196
Chronic granulomatosis, 225
Chronic lung oxidative stress, 104
Chronic obstructive pulmonary disease (COPD), 71
 acute exacerbations of, 154–156
 exacerbation of, 110
 extrapulmonary repercussions of, 111
 mechanisms involved in pathogenesis of, 103
 repercussions on normal physiology of respiration, 101
 structural changes and remodeling, 98
 workplace induced, 237–238
Chronic rhinosinusitis, 273
Chronic thromboembolic pulmonary hypertension (CTEPH), 127, 129
Chrysotile, 225
Churg–Strauss syndrome, 275
Cigarette smoking, on lung immunity, effect of, 103
Circulatory pump, circulatory system, 16
Circulatory system, 16
Clara cells, 8
Classic silicosis, 228
Class III mutations, 261
Class II mutations, 261
Class I mutations, 261
Class IV mutations, 261
Class VI mutations, 261
Class V mutations, 261
Clinical translation, 59
Cloning technique, 45
Clustered regularly interspaced short palindromic repeats (CRISPR), 46
Coating process, 35
Columnar ciliated cells, 7
Community-acquired pneumonia (CAP), 157–158
Compensation mechanisms, 31
Complementary DNA (cDNA), 43

Congenital form PALP, 196
Connective tissue disease, 182–183
Continuous hyperfractionated accelerated radiotherapy (CHART), 217
COP, *see* Cryptogenic organizing pneumonia
COPD, *see* Chronic obstructive pulmonary disease
COPD pathogenesis, 109
Corticosteroids, bronchiectasis, 279
Cryptogenic organizing pneumonia (COP), 190, 191
Cylindrical bronchiectasis, 271
Cysteinyl leukotrienes, 86
Cystic bone defect, 193
Cystic bronchiectasis, 271
Cystic fibrosis (CF), 261, 274
 airway surface liquid volume, regulation of, 263
 CFTR protein, structure and function of, 260
 diagnosis, 266
 genotype and phenotype, correlations between, 261–262
 respiratory tract malfunction, 263–266
 therapeutic interventions, principles of, 266–267
Cystic fibrosis, respiratory epithelial ion flux in, 264
Cystic fibrosis transmembrane conductance regulator (CFTR), 259, 274
 structure and function of, 260
Cytokines, in hypersensitivity pneumonitis, 181

# D

Dead space, 59, 60
Deep vein thrombosis, 131
Dendritic cells, 79
Deoxyribonucleotides, 41

Index 285

Desquamative interstitial pneumonia (DIP), 191–192
Diffusion, respiratory mechanics, 23
DIP, see Desquamative interstitial pneumonia
Direct labeling method, 35
Disease-causing mutations, classification of, 261
DNA fragments, 36
DNAse, bronchiectasis, 279
Drugs, interstitial lung diseases by, 182
Dust fever, 239
Dynamic hyperinflation, 101
during exercise, 102

### E

EBUS bronchoscopy, see Endobronchial ultrasound bronchoscopy
Efferocytosis, reduction in, 106, 107
EGFR, see Estimated glomerular filtration rate
EGPA, see Eosinophilic granulomatosis with polyangiitis
Elastin, 104
Electrical signals, 38
Electrophoresis, 37
ELISA, see Enzyme-linked immunosorbent assay
EMBARC, see European Bronchiectasis Network
Embryonal stage, lungs, 2
Emphysema, 98, 99
ENaC, see Epithelial sodium channel
Endobronchial ultrasound (EBUS) bronchoscopy, 217
Endocrine syndromes, 210
Enzyme-linked immunosorbent assay (ELISA), 35
Eosinophilic granulomatosis with polyangiitis (EGPA), 195
Eosinophilic lung disease, 194
Eosinophils, 77
Epithelial cells, 79–80
Epithelial ion flux, 263–264
Epithelial lesions, 189
Epithelial sodium channel (ENaC), 260
Equal pressure point (EPP), 21
Esophageal endoscopic ultrasound (EUS), 217
Estimated glomerular filtration rate (EGFR), 212
European Bronchiectasis Network (EMBARC), 273
EUS, see Esophageal endoscopic ultrasound
Exchange surfaces, lungs, 9
Exercise-induced asthma, 86
Expiration, sequential unfolding of, 18
Extrapulmonary tuberculosis, 160
Extrinsic allergic alveolitis, see Hypersensitivity pneumonitis
Extrinsic bronchial compressions, 57
Extrinsinc allergic alevolitis, 236

### F

FeNO, see Fractional nitric oxide concentration
Fever metals, 239
Fibronectin, 226
Fibrosing pneumoconiosis, 225
Flow cytometric analysis, 39
Fluorophore, 38
Follicular bronchiectasis, 271, 276
Forced expiratory volume curve, 69
Fractional nitric oxide concentration (FeNO), 90
FRC, see Functional residual capacity
Free silica, 228
Functional residual capacity (FRC), 17

### G

Gas exchange
circulatory system, 17
repercussions on, 102
respiratory system, 16
Gastroesophageal reflux (GOR), 68
GeneChip, 43
Gene-editing method, 46
Gene sequencing, 41
Genetic predispositions, 109
Genetics, 261–262
Genome-wide CRISPR-Cas9 screen, 46
Genotype and phenotype, correlations between, 261–262
Ghon complex, 160
GINA report, see Global Initiative for Asthma report
Global Initiative for Asthma (GINA) report, 68
Globin, 24
GM-CSF protein, in PALP, 196
GOR, see Gastroesophageal reflux
Granulomatosis with polyangiitis (GPA), 183

### H

Haemophilus influenza, 152, 265
Haemophilus parainfluenza, 152
Haldane effect, 64, 102
Hamman–Rich syndrome, see Acute interstitial pneumonia
Hans–Schüller–Christian syndrome, 192
HeLa cells, 48
Hematoxylin-eosin stain, bronchioles, 10
Hemoglobin desaturation curve, 24
Hemoptysis, 277
Henderson–Hasselbalch equation, 30
Hepatopulmonary syndrome, 139, 140

Hereditary pulmonary hypertension (HPAH), 124
HESs, see Hypereosinophilic syndromes
High-resolution chest tomodensitometry (HRCT), 179
Histiocytosis X, see Langerhans cells histiocytosis
Histochemistry, 34
HIV-related bronchiectasis, 275
Hospital-acquired pneumonia (HAP), 157
HP, see Hypersensitivity pneumonitis
HPAH, see Hereditary pulmonary hypertension
HRCT, see High-resolution chest tomodensitometry
Human Genome Project, 40, 41
Humoral and cellular immunity, 150
Humoral immunity, 150
"Hygiene hypothesis" attributes, 70
Hypercapnia, 60, 102
    treatment for, 64
Hypercapnic respiratory insufficiency, 60
Hypereosinophilic syndromes (HESs), 195
Hypermethylation, 41
Hypersensitivity pneumonitis (HP), 180–181, 236
Hypogammaglobulinemia, 275
Hyponatremia, 210
Hypoxemia, 59, 102, 133, 140
    treatment of, 62
    vs. hypoxia, 63
Hypoxemic respiratory insufficiency, 57
Hypoxia, hypoxemia vs., 63

# I

ICS, 91
Idiopathic HES, 195
Idiopathic ILDs
    acute interstitial pneumonia, 192
    cryptogenic organizing pneumonia, 190, 191
    desquamative interstitial pneumonia, 191–192
    idiopathic pulmonary fibrosis, 187–189
    nonspecific interstitial pneumonitis, 189–190
Idiopathic interstitial pneumopathies, 187
Idiopathic pulmonary fibrosis (IPF), 187–189
Idiopathic pulmonary hypertension (IPAH), 124
IgA, see Immunoglobulin A
IgE, see Immunoglobulin E
IgG, see Immunoglobulin G
IgM, see Immunoglobulin M
IHC, see Immunocytochemistry
ILDs, see Interstitial lung diseases
Illumina, 44
IL-12 proteins, 35
Immune defense mechanism, 154
Immune type 1 response, 84
Immunocytochemistry (IHC), 34
Immunoglobulin A (IgA), 152
Immunoglobulin E (IgE), 74
Immunoglobulin G (IgG), 152
Immunoglobulin M (IgM), 152
Indirect labeling technique, 35
Indolent disease, 277
Industrial chronic bronchitis, workplace induced, 237–238
Infection, 265–266
Inflammatory defense mechanism, 154
Innate immunity, 103
Innate lymphoid cells, 78
Innervation, lungs, 12
Inspiration, sequential unfolding of, 18
Interstitial lung diseases (ILDs)
    acute eosinophilic lung diseases, 194
    bronchoalveolar lavage, 179
    causes of, 178
    chronic eosinophilic lung diseases, 194–196
    connective tissue disease, 182–183
    by drugs, 182
    hypersensitivity pneumonitis, 180–181
    idiopathic ILDs, see Idiopathic ILDs
    Langerhans cells histiocytosis, 192–193
    pneumoconiosis, 181
    pulmonary alveolar lipoproteinosis, 196
    pulmonary interstitium, 179
    sarcoidosis, 184–186
    by toxic/physical exposures, 181–182
    vasculitis, 183–184
Intracardiac shunt, 57
Intrapulmonary shunt, 58
Invasive interface, 62
IPAH, see Idiopathic pulmonary hypertension
IPF, see Idiopathic pulmonary fibrosis
Iron recycling (reduction), 105

# K

Kartagener syndrome, 274

# L

LABA, see Long-acting β2-agonist bronchodilators
LAM, see Lymphangioleiomyomatosis
LAMA, see Long-acting muscarinic antagonist bronchodilators
Langerhans cells histiocytosis (LCH), 192–193
Larynx, anatomy of, 5, 6
LCH, see Langerhans cells histiocytosis
Left lower lobar (LLL) bronchi, 4
Left upper lobar (LUL) bronchi, 4
Leukotriene antagonists, 90
Lingula, 5
Löffler syndrome, 194

Long-acting β2-agonist bronchodilators (LABA), 110
Long-acting inhaled β2 agonist (LABA), 86
Long-acting muscarinic antagonist bronchodilators (LAMA), 110
Lower airways, 1
Lower respiratory tract, infections of, 153
Lung adenocarcinoma, histologic patterns of, 211
Lung asbestosis, diagnosis of, 227
Lung cancer, 207
  death rate, 209
  diagnosis and staging, 213–217
  histopathologic classification, 210–212
  molecular events in development, 212–213
  risk factors, 207–208
  signs and symptoms of, 209–210
  treatment and prognosis, 217–220
Lung damage, cause of, 103
Lung hyperinflation, 102
Lung parenchyma, 100
Lungs
  alveolar stage, 4
  bronchopulmonary segments, 6
  canalicular stage, 3–4
  embryonal stage, 2
  exchange surfaces, 9–11
  innervation, 12–13
  lymphatic drainage, 12
  pseudoglandular stage, 3
  ultrastructure, 13–14
  vasculature, 11
Lung with centrilobular emphysema, 100
Lymphangioleiomyomatosis (LAM), 194
Lymphatic drainage, lungs, 12
Lymphocyte activation, 108
Lymphocytes, in hypersensitivity pneumonitis, 180

Lymphoid follicles, 107
Lymphoid tissue, 12

## M

Macrolides, 111
Macrophages, 77
Macroscopic PAVMs
  clinical presentation, 137–139
  overview and pathogenesis, 137
Magnetic resonance imaging (MRI), 215
MAPK, see Mitogen-activated protein kinases
Mast cells, 77
Mean pulmonary artery pressure (mPAP), 120, 122
  and cardiac output relationship, 123
Mechanical ventilation
  hypercapnia treatment, 64
  hypoxemia treatment, 62
Medications, 266
Messenger RNA (mRNA), 36
Metachromatic cells, 77
Metastatic nonsmall-cell lung cancer
  chemotherapy, 217
  paradigm shift in treatment of, 218
Methacholine test, 89
Methylation, 41
  detection of, 42
Microscopic arteriovenous malformations
  clinical presentation, 140
  overview and pathogenesis, 139–140
Middle lobe syndrome, 273
Minute ventilation, 64
Mitogen-activated protein kinases (MAPK), 226
Mixed respiratory insufficiency, 60
Molecular cloning, 45
Monocyte-derived dendritic cell, 153
Monocytes, 77
Mortality
  from PAH, 129

  from pulmonary embolism, 133
MOTT, see Mycobacteria other than tuberculosis
Mounier–Kuhn syndrome, 275
Mouse models, 48
MRI, see Magnetic resonance imaging
mRNA, see Messenger RNA
Mucins, 150
Mucociliary clearance, 150
Mucoviscidosis, 261
  airway surface liquid volume, regulation of, 263
  CFTR protein, structure and function of, 260
  diagnosis, 266
  epithelial ion flux, 263–264
  genetics, 261–262
  infection, 265–266
  therapeutic interventions, principles of, 266–267
Multiple secondary antibodies, 35
Multiplex PCR, 41
Multiplex real-time PCR, 43
Mycobacteria other than tuberculosis (MOTT), 160
Mycobacterium tuberculosis (Tuberculosis bacillus) (MTB) infections, 159

## N

Nasal polyps, 87, 273
Nasal prongs, 62
Neuroepithelial body, 8
Neuropeptides, 234
Neutrophils, 77, 104, 276
Nocturnal hypoventilation, 164
  causes of, 165
  pathophysiology of, 164–165
Nonallergic asthma, 85
Nonatopic asthma, 77
Nonhomologous end joining (NHEJ) mechanism, 46
Nonobstructive respiratory disorders, 169
Non-oneself molecules, 106

# Index

Nonrapid eye movement (NREM) sleep, 164
Nonrespiratory bronchioles, 5, 8
Nonsmall-cell lung carcinomas, 210, 211
  histochemical and immunohistochemical stains, 212
Nonspecific interstitial pneumonitis (NSIP), 189–190
Northern blot technique, 36
Nosocomial pneumonia, 157
NREM sleep, see Nonrapid eye movement sleep
NSIP, see Nonspecific interstitial pneumonitis
Nylon membrane, 36

## O

Obstructive sleep apnea (OSA)/hypopnea syndrome, 165–166
Obstructive sleep-related breathing disorders, 168
Occupational asthma
  bronchial provocation test, 234
  etiology, 231
  evaluation of, 236
  history of, 237
  mechanisms of, 235
Occupational bronchitis, 238
Occupational COPD, 237
Occupational exposure, lung cancer, 208
Occupational infections, 238
Occupational respiratory diseases, 224
  acute inhalation accidents, 238–240
  asbestosis, 225–228
  berylliosis, 230–231
  epidemiology and prevalence, 225
  hypersensitivity pneumonitis, 236–237
  industrial chronic bronchitis, 237–238
  infections, 238
  occupational asthma, see Occupational asthma
  pneumoconiosis, 224–225
  siderosis, 230
  silicosis, 228–230
ODTS, see Organic dust toxic syndrome
Oligonucleotides, 43
Oral mucous telangiectasia, 138
Organic dust toxic syndrome (ODTS), 239
Organized pneumonia, causes and diseases associated with, 190
Oropharyngeal secretions, aspiration of, 152
Overall murine immune system, 48
Overload pneumoconiosis, 225
Oxidative stress, 105, 107
Oxygen carriage, respiratory mechanics, 24
Oxygen therapy
  hypercapnia treatment, 64
  hypoxemia treatment, 62
Oxyhemoglobin dissociation curve, 25

## P

PALP, see Pulmonary alveolar lipoproteinosis
Panlobular emphysema (PLE), 99
Parasitic pneumonia, 195
Parenchymal destruction, 102
Pattern recognition receptors (PRRs), 153
PAVMs, see Pulmonary arteriovenous malformations
PCI, see Prophylactic cerebral irradiation
PCR, see Polymerase chain reaction
PCWP, see Pulmonary capillary wedge pressure
Peribronchiolar plexus, 13
Perimuscular soft tissues, UA muscles and, 168
PET, see Positron emission tomography
PH, see Pulmonary hypertension
Phagocytosis, and inflammatory reaction, 153
pH concept, carbon dioxide, 28–29
Phenotype, 71
  and genotype, correlations between, 261–262
Phosphodiesterase-4 (PDE-4), 111
Phrenic nerve, 56
p$K$, carbon dioxide, 29–30
PLE, see Panlobular emphysema
Pleural plaques, 227
Pleuroparenchymal fibroelastosis (PPFE), 192
Pneumoconiosis, 181
  asbestosis, 225–228
  berylliosis, 230–231
  categories of, 225
  defined, 224
  siderosis, 230
  silicosis, 228–230
Pneumonia, 149
  community-acquired, 157–158
  defined as, 156
  viral pneumonia, 158
Polymerase chain reaction (PCR), 38, 39
Polymorphism, 110
Positron emission tomography (PET), 216
Postexercise bronchial vasodilation, 86
Postradiation organized pneumonia, 181
Potentially immunogenic neo-molecules, 106
PPFE, see Pleuroparenchymal fibroelastosis
Pressure–volume curve, respiratory mechanics, 17
Primary cell lines, 48
Primary ciliary dyskinesia, 273, 274
Primary HES, 195
Primary mucociliary dyskinesia, 273

Prophylactic cerebral irradiation (PCI), 218
Proteases, 104
Proteinases, and antiproteinases, 104
PRRs, *see* Pattern recognition receptors
Pseudoglandular stage, lungs, 3
Pseudomonas aeruginosa, 111, 265, 267
Pulmonary alveolar lipoproteinosis (PALP), 196
Pulmonary arterial hypertension (PAH), 124, 128
   nongenetic anomalies in, 129
Pulmonary arteries, 11
Pulmonary arteriovenous malformations (PAVMs)
   macroscopic PAVMs, 137
   microscopic arteriovenous malformations, 139
Pulmonary capillary wedge pressure (PCWP), 122
Pulmonary circulation, of blood, 11
Pulmonary edema
   clinical manifestations and treatment, 136–137
   overview of, 134–136
   pathophysiology, 136
   pulmonary arteriovenous malformations, *see* Pulmonary arteriovenous malformations
   types of, 135
Pulmonary embolism
   defined as, 131
   diagnosis of, 134
   pathogenesis, 131–132
   pathophysiology, 133
   prognosis and treatment, 133–134
Pulmonary fibrosis, chest tomodensitometry, 227
Pulmonary function
   repercussions on, 101
   tests, 88

Pulmonary hypertension (PH)
   causes of, 124
   chronic thromboembolic pulmonary hypertension, 127
   clinical classification of, 125
   clinical manifestations and diagnosis, 128
   normal pulmonary hemodynamics, 120–122
   physiopathology of, 122–124
   principal categories of, 127
   prognosis, 129
   treatment, 128
   types of, 126
Pulmonary infections, prevalence of, 265
Pulmonary inflammatory response
   effect of pharmacological treatment on, 110
   intensification of, 110
Pulmonary innate immune cells, 103
Pulmonary interstitium, 179
Pulmonary Langerhans histiocytosis, 192
Pulmonary lobule, 9
Pulmonary mycobacterial diseases, 158
Pulmonary vascular diseases, 120
Pulmonary vascular resistance (PVR), 120, 121
   lung volumes influence on, 122
PVR, *see* Pulmonary vascular resistance
Pyrosequencing, 41

## Q

Quantitative flow cytometry analysis, 38

## R

Radiation fibrosis, 181
Radiation pneumonitis, 181
Radiation therapy, lung cancer, 217

Radiological bronchiectasis, 271
Radiotherapy for lung diseases, 181
Radon exposure, lung cancer, 208
RADS, *see* Reactive airways dysfunction syndrome
Rapid eye movement (REM) sleep, 164
Rapidly progressive bronchiectasis, 277
RB-ILD, *see* Respiratory bronchiolitis-interstitial lung disease
Reactive airways dysfunction syndrome (RADS), 231
Reactive oxygen species (ROS), 104
Real-time PCR, 43
REM sleep, *see* Rapid eye movement sleep
Rendu–Osler–Weber disease, 137
Respiratory bronchioles, 5, 8
Respiratory bronchiolitis-interstitial lung disease (RB-ILD), 191–192
Respiratory epithelial ion flux, in cystic fibrosis, 264
Respiratory insufficiency, 56
Respiratory manoeuvres, 22
Respiratory mechanics
   carbon dioxide physiology, *see* Carbon dioxide
   cellular respiration, 24–25
   diffusion, 23–24
   dynamic compression of airways, 21
   inspiration and expiration, sequential unfolding, 18–19
   oxygen transport, 24
   pressure–volume curve, 17–18
   resistive characteristics, 19–20
   respiratory manoeuvres, 22
   tissue oxygenation, 22
   ventilation/perfusion ratio, 22–23
Respiratory syncytial virus (RSV), 70
Respiratory system, 1

air distribution network, 16
anatomic structures of, 2
carbon dioxide physiology, 26
components of, 16
development of, 3
protection mechanism of, 151
resistive characteristics of, 19
Respiratory tract epithelial cells, 152
Respiratory tract infections, 149
  atypical mycobacteria, 160
  chronic obstructive pulmonary disease, 154–156
  community-acquired pneumonia, 157–158
  humoral and cellular immunity, 150–153
  lower respiratory tract infections, 153
  normal host defense mechanisms, 150
  pneumonia, 156–157
  tuberculosis, 159–160
  viral pneumonia, 158
Respiratory tract malfunction, 263–266
Rheumatoid arthritis, 275
Rhinoviruses, 70
Right lower lobe (RLL) bronchus, 4
Right middle lobe (RML) bronchus, 4
Right upper lobe (RUL) bronchus, 4
RSV, see Respiratory syncytial virus

## S

Saccular bronchiectasis, 271
Saccular stage, lungs, 4
Sarcoidosis, 184–186
SDS, see Sodium dodecyl sulfate
Secondary antibody, 35
Secondary form PALP, 196
Secondary HES, 195
Secondary smoking, 208
Secondary tuberculosis, 159
Sequenom iPLEX technology, 41
Serpentine asbestosis, 225

Severe asthma, 86
Shunt, 57, 59
Siderosis, 230
Silicosis
  etiology, 228
  forms of, 228–230
Single-nucleotide polymorphisms (SNPs), 41
Sinus radiograph, chronic rhinosinusitis, 277
Sjögren syndrome, 183
Sleep-related breathing disorders, 163
  central sleep apnea, 169–170
  nocturnal hypoventilation, 164–165
  OSA/hypopnea syndrome, 165–166
  terminology and consequences of, 164
  UA dilating muscle contraction, 166–169
Slowly progressive bronchiectasis, 277
SLPI, 87
Small-cell carcinoma, 211, 212
  chemotherapy, 217
Smoking, 207, 209
SNPs, see Single-nucleotide polymorphisms
Sodium dodecyl sulfate (SDS), 36
Southern blot technique, 36
Spontaneous pneumothorax, 193
Sputum-guided treatment, 88
Squamous cell carcinoma, 211
Staphylococcus aureus, 265
Sulfuric anhydride ($SO_2$), 239
Supplementary oxygen, 64
Surface tension forces, role in UA muscles, 169
Surfactants, in hypersensitivity pneumonitis, 181
Systemic circulation, of blood, 11

## T

Terminal bronchioles, 5
Th2 cells, 85
T "helper" lymphocytes, 158

T helper type 2 (Th2)-type lymphocytes, 70
Therapeutic interventions, principles of, 266–267
Thromboembolic disease, manifestations of, 131
Tissue inflammation, role in UA muscles, 169
Tissue inhibitors of metalloproteinase-2 (TIMP-2) genes, 110
Tissue oxygenation, respiratory mechanics, 22
Tissues, traditional staining methods in, 34
T-lymphocyte chemotaxis, 109
T-lymphocytes, 78
TNF-related apoptosis-inducing ligand (TRAIL), 109
TNM staging system, see Tumor, node and metastases staging system
Tobacco smoke, 103
Tomodensitometry, chronic rhinosinusitis, 277
Tracer, 35
Trachea, anatomy of, 5, 6
Traditional staining methods, in tissues, 34
Transbronchial biopsies, interstitial lung diseases, 179
Transforming growth factor-β (TGF-β), 77
Tropical pulmonary eosinophilia, see Parasitic pneumonia
Tuberculosis, 159–160
Tumor, node and metastases (TNM) staging system, 213, 214
Type II pneumocytes, 10, 14, 150
Type I pneumocytes, 150

## U

UACS, see Upper airway cough syndrome
UA dilating muscle contraction, 166–169

Ultrastructure, lungs, 13
United airways disease, 74
Upper airway colonization, risk factors for, 152
Upper airway cough syndrome (UACS), 68
Upper airway (UA) muscles
  activity level fluctuations of respiratory, 168–169
  clinical applications, 169
  closing and reopening mechanisms, 167
  interfering factors, muscle physiological properties, 167–168
  mechanical coupling, muscles and perimuscular soft tissues, 168
  shape and cross-sectional area, 166
Upper airways obstruction, 56–57
Upper respiratory tract
  anatomical and mechanical barriers of, 150
  infections of, 153

## V

VAP, *see* Ventilation-associated pneumonia
Varicose bronchiectasis, 271
Vascular endothelial growth factor (VEGF), 109
Vascular pressure waves, measurement of, 121
Vasculature, lungs, 11
Vasculitis, 183–184
VEGF, *see* Vascular endothelial growth factor
VEGFR2 receptors levels, 109
Ventilation, 56
  respiratory mechanics, 22
Ventilation-associated pneumonia (VAP), 157
Ventilation interfaces, 63
Ventilation/perfusion (V/Q) imbalances, 158
Ventilation/perfusion ratio, respiratory mechanics, 22, 23
Ventilatory pump, respiratory system, 16
Venturi mask, 62
Viral pneumonia, 158
Viral respiratory infections, 158
Vitamin D deficiency, 276
V/Q ratio abnormalities, 58

## W

Wegener's necrotizing granulomatous vasculitis, *see* Granulomatosis with polyangiitis
Western blot technique, 36, 37
Workplace induced COPD/industrial chronic bronchitis, 237–238

## Y

Yellow nail syndrome, 275
Young's syndrome, 274